Feeding Problems in Children

PEDIATRIC PSYCHOLOGY

Feeding Problems in Children

A practical guide

Second Edition

Edited by

ANGELA SOUTHALL

Consultant Clinical Psychologist
Director of Services, Midlands Psychology CIC, Birmingham

and

CLARISSA MARTIN

Consultant Clinical Psychologist in Paediatrics
Honorary Research Fellow
Centre for Research in Eating Disorders, Loughborough University

Foreword by

William B Crist PhD

Psychologist
Nutrition and Feeding Clinic
IWK Health Centre
Halifax, Nova Scotia
Canada

Radcliffe Publishing
Oxford • New York

Radcliffe Publishing Ltd
18 Marcham Road
Abingdon
Oxon OX14 1AA
United Kingdom

www.radcliffepublishing.com

Electronic catalogue and worldwide online ordering facility.

First Edition 2000

British Library Cataloguing in Publication Data

A catalogue record for this book is available from the British Library.

ISBN-13: 978 184619 386 6

Typeset by KnowledgeWorks Global Ltd, Chennai, India
Printed and bound by Cadmus Communications, USA

Contents

Series introduction

Whenever a child receives a diagnosis of a medical condition, numerous considerations are immediately brought to the fore, many of which are unique to children, including, of course, developmental, family and parenting issues. A child's cognitive, emotional, behavioural and social functioning may be significantly affected by their illness. Most significantly, just as the child is affected by their illness, so is the course of the illness affected by the child. This simple understanding and the success of paediatric psychologists in communicating and demonstrating it has led to the growth of paediatric psychology in children's wards, out-patient departments, community clinics and health centres around the world. Indeed, it is the propensity of the paediatric psychology team to make a difference to the child and their treatment that has led to widespread acknowledgement of the value that paediatric psychology brings.

Paediatric psychology is essentially the application of psychological theory, research and practice to children with medical conditions and health-related concerns. It takes a 'whole child' approach and is developmentally focused. Practice is most often multi-disciplinary and focuses on the understanding of physical, psychosocial and neuropsychological aspects of health and illness, and how these impact on each other. The scope of paediatric psychology is extensive and encompasses many treatment areas ranging from adjustment to illness, coping with invasive medical procedures and pain management to adherence to treatment, children with chronic conditions and palliative care, to name just a few, as well as the prevention of illness among healthy children (Roberts et al., 1984).

As a specialty, paediatric psychology has a surprisingly long history. Soon after the emergence of psychology as a discipline in the 19th century, it was suggested that psychologists and paediatricians would benefit from mutual collaboration (Witmer, 1907). These psychologists worked alongside paediatricians and shared with them a developmental perspective; they came to be described as 'paediatric psychologists' (Wright, 1967). These early paediatric psychologists helped establish that children with health and developmental problems had significant needs, which though similar to one another were different to those with psychiatric diagnoses. In the United States the *Society of Pediatric Psychology* was founded to meet those needs

(Wright, 1967). In the United Kingdom, paediatric psychology developed out of the discipline of clinical psychology and continues to be located within the category of *clinical child psychologists working in medical healthcare settings*, under the auspices of the British Psychological Society (BPS).

Recent policy emphases in the United Kingdom have highlighted the needs of children and young people with long-term conditions and the importance of providing them with good mental health input to maximise emotional well-being and minimise problems.[1] These polices emphasise that such support should be an integral part of the service a child receives in hospital and highlight the imperative on hospitals to ensure staff have an understanding of how to assess the emotional well-being of children and address any needs that are identified.[2] Elsewhere in Europe, mental health has also come to be emphasised as an essential ingredient in health and well-being, not just for children but for everyone. This is perhaps best exemplified by the European Union's slogan, 'there is no health without mental health' (Lavikainen *et al.*, 2000).

The *Paediatric Psychology Series* to which this book belongs was conceived as a way of sharing with readers salient ideas from applied research and practice that would be experienced as helpful to others in their own practice. A series of books was planned, each focusing on a different topic within paediatric psychology, with the overall aim of raising awareness among health professionals of the concomitant psychological and psychosocial aspects of child ill-health and chronic illness.

The series has a deliberately international focus, which reflects the paediatric psychology community and brings together material which is otherwise unavailable in this form. The accompanying electronic toolkit offers practical, useable support to practitioners, as well as an opportunity to contribute to the developing knowledge base. It is our hope that the books will prove to be an inspiring and reliable resource for day-to-day paediatric practice.

Angela Southall
Clarissa Martin

REFERENCES

Lavikainen J, Lahtinen E, Lehtinen V, editors. *Public Health Approach on Mental Health in Europe.* National Research and Development Centre for Welfare and Health, STAKES Ministry of Social Affairs and Health; 2000.

Roberts MC, Maddux JE, Wright L. Developmental perspectives in behavioral health. In: Matarazzo JD, Miller NE, Weiss SM, *et al.*, editors. *Behavioral Health: a handbook of health enhancement and disease prevention.* New York: Wiley; 1984.

Wright L. The pediatric psychologist: a role model. *Am Psychol.* 1967; **22**: 323–5.

Witmer L. Clinical psychology. *The Psychol Clinic.* 1907; **1**(1): 1–9.

---

[1]Department of Health (2004) *National Service Framework (NSF) for children young people and maternity services: children and young people who are ill. Standard 6.* London: DoH.
[2]Department of Health (2003) *National Service Framework (NSF) for children at hospital. Standard 7.* London: DoH.

Dedicated to Dr J Houghton PhD

This series is dedicated to Dr Judith Houghton PhD, Consultant Clinical Psychologist and first elected chair (2001–06) of the British Psychological Society – Paediatric Psychology National Committee (BPS-PPNC) in gratitude and acknowledgment for her outstanding contribution to the development of Paediatric Psychology in the UK.

Foreword

Twenty-five years of practice and 2500 patients later, I find myself reflecting about the surprising twists and turns that my career has taken. When I was a graduate student, the clinical area of feeding problems in young children was largely unknown. There were a few papers out, but nothing that would have caught the attention of a graduate student. Shortly after accepting a position as staff psychologist at a pediatric teaching hospital, my first patient with a feeding problem, however, certainly caught my attention. She was a cute-as-a-button 14-month-old with cystic fibrosis who had significant gastrointestinal complications at birth and was now being tube-fed. Her mother had been battling with her to accept a spoonful of food. In tears she asked, "What will I do if I can't feed my child?" And with that simple question, she conveyed how vitally important the ability to nurture one's own child is to the parent–child relationship and I was hooked.

For another surprise I have the internet to thank. When I began my career, receiving requests for an article that I had written or a questionnaire that I had developed was, of course, done through regular mail and replying was a task delegated impersonally to a secretary. But when the requests started being delivered by email, somehow the immediacy and the interactive nature of the internet changed all that – now those requests led to exchanges and sharing of information and ideas with colleagues in far distant countries. I call them my internet colleagues. It is the internet that I have to thank for introducing me to the work of Angela Southall and Clarissa Martin, the Editors of this book, for which I shall forever be grateful.

Their vision in compiling this edition reflects this new social reality – it is truly an international edition. In order to bring the reader the best, most up-to-date information about feeding problems in young children, they invited experts in their field from around the world to contribute to this edition. With chapters that cover the basic biological and psychological aspects of feeding skill development in babies and young children this book provides an excellent orientation for newcomers to the field. For the more experienced professional recent advances in the treatment of severe feeding difficulties in the neurologically impaired, chronically ill, and tube-fed child are summarized clearly and succinctly. And given the multi-cultural composition of today's communities, the decision by Southall and Martin to include a chapter on cultural aspects to feeding was most insightful.

Comparing the knowledge and understanding of feeding problems in young children that is contained in this edition to what was known when I first started in this area 25 years ago is a dramatic testament to how rapidly fields can evolve. The challenge with such rapid evolution is how to get up-to-date information to frontline clinical workers. This book, with its comprehensive coverage of the issues and a practical Toolkit with examples of materials from a multi-disciplinary practice, makes an essential contribution to the education of frontline clinicians dealing with feeding problems in young children.

William B Crist PhD
Psychologist
Nutrition and Feeding Clinic
IWK Health Centre
Halifax, Nova Scotia
Canada
August 2010

About the editors

Angela Southall has a long experience of working as a clinical psychologist with children, young people and families and was for many years head of child psychology and psychological therapies in Staffordshire, UK. Throughout this time, her primary focus has been the development of psychological services for children and the promotion of the psychosocial understanding of children's mental health. Her commitment to community psychology has led to the initiation and development of a number of innovative services and partnerships and to new ways of working. Her specialist field is parenting, attachment and trauma. She has contributed to the literature through several books and papers.

Clarissa Martin is consultant clinical psychologist in Paediatrics and Honorary Research Fellow at the Centre for Research in Eating Disorders at Loughborough University (LUCRED) in the United Kingdom. She is a specialist in children's feeding disorders and has pioneered multi-disciplinary intensive intervention for children with severe feeding disorders in a general hospital setting. She has run extensive programmes on training and support for other professionals in the field and is active in collaborative, interdisciplinary work in both community and acute settings. She has presented at both national and international conferences and is the author of a number of peer-reviewed papers.

List of contributors

Professor Stephen Briggs is associate dean and specialist in Adult Mental Health Services at the Tavistock and Portman NHS Foundation Trust, where he is also consultant social worker in the Adolescent Department. He is professor of social work and director of the Centre for Social Work Research in the University of East London. He has a wide range of research interests, including adolescent mental health and suicidality, but his PhD and subsequent research has focused on infant mental health and problems in the infant–parent relationship. He has written widely on psychodynamic work with children and adolescents.

Dr Mandy Bryon is a clinical psychologist and joint head of the Paediatric Psychology Service at Great Ormond Street Hospital for Children, London, the United Kingdom, where she is a specialist in cystic fibrosis. She lectures extensively within the United Kingdom on psychosocial aspects of childhood illness and is a regular presenter at national and international conferences. Mandy has been invited to join the Scientific Committee of the European Cystic Fibrosis Society and is a member of the Medical Advisory Committee for the Cystic Fibrosis Trust. She has published widely on several child health topics and is also a regular advisor to the BBC.

Dr Suzanne Colson is co-founder of The Nurturing Project, a company created to disseminate biological nurturing research. She is an honorary senior lecturer at Canterbury Christ Church University, a Royal College of Nursing Akinsanya Scholar and a member of the LLL panel of professional advisors in the United Kingdom and France.

Jo Douglas is a clinical psychologist who has specialist experience in treating young children with eating and feeding difficulties over a considerable time. She worked at Great Ormond Street Children's Hospital, London, the United Kingdom, for many years, where she established the first psychological treatment programme in the Day Center of the Department of Psychological Medicine in 1985. She has written and lectured extensively over the years on the psychological approaches to these problems, as well as the wider range of behavioural and emotional problems in young children and their families. She now runs a private practice where she continues to work with eating and feeding difficulties.

Dr Terence M Dovey is a psychologist specialising in eating behaviours and disorders based at Loughborough University's Centre for Research into Eating Disorders (LUCRED). He is also an Honorary Research Fellow at the Kisseleff Laboratory for the Study of Ingestive Behaviour at Liverpool University. Terry has published numerous works including books and peer-reviewed papers on the subject of childhood feeding disorders and adult eating behaviour and has given many presentations at the United Kingdom and international conferences.

Professor Kedar Nath Dwivedi, London Metropolitan University and director of the International Institute of Child and Adolescent Mental Health, previously assistant professor in social and preventive medicine and consultant in child, adolescent and family psychiatry in Northampton, the United Kingdom. He also served the British Council as the UK Link Coordinator for the Higher Education Link in Child and Adolescent Psychiatry in India. He has contributed extensively to the literature and has a special interest in Eastern, particularly Buddhist, approaches to mental health.

Dr Charles Essex is a consultant neurodevelopmental paediatrician based in Coventry, the United Kingdom, specialising in child development.

Dr Anthony P Messer is a clinical psychologist who worked for many years in the field of children's feeding problems in the Department of Paediatric Psychology & Social Work of the University Medical Center Utrecht/Wilhelmina Children's Hospital in Utrecht. His pioneering work in behaviourally oriented and evidence-based treatment for severe food refusal and eating difficulties led to the current integrated feeding difficulties programme at the University Medical Centre, led by Monique Thomas-Holtus. Dr Messer continues to consult on specialist cases.

Dr Angela Morgan is a Research Fellow at the Murdoch Children's Research Institute and senior speech pathologist at the Royal Children's Hospital, Melbourne, Australia. Her research program is focused on the study of genes, brain and behaviour in childhood speech and swallowing disorders. A central tenet of her work is the translation of research findings into clinical practice. Her current program is funded by the National Health and Medical Research Council of Australia.

Dr Cathleen C Piazza is a professor and the director of the Pediatric Feeding Disorders Program at the University of Nebraska Medical Center's Munroe-Meyer Institute in the United States. Her research has focused on the assessment and treatment of severe behaviour problems, including feeding disorders, in children, and she has published a large number of data-based, peer-reviewed studies on the topic in addition to numerous book chapters and is the editor of the *Journal of Applied Behavior Analysis*.

Dr Lynn Priddis is a counselling and clinical psychologist who has a long history of working with children and families in health, education and private practice contexts. Her academic interests are in the field of attachment theory and parent–infant psychotherapy. Lynn teaches in the Master of Counselling Psychology programme at Curtin University of Technology in Western Australia.

Professor Sheena Reilly is professor of speech pathology at the Royal Children's Hospital and the University of Melbourne, Australia, and is director of the Healthy Development research theme at the Murdoch Children's Research Institute.

Dr Anthony Schwartz is a clinical and health psychologist who worked for many years in the field of paediatric psychology, specialising in children with chronic illnesses. Anthony's work with various healthcare professionals and his specialism in the psychological aspects of stress and coping has led to an applied focus across the age range. He currently specialises in Mindfulness training and developing resilience. Anthony is a visiting professor at the Staffordshire University, the United Kingdom. He is a regular speaker at conferences, both in the United Kingdom and abroad, and has written a number of peer-reviewed articles and books.

Dr Gerben Sinnema is professor of clinical child psychology at the University of Utrecht. He is also a consultant clinical psychologist and head of the Department of Paediatric Psychology & Social Work of the University Medical Center Utrecht/ Wilhelmina Children's Hospital. His clinical and research interest is in the field of chronic illness in childhood. He has contributed extensively to the literature through many peer-reviewed studies, as well as chapters in handbooks of paediatrics and behavioural medicine.

Dr Alan Silverman is an assistant professor of pediatrics at the Medical College of Wisconsin, and the Medical Staff Section Chief of Pediatric Psychology for Children's Hospital of Wisconsin, USA. His primary clinical services are provided through the section of Gastroenterology and Nutrition working with families of children diagnosed with Feeding Disorders of Childhood. He also leads the research efforts of the interdisciplinary feeding program at the Children's Hospital in Wisconsin, which includes studies of disease etiology, treatment efficacy and telemedicine interventions. He is the author of a number of publications, including a review of feeding and vomiting disorders for the *Handbook of Pediatric Psychology*.

Monique Thomas-Holtus is a feeding counsellor at the Department of Paediatric Psychology & Social Work of the University Medical Center/Wilhelmina Children's Hospital in Utrecht. Monique has a long association with the hospital and extensive experience of treating young children with feeding problems. She advises a number of professionals, including paediatricians, dieticians and nurses.

Dr Petula CM Vaz is an assistant professor at the Center for Autism Spectrum Disorders, Munroe-Meyer Institute at the University of Nebraska Medical Center in the United States. Her primary research interests are in the area of paediatric feeding disorders. Dr Vaz is a licensed and certified speech-language pathologist. She received her PhD from Ohio University specialising in dysphagia and voice disorders. She has extensive predoctoral, doctoral and postdoctoral research and clinical training in swallowing and feeding disorders and has several years of graduate- and undergraduate-level teaching and clinical mentoring experience.

Dr Mary Wickenden worked clinically as a specialist speech and language therapist in under 5s special needs and paediatric dysphagia before moving into an academic teaching and research career. She now works at the Institute of Child Health, University College London, the United Kingdom, as a medical anthropologist. Her main interests include broad aspects of training and skills development of international health workers working in disability, cultural and social aspects of disability and the experiences of children with disabilities and their families.

Alison Wisbeach is an occupational therapist and honorary research occupational therapist, Great Ormond Street Hospital for Children, the United Kingdom.

Dr Jeremy Woodcock is a family and couples psychotherapist in independent practice in the Cotswolds, the United Kingdom. For many years, he was a senior psychotherapist in a human rights organisation that worked with families from all over the world. He continues to consult and advise organisations and psychotherapists that engage with human rights issues and cultural difference.

Kim Woolliscroft is an advanced nurse practitioner in general paediatrics and Head of Children's and Neonatal Services in Staffordshire, the United Kingdom. Kim has more than 30 years experience working with children and their families and is particularly interested in gastroenterology and parent–child relationships. She is an honorary tutor at Staffordshire University. Her research interests are mainly in gastroenterology and quality of life, the results of which Kim has presented at both national and international conferences.

Zuzana Rothlingova works as an assistant psychologist in health psychology in Dudley, the United Kingdom, where she works with people with physical health conditions.

Introduction

We are delighted to introduce the second edition of this book, which we hope you will find as helpful and stimulating as the first. Every chapter has been updated and has undergone some revision or re-writing; in some cases new authors or co-authors have added fresh perspectives. In keeping with the 'real world' of paediatric psychology, this edition offers an international overview with chapters from the United Kingdom, Europe, North America and Australia. It also has a third part, a 'toolkit', comprising check lists, questionnaires, handouts and other resources that may be used by practitioners working in the field.

Feeding is a fundamental process, essential to survival. The taking of food serves an important biological function, enabling the child to grow and develop both physically and psychologically. Feeding and eating have important psychosocial functions too. From the onset, feeding experiences are central to the development of relationships with the primary care-givers, especially the mother. Later, eating forms an important and integral part of family and wider social interaction. When things go wrong with this process, it is understandable that anxiety levels in parents, not to mention professionals, become raised. Consequently, there are inevitable difficulties not only for the child but also for the parents and often for the whole family.

This book is about the different approaches to feeding problems and the various applications of some of the theoretical perspectives. It takes as its starting point the premise that feeding problems are distinct from eating disorders. This understanding is reflected in the emphasis on the feeding process and the link between parents and children in defining feeding problems (Lindberg *et al.*, 1991). The term 'feeding' implies a relationship – there is one who feeds and one who is fed. A focus on the process of feeding inevitably calls into question traditional notions of 'disorder', applied to a child who is only part of the equation, while challenging us to think differently about these complex problems.

Feeding problems that remain below the clinical threshold tend to be quite common in children. Most children will go through periods of food refusal or faddiness and this is entirely within the range of normal behaviours during the early years. With appropriate management, these difficulties usually resolve themselves. For some children, however, this is not the case; the problems do not resolve themselves and can prove very resistant to change. In some cases, without skilled intervention they can become life-threatening. These cases may be thought of as lying further towards the 'clinical' end of the feeding problems continuum. They are usually identifiable by a complex matrix of professionals and interventions. At the extreme end, children may be maintained on nasogastric tube feeding in the community for long periods, sometimes years, requiring considerable involvement of community and acute paediatrics, dietetics, community paediatric nursing, speech and language therapy and psychological services. The inherently multidisciplinary nature of feeding problems means that there are typically a number of professionals involved, each focusing on a different aspect of the problem. Those involved often find themselves taking conflicting positions or representing different interests. Coupled with the very emotive nature of the problem, this adds to the overall complexity of the work. It also limits possibilities for the well-coordinated response, which many see as an essential pre-requisite for successful therapeutic intervention, a view echoed by current child health policy which emphasises the need for teamwork and collaboration.

Despite the scale of the problem and the scope for useful intervention, there is still remarkably little literature on the subject. That which exists tends either to equate feeding problems with eating disorders or to assume a developmental continuum between the two, despite a lack of evidence for any such relationship. At the time of writing there continues to be confusion about terminology and classification, with little attempt to integrate the various perspectives within clinical paediatrics. This book addresses this issue, both by exploring the interrelationship of various aspects of feeding within a multidisciplinary perspective and by focusing on clinical issues. In doing so, it aims to increase understanding about feeding problems, thereby helping us to move towards greater clarification of some of the key issues. An applied emphasis will be maintained throughout.

The chapters contained in this book concern the nature, development, maintenance and treatment of feeding problems. The terminology used by the authors varies between feeding 'problems', 'difficulties' and 'disorders'. We have resisted the temptation to homogenise the language and have instead chosen to preserve these differences. We think this reflects not only the various positions of the authors but also the state of play within the field in terms of terminology. The text is divided into two parts: Part I, 'approaches', where the theoretical frameworks will be discussed, and Part II, 'applications', focusing on clinical or applied research aspects of children's feeding. Together they provide a 'whole child' perspective.

Mary Wickenden's chapter begins, and serves as an important foundation for the chapters to come by providing an overview of the development of feeding skills from conception to three years, and how these processes can become disrupted. This is followed by Charles Essex and Kim Wooliscroft's exploration of the medical contribution through their work in community and acute paediatrics, with a valuable nursing perspective added by Kim. Since this is the first point of contact for many children with feeding problems, as well as those who help them, this chapter provides an appropriate backdrop for further exploration of frontline health professional involvement. Petula Vaz and Cathleen Piazza follow this with a new chapter on behavioural approaches to the assessment and management of feeding disorders, which gives a flavour of some of the work within the Paediatric Feeding Disorders Program at the Munroe–Meyer Institute, Nebraska, USA.

Chapter 4 sees Stephen Briggs joined by co-author Lynn Priddis to present psychoanalytic perspectives on the dynamics of feeding difficulties, with a primary focus on the infant–parent relationship. In Chapter 5, Terry Dovey and Clarissa Martin re-examine the psychophysiological and regulatory mechanisms in the aetiology of feeding, presenting an interactional model in which cognitive and developmental factors are considered. Cultural aspects of feeding are introduced in a revised and extended Chapter 6 by Kedar Dwivedi and Jeremy Woodcock, who, through examples drawn from India, Africa, the Middle East and the Caribbean, demonstrate the important and pervasive influences of culture on human behaviour and practices, and, critically for this text, on feeding. The 'approaches' section concludes with Angela Southall's overview of the contribution of family and wider system perspectives in feeding problems.

Part II, the 'applications' part of the book, comprises a number of applied clinical and research examples, which may be seen as developing out of the theoretical and conceptual perspectives discussed in Part I. Again, there have been some new additions to this second edition, which we believe add considerably to the book, not only in terms of updating but also in achieving greater inclusiveness and a sense of connectedness with the international paediatric community. Suzanne Colson's chapter introduces biological nurturing for the nursing mother and infant, not only as an intuitive and natural process but also as offering remedial benefits where there are difficulties. This chapter serves as an important reminder of the importance of facilitating effective feeding from the onset and provides the reader with a normative standpoint from which to think about feeding and feeding-related issues as they are discussed in the following chapters. Jo Douglas provides an illustration of how the behavioural approach lends itself to interventions with children who are selective eaters. Sheena Reilly and Alison Wisbeach are joined in Melbourne, Australia by Angela Morgan in an updated distillation of their previous two chapters (now one) on the assessment and treatment of children with neurological impairments. As in edition one, specific interventions with children who are tube fed are explored by Mandy Bryon, while the area of feeding problems in children with chronic conditions is covered by Anthony Schwartz. A new chapter by Monique Thomas Holtus and colleagues from the Wilhelmina Children's Hospital in Utrecht, introduces the role of the Feeding Counsellor and looks at the use of an intensive coaching protocol in both acute and community settings. Alan Silverman and colleagues in Wisconsin (USA) present Telemedicine as a vehicle for supporting families in their own homes or in satellite facilities. Finally, Clarissa Martin and Terry Dovey discuss intensive interventions in the UK and elsewhere.

We hope these chapters provide much 'food for thought' for the interested reader and, for those who work in the field, ideas and inspiration for your own practice.

Angela Southall and Clarissa Martin
August 2010

REFERENCE

Lindberg L, Bolin G, Hagekull B. Early feeding problems in a normal population. *Int J Eat Disord.* 1991; **10:** 395–405.

PART I

Approaches

CHAPTER 1

The development and disruption of feeding skills in babies and young children

Mary Wickenden

INTRODUCTION

This chapter outlines the normal development of feeding skills from conception to 3 years as a foundation for looking at the ways in which this development may be disrupted either during these early stages or subsequently. It examines a number of situations where multi-disciplinary intervention may be necessary to help the child to eat and drink as normally as possible, and thus thrive. Feeding is of course a complex and biopsychosocial process that can be disrupted in a number of ways throughout childhood. However, in the early months and years, it is important to understand the normal development of oromotor and oral sensory skills, and where appropriate assessment of these skills, in order to gain an overall picture of the child with possible feeding problems. Additionally, specific assessment of the child's parallel overall development, in particular gross motor and communication skills, may reveal important factors that contribute to a wider view of the problem. Sometimes assessment of a child's oromotor skills is necessary to exclude neurological difficulties, and so enable a focus on sensory and experiential, or move overtly psychological or environmental aspects of the feeding problem.

It is often difficult to isolate any specific oral problems from the perhaps much more obvious developmental and or behavioural difficulties that may abound and this is when a multi-disciplinary approach becomes crucial. Previously, there was a tendency to categorise children with no obvious oromotor problems as having a 'behavioural feeding problem'. However, this dichotomous categorisation has not proved very helpful, as it immediately raises further questions about why these children are apparently poor feeders or actively 'anti-feeding'. The possibility of very real sensory disturbance either as a soft neurological effect or as a result of experience is now acknowledged as contributing to some children's feeding problems. Thus, the child's inability to respond normally to sensation (i.e. either over or under-responding or both) needs to be considered as the possible, less easily identified root of the difficult behaviour, which is more obvious. This is not to say that primary psychological causes of feeding problems do not exist (and they are discussed amply elsewhere in this book) but that caution should be exercised when ruling out subtle oral-motor or oral-sensory disorders. 'Behavioural' resistance to mealtimes may have its origins in difficulty with the movements and sensations of eating and drinking and may be linked to particular medical diagnoses and experiences.

In order to appreciate the often multi-factorial nature of feeding problems, it is necessary to understand something of the development of the skills needed for eating and drinking. An overview of the normal development of feeding skills up to 3 years is presented. In addition, the ways in which this development can be disrupted in the context of various medical conditions and interventions are discussed.

NORMAL DEVELOPMENT OF ORAL SKILLS
Conception to birth

The process of taking in and swallowing food or drink involves three linked anatomical and physiological regions connected to each other anatomically and by neurological systems. These are:

- the oral cavity (including activity of the lips, tongue and palate)
- the pharynx (where food is directed safely backwards and down during the swallow)
- the oesophagus leading to the stomach.

Oral activity begins very early in life, well before it is needed for feeding proper. Mouth opening in response to perioral stimulation can be seen in the foetus from around 9.5 weeks gestation, and between 10 and 17 weeks swallowing is evident. The foetus is swallowing amniotic fluid at this stage (500–1000 mL/day), and problems with swallowing can be indicated by polyhydramnios (excess amniotic fluid) during pregnancy. By 26–28 weeks, the main reflexive pathways are established. At 32 weeks a clear gag reflex is observable, quickly followed by the emergence of the cough reflex. These two reflexes are essential for airway protection immediately after birth and throughout life.

Sucking is a reflex that also begins in utero, although it has little nutritional purpose apart from hydration at this stage. It is important to distinguish between the two different types of suck. The non-nutritive suck is first seen in the foetus between 18 and 24 weeks. This is a fast (two sucks per second), 'non-feeding' suck that although rhythmical does not need to be coordinated with swallowing.

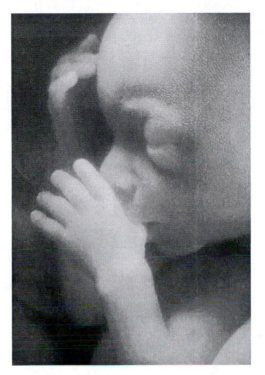

FIGURE 1.1: Human foetus male 19 weeks.

Breathing after birth is through the nose and is not interrupted by non-nutritive sucking because no fluid is being taken in. There is substantial evidence that this suck has comforting, settling and organising effects on the baby (Field *et al.*, 1982; Law-Morstatt *et al.*, 2003; Measel and Anderson, 1979).

In most neonatal care units, non-nutritive sucking is actively encouraged by the provision of dummies. It is this fast, shallow action that is observable when babies suck their thumb in utero and on a dummy or other object once born. Sometimes they will also suck non-nutritively on a breast nipple or bottle teat in between bursts of nutritive sucking. The second type of suck is the nutritive or 'active feeding' suck, which is more mature and complex and is designed to deal with fluid. This type of suck can be seen first in the 34–37-week-olds, and it necessitates coordination of the suck, swallow and respiration. Again, it is strongly rhythmical, but is much slower (one suck per second) and appears more effortful. The usual pattern is for suck and swallow to be in a one-to-one relationship (i.e. suck and swallow alternating). Again, breathing is nasal and remains smooth and rhythmical, although there is a momentary pause in respiration during the swallow. Normally, a swallow is always followed by expiration, and this makes good sense, as it protects the baby's airway by expelling any material that might be in the laryngeal region threatening to be aspirated into the airway. After 40 weeks gestation, the number of sucks per swallow normally increases to two or three so that feeding will be faster and more efficient.

Sucking occurs in a 'burst-pause' pattern, where a series of nutritive sucks is followed by a rest period. Babies under 37 weeks manage three to five sucks in a burst and then pause for an equal interval before starting up again. They often delay swallowing and breathing until the pauses rather than integrating them into the sucking sequence. They may therefore have periods of apnoea during feeding and may appear breathless and in need of rests. Babies more than 37 weeks usually sustain nutritive sucking in bursts of 10–30 sucks and then pause for a shorter time, before another burst (more than 2 seconds between sucks counts as a pause). This is obviously more efficient as swallowing and breathing are integrated into the sequence, and there is proportionately more feeding time and less resting as the baby matures.

Babies will sometimes change to non-nutritive sucking during feeding, presumably to rest and breathe without the interruption of swallowing. Sucking is a *flexion* activity, the body being curled up with the limbs held bent and in towards the body. The ideal position for efficient feeding both in utero and post-delivery is therefore a flexed one. Premature babies are often unable to maintain this position and need help to stay flexed through careful handling by the carer. For more on feeding position in relation to breastfeeding infants and their mothers, refer to Chapter 8.

Birth to three months

Efficient feeding is usually established within a few hours or days of birth in the normal term baby weighing 1900 grams. At this stage, it is a reflex-driven activity, is coordinated, smooth, rhythmical and regulated by the baby whether breast or bottle-fed. Non-nutritive sucking can be seen at non-feeding times, particularly in the 30 minutes before a feed when the baby is hungry. The baby is easily able to make the transition from non-nutritive activity to a nutritive suck within a matter of seconds on receiving a nipple or teat in the mouth. The jaw and cheeks are very active in sucking and can be seen vigorously pumping up and down. The tongue makes predominantly forwards and backwards movements, with most activity in the body and back of the tongue, the tip being tucked under the teat. The tongue forms a central groove that helps to propel the milk back towards the pharynx. The lips are open but not very active at this stage. There are two phases to the suck, expression and suction. This early sucking pattern is often referred to as 'suckling'. Both motor and sensory components are important in facilitating control of the bolus and timing the trigger of the swallow. For more detailed information about early feeding development, the reader is referred to Arvedson (2006).

The development of these complex, coordinated skills is rapid. Physiological, neuroanatomical and psychological aspects of feeding interweave in a dynamic and fast-changing way. The more experience the baby has, the more refined and efficient the system becomes. During the first few months of life, patterns of feeding behaviour become established. A typical normal baby will manage about 113 grams of milk in 5 minutes and 227 grams in 10–15 minutes. The baby controls the speed, volume and timing of bursts and pauses during feeding. The burst-pause pattern is very obvious on observation and has been likened to early conversation, as it has a turn-taking element. Often the mother will say something to the baby during the pauses, and eye contact seems to be maintained. This is felt to be an important foundation for the mother–child relationship (*see* Chapter 4). The mother quickly becomes an expert at interpreting the baby's feeding activity and is able to make judgments about whether he or she is hungry, full or uncomfortable.

Three to six months

During the second 3 months of life, the dynamic feeding system continues to change and develop. The baby will now be fast and efficient at sucking and will probably also be getting very good at expressing hunger, discomfort or satiation clearly. The amount of milk taken in per suck increases and so the volume of feed taken gradually increases over time, and the frequency of feeds decreases. By 6 months the baby has three or four 240 mL feeds per day.

The physical position in which young babies are fed complements their anatomy at this stage. Up to about 3 months the proportions and arrangement of structures in the pharynx are different from those of older infants, children and adults. The small baby effectively has anatomical protection from the dangers of aspiration (penetration of food into the airways) by virtue of the position of the larynx and tongue. The larynx is much higher up in the neck, tucked under the tongue, and the epiglottis and soft palate can make contact. Thus, the normal position in which to feed a young baby is a supine one. Aspiration, even in the neurologically compromised child, is unlikely. However, between 3 and 6 months, this arrangement evolves so that the proportions and relationships become more like those of an older child. The chance of penetration of material into the airway is actually greater in the mature anatomy, and the position of the head becomes important, especially in the child with possible dysphagia.

As the child develops good head control and then sitting balance, the mother automatically starts to adapt the feeding position to a more upright, semi-sitting one. The sucking pattern matures as the tongue begins to move up and down as well as backwards and forwards and the lips become more active in sealing around the teat.

At some time during this stage, the mother will wean the baby on to runny, pureed food from a spoon. Initially the baby takes this new food texture using old oral motor skills, that is continuing to suck. However, over a few weeks or months, many of the early feeding reflexes fade away and the child learns to have more volitional control over oral movements and develops a new range of movements, particularly of the jaw and tongue. The mother gradually expands the range of tastes and textures that the baby will accept and enjoy. The development of taste preferences is discussed elsewhere in this book (*see* Chapter 5). Different textures of food provide valuable learning opportunities for the baby, from both the sensory and motor points of view. The sensations of different textures and tastes (e.g. slimy, granular, hot and cold) stimulate the child to perceive, tolerate and habituate to a variety of foods.

The perception of the differences between textures seems to stimulate the development of a broader range of motor skills. The absence of a teat or nipple in the mouth leaves more space for tongue-tip movement. The child gradually learns to control food coming off the spoon with more discrete jaw, lip and tongue movements. There is a suggestion in the literature that the introduction of an increasing range of textures of food at this developmental stage is an important critical period, which if missed, may lead to greater difficulty with textures and faddiness later (Arvedson, 2006).

Six months to one year

During the next 6 months the infant will play an increasingly active part in mealtimes. They will be learning early self-feeding skills, such as holding a biscuit and grabbing at the spoon. The range of tastes and textures eaten will expand greatly during this time. Children will manage to eat quite hard foods, such as breadsticks and carrots, mainly by sucking them and breaking pieces off. They are unlikely to choke, as large lumps will easily be ejected by a strong cough and a push out by the tongue. Chewing is at a preliminary stage, effectively an up and down 'munching' movement. Many babies may be weaned on to drinking from a cup or spouted beaker at this stage, although they may continue to have breast- or bottle-feeds as well. Drinking from a cup involves moving on from sucking to more controlled lip, jaw and tongue-tip activity.

Non-feeding oral activity continues to be important and normal at this stage. Many babies enjoy non-nutritive sucking on a dummy or other favourite object, and there are no reasons to discourage this at this age. Many of the early oral reflexes begin to fade out as voluntary control takes over, but spontaneous oral activity continues throughout life and performs the function of keeping the mouth clean and washed with saliva. Children learn to control saliva by closing their lips and swallowing as necessary. They may be quite dribbly at this age, as they are learning to control food and saliva effectively.

Eating and drinking is a messy business, as children often want to feel the food with their fingers both before and after committing it to the mouth. When eating difficult textures, many children will help themselves by moving the food around their mouth with their fingers. This is an important experience, and links between manual and oral activity are regarded as part of the normal development of an integrated sensory system.

The second year

Between 12 and 24 months, the toddler becomes a more skilled eater and learns to chew and bite with control. The oral and pharyngeal stages of swallowing become separable, so that the child can decide not to swallow something and can hold it tantalisingly in their mouth, while looking for an opportunity to spit it out. The tongue develops a range of more complex movements, including tipping and side-to-side movements, and a more defined use of the tip. Children become able to eat mixed textures, which requires more sorting in the mouth of the various constituents (e.g. meat, gravy and soft vegetable in one spoonful needs skilled sorting and control by the tongue). The child may be fiercely suspicious of new experiences generally and this includes new tastes and textures. However, they enjoy exploration of new foods, if given an atmosphere in which they are in control.

SUBSEQUENT DEVELOPMENTS IN CHILDHOOD

The fine-tuning of eating and drinking skills continues over the next 2 years or so. The child learns to bite, chew and swallow a complete range of textures, including very chewy, very hard and mixed foods. They learn to keep their lips closed during eating, which is mainly a social convention but does cut down on spillage. The tongue is able to move accurately to retrieve food lost outside the lips or stuck around teeth and cheeks. The time taken by a child to eat a meal can be an important indication of normal feeding skills, and as a general rule feeds in babies, and meals in toddlers and children should not take more than 30 minutes. Gradually children learn to tolerate and enjoy changes in tastes and learn to express their preferences verbally. Social aspects of meal times become more important as the child has increasing opportunities to eat outside his or her own home and family. Thus, we can see the process of learning to eat and drink is indeed a *biopsychosocial* process.

TYPES OF FEEDING DIFFICULTY

Causes of feeding difficulties may be many and varied, depending on the medical and experiential history of the child. Nevertheless, the actual effects on the child's feeding behaviour can be described and categorised functionally, as opposed to by medical diagnosis *per se*. This is helpful, in that it leads more clearly to practical intervention approaches that match the child's difficulties, often irrespective of their health condition.

PATTERNS OF DIFFICULTY IN PREMATURE BABIES AND NEONATES

In young babies, the distinction between 'dysfunctional' and 'disorganised' feeding as described by Palmer and Heyman (1993) is important. Very often these categories map consistently onto possible oral and/or sensory difficulties in older children. Thus, these early patterns of difficulty appear to be predictive of later types of feeding problems, at least for some.

Palmer *et al.* (1993a) suggest that there are two distinct and distinguishable groups of difficulty, and that it is useful to aim for a differential diagnosis between them. Palmer's work with premature and young babies suggests that those with evident feeding difficulties can be grouped as either dysfunctional or disorganised (*see* Table 1.1). The NOMAS assessment records in detail the activity of the

TABLE 1.1: Features of normal, dysfunctional and disorganised feeding (Palmer, 1993a)

Normal	Disorganisation	Dysfunction
Jaw		
• Consistent degree of jaw depression	• Inconsistent degree of jaw depression	• Excessively wide excursions that interrupt intra-oral seal on nipple
• Rhythmic excursions	• Arrhythmic jaw movements	• Minimal excursions; clenching
• Spontaneous jaw excursions occur on tactile presentation of nipple up to 30 minutes before a feeding	• Difficulty initiating movements: — inability to latch on — small, tremorlike start-up movements noted — does not respond to initial cue of nipple, until jiggled	• Asymmetry; lateral jaw deviation • Absence of movement (% of time)
• Jaw movement occurs at the rate of approximately 1/second (half rate of non-nutritive suck)		• Lack of rate change between non-nutritive suck and nutritive suck (non-nutritive suck = 2/second; nutritive suck = 1/second)
• Sufficient closure on nipple during expression phase to express fluid from nipple	• Persistence of immature suck pattern beyond appropriate age	
Tongue		
• Cupped tongue configuration (tongue groove) maintained during sucking	• Excessive protrusion beyond labial border during extension phase of sucking without interrupting sucking rhythm	• Flaccid; flattened with absent tongue groove
• Extension-elevation-retraction movements occur in anterior-posterior direction	• Arrhythmic movements	• Retracted; humped and pulled back into oropharynx
• Rhythmic movements	• Unable to sustain suckle pattern for 2 minutes because of: — habituation —poor respiration — fatigue	• Asymmetry; lateral tongue deviation
• Movements occur at the rate of 1/second	• Incoordination of suck or swallow and respiration, which results in nasal flaring, head turning, extraneous movement	• Excessive protrusion beyond labial border before or after nipple insertion with out and down movement
• Liquid is sucked efficiently into oropharynx for swallow		• Absence of movement (% of time)

Assessment:

Recommendations:

Therapist:

jaw, lips and tongue in both non-nutritive and nutritive sucking. It has achieved good inter-rater reliability judgments of these features, and the overall profile of the child across a range of features provides a picture of normal, dysfunctional or disorganised feeding. Recent studies have confirmed the usefulness of the tool, but have also suggested that its robustness could be improved (Howe *et al.*, 2007; Da Costa and Van der Schans, 2008). Follow-up suggests that dysfunctional feeding as a baby does not resolve over time and later attracts diagnoses of neurological involvement and continued motor difficulties. Indeed dysfunctional feeding may be an earlier indication of possible cerebral palsy. Disorganised feeding either resolves to normal feeding with time or may go on to show sensory-type feeding disorders.

Research continues to suggest that this dichotomy can be useful and suggests different interventions and an indication of different prognoses (Palmer *et al.*, 1993b). Thus, the question 'does the child have an oral motor difficulty?' is an important one, but so also is 'does the child have oral sensory difficulty'. There may not be a diagnosis of frank cerebral palsy or other neurological disorder but a more subtle movement and coordination problem with oral movement, or a disturbance of sensation.

Of course, any detailed assessment of this kind is only as good as the assessor who administers it. Although Palmer achieved reliable results with her researchers, it has to be said that this is by no means an easy skill to acquire. Little research has thus far confirmed the diagnostic power of these early categories, although the NOMAS is quite widely used. If the link between dysfunctional features and later neurological difficulties is reliable, then the skilled use of this tool is an important addition to infant assessment and a useful way to view a complex problem. However, this kind of detailed oral assessment does require rigorous training before it can be relied upon. It is usually carried out by specialist speech and language therapists or by nurses specialising in neonatal feeding.

TYPES OF INTERVENTION FOR OROMOTOR AND ORAL SENSORY DIFFICULTIES

Once the main processes that are maintaining the feeding problem have been identified, there are a number of different approaches and elements to any intervention. If a child has a motor-based problem in particular, changes to the positioning and physical support of the child will be crucial, and here input from a physiotherapist is likely to be important. Specific help with jaw, tongue and lip movements may be suggested. Decisions about the textures of food offered, both to prevent difficulties and encourage development of skills, will be important. There is also a balance to be struck between the nutritional needs of the child, possibly met by *easy* foods (e.g. yoghurt), and the need to challenge and stimulate new skills with more difficult (hard, lumpy and chewy) foods. Thus, input from a dietician about the child's nutritional status and needs will be crucial in order to maintain appropriate weight or weight gain during interventions to change feeding skills and behaviours. Taste and temperature can also play an important part in stimulating oral activity and increased movement. For more information about children with neurological involvement, refer to Chapter 11.

Sensory problems (where the child has no difficulties with motor coordination of oral movements, but will only eat a very restricted range of foods) are likely to be tackled through a combination of carefully planned changes to tastes, textures and meal-time situations, the aim being to build in confidence and enjoyment of food and an expanded range of skills and experiences. The timing and type of meals may be changed and there may be the addition of *food-based play* and more social reinforcement of positive feeding behaviours. The child may need to build up tolerance of new sensations. Often not all the changes that need to be made can be implemented at once and a planned approach is crucial so that the child does not feel unduly rushed or pressurised. The child may need to continue to be fed on 'easy' foods for some time in order to thrive, with changes and variety being introduced gradually.

Methods for overcoming sensory difficulties vary in approach. Some practitioners adopt a behavioural approach and encourage the pairing of the feeding experience with positive feedback and social reinforcement; others emphasise the need to give the child as much control and choice as possible, so that he or she is in charge of trying new foods but with adult encouragement. Some clinicians advocate sensory bombardment techniques, such as stuffing the mouth, massaging and playing around the face and mouth, to desensitise the child and to gradually normalise their response to sensations.

In all cases, the approach should be tailor-made for the individual, in collaboration with the parents and all the professionals involved. Advising medical and nursing staff about reducing the aversive effects of some procedures is valuable (e.g. administering unpleasant drugs by tube, encouraging non-nutritive oral activity, encouraging the child to self-feed, using consistent feeders, the role of social reinforcement and interaction in feeding, and the use of appropriate utensils). Often a combination of the methods mentioned above will be adopted though it is important not to instigate too many changes at once. In all cases, it is important for everyone concerned to be clear about the techniques and aims adopted and for them to be systematically used.

MOTOR VERSUS SENSORY PROBLEMS

Motor and sensory aspects of feeding obviously develop simultaneously and interact with each other in the normal development of feeding skills. However, it can be helpful to think about motor and sensory difficulties separately, although of course in many children both may be in evidence and may exacerbate each other.

For instance, children who have difficulty with movements generally may have less experience of sensation, for example because they cannot get their hands to their mouths to explore at the normal stage. This may then lead to a dislike of touch around the face and mouth and refusal to try new foods, as well as poor oral movement. Conversely, children who have essentially normal motor skills but have had many aversive sensations around the mouth as a result of suction, passing of tubes or medicines may be unwilling to try new experiences and thus do not practise new motor skills, such as coping with lumps, chewing or biting.

Gisell (1991) has shown that children will use the easiest motor skills possible for any food. This suggests that if children can manage a meal by sucking (e.g. pureed vegetable and yoghurt), they will, and therefore will not be precipitated into developing more mature oral movements required by more challenging food textures. Thus there is a subtle interaction between movement and sensation, and between experience and learning new skills. It can sometimes be difficult to work out which is the primary problem, the movement or the sensation. Careful analysis of the child's willingness and ability to manage different tastes and textures can often clarify this issue. Palmer and Heyman (1993) have summarised this neatly in Table 1.2.

CHILDREN AT RISK OF ORAL-MOTOR OR ORAL-SENSORY PROBLEMS

There are a number of medical conditions which place children at risk of feeding difficulties. Of course any child may fall into more than one category, in which case their problems may be compounded and the presenting difficulty may be complex and multi-factorial in aetiology. There will almost certainly be a mixture of physiological, psychological and experiential factors at play.

PREMATURITY

Premature babies do not necessarily have a problem with feeding; they are just at an earlier stage, as described earlier. A baby delivered at under 34 weeks will have a non-nutritive suck but is not yet neurologically ready to suck nutritively.

TABLE 1.2: Features that differentiate sensory from motor difficulties

		Sensory	*Motor*
1	Normal oral-motor patterns	Yes	No
2	Liquids are easier to manage than textured or strained food	Yes	No
3	Mixed consistencies are difficult	No	Yes
4	Able to chew solids well	Yes	No
5	Gags when food approaches or contacts lip	Yes	No
6	Holds food to avoid swallowing	Yes	No
7	Hypersensitive gag for solids with normal liquid swallow	Yes	No

He or she may have additional complications, such as cardiac, respiratory or gastrointestinal problems, which can affect feeding, but in the absence of these, appropriately timed introduction of oral feeding should lead to normal feeding development. The premature baby is at risk of developing sensory feeding difficulties because of the likelihood of experiencing potentially aversive experiences, such as tube-feeding, suction or exhaustion. Careful and sensitive management of the very young baby's feeding development is increasingly being recognised as important (Field *et al.*, 1982; Hawdon *et al.*, 2000; Law-Morstatt *et al.*, 2003). The provision of opportunities for non-nutritive sucking has been shown to be beneficial even when oral feeding *per se* is not yet expected. Thus a distinction in intervention can be made between *oral therapy* and *feeding therapy*, the former being appropriate when the child is not developmentally ready for the latter (Morris and Klein, 1987).

Joshua: a disorganised feeder

Joshua was born at 32 weeks and weighed 1600 grams. He had bronchopulmonary dysplasia. He appeared distressed and easily tired if handled but sucked well on a dummy. He was tube-fed for 3 weeks with use of the dummy between feeds. When started on oral feeds at 35 weeks, he took only 10 mL before tiring and appeared irritable. He took a few seconds to initiate sucking and paused after three to four sucks for a rest. Over the next 4 weeks, there was a gradual increase in the amount taken per feed. Feeding was carried out in low stimulation surroundings and timing of pauses between bursts of sucking was structured by the feeder to allow rests and respiratory recovery. He increased his burst length to 15–20 by 38 weeks and continued to do well subsequently.

ORAL OR FEEDING THERAPY INVOLVEMENT IN SPECIFIC MEDICAL CONDITIONS

Speech and language therapists are involved in the assessment and treatment of feeding problems in children with a wide range of medical conditions, working in collaboration with the multi-disciplinary team. They usually take the lead in assessing oromotor and oral sensory skills and in planning intervention for difficulties with these. Much of the description of assessment and ideas about intervention described above are applicable to a number of different medical conditions. However, there are some specific issues for each broad group outlined below. It should be remembered that individual presentations can vary greatly and may defy the expected pattern for that condition.

CARDIAC AND RESPIRATORY CONDITIONS

In cardiac and respiratory disease, the main challenge for children is the coordination of feeding and respiration. They can easily become breathless, apnoeic and exhausted during feeding, which may compromise the whole process, and thus an efficient and effective feeding regime may not be easily established. Their feeding pattern is quite likely to fall into the disorganised category (Palmer *et al.*, 1993b), and they are then at risk of disruption to sensory aspects of feeding. They need careful management of the quantity and timing of feeding so that they do not become anoxic, overtired or anxious. Children who have experienced breathlessness, exhaustion or aspiration because of mistimed breathing and swallow can become fearful of the feeding process. Their capacity to take enough feed orally may be reduced, so supplemental tube-feeding is often used as a backup and to save energy. The gradual increase in oral feeding and reduction of tube-feeding requires careful staging and team discussion. Changes to feeding practice, such as maximising the positive effect of positioning, using special teats, and feeding little and often, can also contribute to success for this group. Parents often report remarkable improvements in feeding once a child waiting for cardiac surgery has had his or her operation. They may, however, need subsequent advice to help them gradually increase the volume and textures of food subsequently.

GASTROINTESTINAL CONDITIONS

Similarly, assessment of feeding skills may be needed for children with abnormalities of gut structure or function, such as necrotising enterocolitis, coeliac or Crohn's disease, gastroschisis and various malabsorption and dysmotility disorders. These children are often reluctant or difficult feeders. In the absence of neurological complications, they do not usually have oromotor problems but are prone to disturbances of appetite and sensation. They are a group who are likely to have had extensive medical and/or surgical intervention and prolonged hospital stays. The chances are high that experiences such as vomiting, constipation, diarrhoea, gastro-oesophageal reflux, oesophagitis, tube-feeding, medication by mouth and operative procedures will have an aversive effect on oral feeding in particular. Children may need supplemental feeding by nasogastric or gastrostomy tube or total parenteral nutrition (central line into vein). The amount, timing and type of oral feeding needs sensitive planning within the multi-professional team. Even though the team may be anxious to get the child eating and drinking quickly, for a child with significant sensory difficulties, this may be unrealistic in the short term. It may take many months to build up the child's confidence with, and enjoyment of, eating and drinking, and it is important that the total nutritional regime for a child is planned to foster a positive attitude to oral activity and feeding as well as adequate intake (Gryboski, 1975; Link and Rudolph, 2003; McKirdy *et al.*, 2008).

Catherine: an example of sensory feeding difficulty

Catherine was an 18-month-old baby with gastroschisis (malformation of the gut, with part of it outside the abdominal wall at birth). She had been in hospital and fed by a combination of nasogastric tube and central line from birth. She responded well to non-nutritive and oral activities, including sucking, licking, vocalising and food-related play with dolls. She was, however, very fussy about textures, both in her mouth and on her hands. Through play she was introduced to a variety of sensations of both foods and non-foods. She showed potentially normal oromotor skills but was resistant to any foods except a bottle and pureed fruit. She was very unwilling to try a new food unless left by herself to try it without adult persuasion. She was not permitted to eat more than a small quantity of food by mouth because of her gut abnormalities, but therapy (carried out by the Speech and Language Therapist, nurses and her mother) did result in a wider range of tastes and textures and an increased range of oromotor skills, appropriate for her age.

NEUROLOGICAL DISORDERS

Neurological disturbance, whether as a result of congenital, degenerative or acquired conditions, will clearly predispose the child to both oromotor and swallowing dysfunction (dysphagia) and to sensory abnormality (Tuchman, 1989). The largest group of children presenting with neurologically based feeding difficulties are those with cerebral palsy (discussed in detail in Chapter 10). It should, however, be remembered that there are more specific conditions, such as Moebius syndrome and Worster-Drought, affecting the oral musculature only. Many clinicians would agree that children with syndromes such as Retts, Williams and autism have increased incidences of feeding problems, though detailed research about these is sparse, and often it is unclear whether these have a clear neurological component. Some interesting work on the specific problems for children with Down's syndrome has been carried out recently by Bolders Frazier and Friedman (1996) and Spender *et al.* (1996), suggesting that their hypotonicity and hypersensitivity are likely to cause problems.

Children with degenerative conditions, or who have survived anoxia or head injury, often have marked oromotor feeding difficulties as part of their neurological disorders and may also have sensory disturbances. Children with less easily defined and more subtle motor dysfunction, such as those with dyspraxia and soft neurological signs, are among the most difficult to assess and define from the feeding point of view. Abnormal tone (increased, decreased or fluctuating) leads to postural problems and reduced control and muscle power for feeding. Gastro-oesophageal reflux is also a complicating factor for many children in this group (*see* Chapter 10). There are several good publications that cover intervention for neurologically disordered children in particular (*see* Further reading).

DEVELOPMENTAL DELAY

Mild, moderate or severe developmental delay and learning difficulties are often precursors of a range of difficulties with feeding development. This may be in the absence of obvious anatomical or physiological abnormality or in parallel with motor delay. If cognitive, social and communication development are delayed, then it is likely that feeding development will also be delayed. Recognition that the child's feeding skills may appear poor but are actually in line with their overall development can be important in planning management and in reassuring and advising carers. Unrealistic expectations about a child's feeding skills can cause problems in themselves.

Philip: a boy with Down's syndrome

Philip was referred for help with feeding at 2 years of age. He had delayed motor skills and was not yet sitting well without support. He was unable to eat any textures other than liquids and purees. Lumps of solid foods were dropped out of his mouth, and his mother interpreted this as he is rejecting the taste. He had marked hypotonicity of his tongue, lips and jaw. Explanation that his level of oral ability was reflective of and in parallel with his general development and low tone was reassuring to his mother. This reduced her anxiety and helped her to understand that his apparent resistance to harder foods was probably not because of dislike but because of physical difficulty and possibly some hyper-sensitivity to the textures. She was given advice about oral activities to increase Philip's tone and range of movements and to normalise sensation by giving him a variety of tastes and textures very regularly.

PROLONGED AND COMPLEX MEDICAL INTERVENTIONS

Children who are very sick have undergone major surgery or other invasive medical treatment, and prolonged hospital stays are at risk of feeding problems (*see* Chapter 12). These can be sensory or motor in nature, quite apart from any psychological effect such experiences may have. The age at which medical or surgical intervention has taken place is important. A child who has been in and out of hospital from infancy may never have established appropriate feeding routines and skills. The normal development of oral skills in the home environment, accompanied by social context and enjoyment, may have been disrupted, and thus important critical periods for feeding missed. Other children may have learnt to eat normally and then developed a condition, the treatment of which exposes them to potentially aversive experiences.

If the child is neurologically intact they are unlikely to have any frank oromotor problems. However, he or she may then appear to regress, for instance refusing all but pureed textures having previously been a competent eater of mixed foods. Children can become very fussy about both tastes and textures. This can be seen as a logical response to discomfort (such as nasogastric tube, unpleasant medicine given by mouth, frequent nausea and vomiting, intubation). Assessment of the child's oromotor skills is important in order to exclude a neurological aetiology and so focus on sensory and experiential aspects as the most likely precipitating factors. Children who are likely to fall into this group include those undergoing chemotherapy, those exposed to drugs in utero or later and those undergoing major surgery.

Tara: an example of conditioned aversive response

Tara was a 2½-year-old with previously normal feeding skills, undergoing treatment for leukaemia, including chemotherapy and bone marrow transplant. While in hospital, she was fed mainly by nasogastric tube to keep her weight up and although she was encouraged to eat as well, this was reduced to very occasional soft foods. She was happy to touch and explore other foods, but if it were suggested that she put them in her mouth, she would gag long before the food reached her mouth (conditioned gag). She was encouraged to feed herself and gradually gained confidence with a wide range of purees, mousses, etc. However, she did not make major improvements until she was at home and had some meals without the tube *in situ*. She quickly showed very good oromotor skills but remained fussy about new textures and mixed textures for one more year.

ENT DISORDERS AND UNUSUAL STRUCTURE OR FUNCTION
Cleft of the lip and/or palate

There are a number of abnormalities of the oral, nasal and pharyngeal regions that may disrupt feeding. The most common of these are the various types of cleft of the lip and/or palate, which as a group occur in one in 600 births. As a general rule, cleft just of the lip alone does not cause great problems; indeed, mothers who wish to breastfeed these babies are often successful. Cleft palate occurs in various forms. These range from sub-mucous cleft where there is no obvious 'hole', as it is the underlying bone and muscle which has failed to fuse despite an intact mucosal layer, through unilateral cleft of the hard and/or soft palate to bilateral cleft, where the child has very little effective roof to the mouth. This lack of intact palate may affect the posture and function of the tongue and thus feeding efficiency. Without an efficient soft palate, which would normally elevate to close of the nose during sucking and swallowing, there is a tendency for food to enter the nose. Some cleft babies learn to direct milk backwards with relatively little leakage into the nose. Others are troubled by a very inefficient suck and marked nasal regurgitation, particularly of liquids.

In the absence of any neurological problems, the muscle power and control of cleft babies is normal, but because of the lack of palate closure, they have difficulty building up pressure in the mouth. This results in a weak suck and often also the swallowing of air. Babies with clefts may therefore have discomfort from wind, sneezing, very long feed times and sometime a general disinclination to feed. In the early days, much can be done to help by using specialist teats, cup and spoon feeding, and careful positioning. Once the cleft lip and/or palate have been repaired, an improvement in feeding skills can usually be expected. But this may not be immediate as the effect of negative learning about feeding, alongside the physical difficulties, may have taken its toll. Children with cranial facial syndromes, such as Crouzons, are likely to have more complex feeding problems because of the combination of clefting, airway and other difficulties (for further information, refer to Bannister, 2001).

Pharyngeal and laryngeal malformations

Much less common are the various pharyngeal and laryngeal malformations that are usually of congenital aetiology but can also arise through trauma. Laryngomalacia (literally malformed larynx) causes problems because the baby has a compromised (inefficient or blocked) airway. This will inevitably affect feeding, particularly if the child has a tracheostomy fitted in order to ensure an adequate airway. Children with compromised airways often adopt a characteristic extended neck position, and this is an exception to the general rule that the best head position for swallowing is one where the chin is at 90° to the neck. Many tracheostomised children will be neurologically intact and can quite safely swallow with an extended head. However, it is important that the efficiency of the swallow is assessed. If it is not safe they may need to be fed by tube for some time. In older children, the presence of the tracheostomy may result in 'tethering' of the larynx, preventing it from elevating normally during swallowing. A marked improvement in swallowing may therefore be seen once the trachae tube is removed. A videofluoroscopic view of the oral and pharyngeal mechanisms during feeding can be very useful in these cases (Griggs et al., 1989). The child may be able to swallow some textures easily but have difficulty controlling liquids safely, and this can be demonstrated by using X-ray.

Bhupinder: a child with congenital laryngomalacia

Bhupinder was referred at 10 months with congenital laryngomalacia. He had had a tracheostomy in place since birth and had undergone two operations to try to remodel his larynx to ensure a safe airway. He was tube-fed until 6 months and then intermittently whenever he had a chest infection. He tended to be congested and short of breath and needed frequent suction, which his mother was able to do at home. He had normal oromotor skills and could drink well from a bottle for short periods before becoming tired and breathless. He tended to adopt an extended head position but had a safe swallow. He was interested in solid food but was tentative about new foods. Once he had tasted them he usually indicated that he wanted more. He needed to be sucked out during meals as he produced lots of mucus during oral activity and then became breathless. He enjoyed munching on breadsticks and other finger foods. His mother was encouraged to feed him little and often and offer a wide variety of different textures and tastes. He showed slow but steady improvement over the following 18 months, and once his trachae was removed at the age of 2 years and 10 months, he showed increased willingness to experiment with a variety of food types.

Tracheo-oesophageal fistula

Children with various types of tracheo-oesophageal fistula (TOF) also have difficulties, usually with swallowing rather than oral skills. These children have a malformation of the trachea and or the oesophagus such that there may be a danger of food entering the trachea. This malformation is identified within the first few hours or days of life, and the child will probably then be fed by tube for some months or occasionally years. After surgical repair of the anatomy, the child has gradually to be weaned on to oral feeding and has to get used to the associated sensations both in the mouth and in the thorax and abdomen. Some hospitals advocate 'sham feeding', which is the use of oral feeding to provide practice at eating, but with the food re-routed out through a stoma in the neck rather than going into the oesophagus and gut. Thus, the child is experiencing at least some aspects of oral feeding, while awaiting surgery or healing of the repair. Some TOF children continue to be reluctant feeders for many years, and some are bothered by recurrent strictures around the repair site, which cause discomfort and discourage the child from eating lumpy foods. Strictures can be dilated surgically but in the meantime some adverse learning about eating may have taken place. Similar types of problems sometimes occur in children who have acquired damage to the larynx, pharynx or oesophagus through swallowing acid, physical trauma or similar accidents (Puntis *et al.*, 1990).

THE EFFECTS OF EARLY AVERSIVE EXPERIENCES ON FEEDING SKILLS

Any aversive experiences that involve the oral structures or the feeding situation may affect feeding skills subsequently. These include aspiration, gastro-oesophageal reflux, oral medication, intubation, tube-feeding, breathlessness, suction, ventilation, force-feeding, etc. If early experiences of eating and drinking have been traumatic or difficult and have involved physical discomfort, such as coughing, choking or pharyngeal irritation, then the likelihood of feeling positive about mealtimes is reduced. A child who aspirates on liquids will associate drinking with the discomfort and panic involved rather than the pleasure of the drink. Feelings of breathlessness and exhaustion during feeding will also disincline the child to persevere even if they enjoy the taste of the food.

Similarly, children who have experienced regular medical procedures involving their mouth, such as passing of tubes, ventilation or taking unpleasant medicine, may develop abnormal sensory responses to any kind of activity in the oral and facial area. This often presents in the form of fussiness about taste and texture of food or more extreme refusal. In addition to the actual negative response to the food, it should be remembered that, for many children, there is also the simple matter of lack of practice. If they have had problems from infancy, they may never have built up the routine and skills needed to be consistently good feeders in a variety of situations. Tube feeding is discussed in detail in Chapter 11.

INTERACTION BETWEEN DIFFERENT TYPES OF FEEDING PROBLEMS

Of course there can be coexistence of several types of feeding problem, as well as between the bio, psycho and social aspects of eating and drinking. In fact, it is likely that several important factors will combine to create a marked difficulty rather than there being a single cause. Sometimes it is difficult to be sure where the boundaries between, say, a motor and sensory problem or a sensory and a behavioural difficulty lie. In a sense, it is an artificial boundary of only academic interest. The question of cause or effect of a resulting problem looms often and is frequently intractable in practical terms. For instance, most children who have experienced tube-feeding probably have some elements of both sensory and motor difficulty. Recognition that problems are often multi-factorial is important when planning intervention and underlines the importance of the contributions of many members of the multidisciplinary team.

SUMMARY

Normal feeding development begins in utero and is a dynamic physiological as well as psychological process. Progression through the stages of sucking and weaning on to more mature eating and drinking is usually smooth and unproblematic, and proceeds in parallel with other aspects of the child's motor, cognitive, communication and social development. Both the motor and sensory components of feeding development are important. The integration of movement and sensation with experience can be easily disrupted by a number of disease processes and/or any intervention that follows them. The reasons for feeding problems can be many and varied if a child has had a significant medical condition in infancy or childhood. In some ways, it is surprising that so many children who have aversive experiences early in life eat and drink well. Progress has been made in recent years with the recognition of the existence of subtle oral-motor and oral-sensory difficulties, which can have a major effect on feeding behaviour. Some of these effects may be preventable as there is some evidence that early aversive experiences and subtle oral-motor difficulties can have significant effects on later skills and attitudes at meal times. More research is needed into the most beneficial early preventative interventions to minimise the chances of long-term feeding difficulties in children with complex medical conditions. It is clear that careful assessment of children's oral-sensory and oral-motor skills and experiences, and specific intervention advice, form an important part of the bigger picture.

REFERENCES

Arvedson JC. Swallowing and feeding in infants and young children. *GI Motility Online*; 2006. Doi:10.1038/gimo17.

Bannister P. Early feeding management. In: Watson ACH, Sell DA, Grunwell P, editors. *Management of Cleft Lip and Palate*. London: Wiley; 2001.

Bolders Frazier J, Friedman B. Swallow function in children with Down syndrome: a retrospective study. *Dev Med Child Neurol*. 1996; **38**: 695–703.

Da Costa SP, Van der Schans CP. The reliability of the Neonatal Oral-Motor Assessment Scale. *Acta Paediatr*. 2008; **97**(1): 21–6.

Field T, Ignatof E, Stringer S, *et al*. Non-nutritive sucking during tube feedings: effects on preterm neonates in an intensive care unit. *Paediatrics*. 1982; **70**: 381–4.

Gisell EG. Effect of food texture on the development of chewing of children between six months and two years of age. *Dev Med Child Neurol*. 1991; **33**: 69–79.

Griggs CA, Jones PM, Lee RE. Videofluoroscopic investigation of feeding disorders of children with multiple handicap. *Dev Med Child Neurol*. 1989; **31**: 303–8.

Gryboski J. Gastrointestinal problems in the infant. *Major Problems in Clinical Pediatrics*. Philadelphia, PA: Saunders; 1975.

Howe TH, Sheu CF, Hsieh YW, *et al*. Psychometric characteristics of the Neonatal Oral-Motor Assessment Scale in healthy preterm infants. *Dev Med Child Neurol*. 2007; **49**(12): 915–19.

Law-Morstatt L, Judd DM, Snyder S, *et al*. Pacing as a treatment technique for transitional sucking patterns. *J Perinatol*. 2003; **23**: 483–8.

McKirdy LS, Sheppard JJ, Osborne ML, *et al*. Transition from tube to oral feeding in the school setting. *Language, Speech Hearing Ser Schools*. 2008; **39**: 249–60.

Measel CP, Anderson GC. Non-nutritive sucking during tube feedings: effect on clinical course in premature infants. *J Obs Gynecol Neonatal Nursing*. 1979; **8**: 265–72.

Palmer MM, Crawley K, Blanco I. NOMAS: nutritive suck: tongue. *J Perinatol*. 1993a; **xiii**(i): 30.

Palmer MM, Crawley K, Blanco I. The Neonatal Oral-Motor Assessment Scale: a reliability study. *J Perinatol*. 1993b; **13**: 28–35.

Palmer MM, Heyman MB. Assessment and treatment of sensory-versus motor based feeding problems in very young children. *Infant Young Child.* 1993; **6**(2): 67–73.

Puntis JW, Ritson DG, Holden CE. *et al.* Growth and feeding problems after repair of oesophageal atresia. *Arch Dis Child.* 1990; **65**: 84–8.

Spender Q, Stein A, Dennis J, *et al.* An exploration of feeding difficulties in children with Down syndrome. *Dev Med Child Neurol.* 1996; **38**: 681–94.

Tuchman DN. Cough, choke, splutter: the evaluation of the child with dysfunctional swallowing. *Dysphagia.* 1989; **3**: 3.

FURTHER READING

- Arvedson JC. Evaluation of children with feeding and swallowing problems. *Language, Speech, and Hearing Services in Schools.* Vol. 31. 2000. pp. 28–41.
- Braun MA, Palmer MM. A pilot study of oral-motor dysfunction in 'at-risk' infants. *Phy Occup Ther Pediatr.* 1985; **5**(4): 13–25.
- Bosma JF. Development of feeding. *Clin Nutrition.* 1986; **5**: 210–18.
- Bu'Lock F, Woolridge MW, Baum JD. Development of co-ordination of sucking, swallowing and breathing: ultrasound study of term and preterm infants. *Dev Med Child Neurol.* 1990; **32**: 669–78.
- Caeser P, Daniels H, Devleiger H, *et al.* Feeding behaviour in preterm neonates. *Early Hum Dev.* 1982; **7**: 331–46.
- Hawdon JM, Beauregard Slattery NJ, Kennedy G. Identification of neonates at risk of developing feeding problems in infancy. *Dev Med Child Neurol.* 2000; **42**: 235–9.
- Kramer SS. Radiological examination of the swallowing impaired child. *Dysphagia.* 1985; **3**: 117–25.
- Link DT, Rudolph CD. Gastroenterology and nutrition: feeding and swallowing. In: Rudolph CD, Rudolph AM, editors. *Rudolph's Pediatrics.* 21st ed. New York, NY: McGraw–Hill; 2003. pp. 13–82.
- Mathisen B, Skuse D, Wolke D, *et al.* Oral-motor dysfunction and failure to thrive among inner-city infants. *Dev Med Child Neurol.* 1989; **31**: 293–302.
- Morris SE. *Pre-speech Assessment Scale.* New Jersey: JA Preston Corporation; 1982.
- Morris SE, Klein MD. *Pre-feeding Skills: a comprehensive resource for feeding development.* Tucson, AZ: Therapy Skill Builders (available from Winslow Press, Buckingham); 1987.
- Reilly S, Skuse D, Mathisen B, *et al.* The objective ratings of oral-motor functions during feeding. *Dysphagia.* 1995; **10**: 177–91.
- Skuse D, Stevenson J, Reilly S, *et al.* Schedule for oral motor assessment (SOMA) methods of validation. *Dysphagia.* 1995; **10**: 192–202.
- Sullivan PB, Lambert B, Roe M, *et al.* Prevalence and severity of feeding and nutritional problems in children with neurological impairment: Oxford feeding study. *Dev Med Child Neurol.* 2000; **42**: 674–80.
- Van den Berg KA. Nippling management of the sick neonate in the NICU: the disorganised feeder. *Neonatal Network.* 1990; **9**(1): 9–16.

- Winstock A. *The Practical Management of Eating and Drinking Difficulties in Children*. Buckingham, UK: Winslow Press; 1994.
- Wolf PH. The serial organisation of sucking in the young infant. *Pediatrics*. 1968; 42(6): 943–56.
- Wolf S, Glass R. *Feeding and Swallowing Disorders in Infancy*. Tucson, AZ: Therapy Skill Builders; 1992.

CHAPTER 2

Children with feeding difficulties: medical and nursing perspectives

Charles Essex and Kim Woolliscroft

INTRODUCTION

About 25%–40% of infants and toddlers are reported by their caregivers to have feeding problems (Reau *et al.*, 2006). Although most of these difficulties are transient, they become persistent in 3%–10% of the children (Mitchell *et al.*, 2004), and these are the cases that bring families into contact with medical professionals. Many children are seen in clinic and hospital out-patient facilities by doctors and nurses who manage their feeding difficulties, often alongside their multi-disciplinary colleagues. Others are seen on the paediatric ward, either because they require a more intensive or specialist approach or because their need is acute; at such times, their feeding difficulties can be life-threatening.

This chapter focuses on medical and nursing approaches to feeding problems through exploration of the involvement of doctors and nurses as they collaborate in the assessment and treatment of children with a range of feeding difficulties. It looks at the role of the paediatrician in coordinating information, conducting investigations, making diagnoses and prescribing certain types of treatment. It integrates this with principles of nursing assessment, care and evaluation, outlining the contribution made by the paediatric nurse, much of whose work may be spent engaged in on-going assessment work, implementing treatment protocols and supporting families whose children have some form of feeding difficulty.

COLLABORATION ON THE PAEDIATRIC WARD

Doctors and nurses are engaged everyday in collaborative work, much of which involves their multi-disciplinary colleagues in various configurations according to the needs of the child. In recent years, much attention has been paid to the nature of this collaboration. This is acknowledged in the UK National Institute for Health and Clinical Excellence (NICE) guidelines, which recognise that the pace of organisational and clinical change makes it imperative to work collaboratively in order to stay at the forefront of knowledge. Nevertheless, it is a challenge to all professions, not least to nursing and medical traditions that have in the past been role-bound and hierarchical. New models emphasise specialisation, delegation and joint decision-making as improving collaborative relationships and leading to improved patient care. Rather than focusing on what doctors and nurses can do that are *the same*, these models focus on *difference* and the important contributions difference can bring.

It's the differences that matter

What characterises the new models of collaboration is the recognition that it is not what people have in common but their differences that make collaborative work more powerful than working separately. Working together means acknowledging that all participants bring equally valid knowledge and expertise from their personal and professional experience. Affirmations, acknowledgement and recognition are important, but it is the questions and challenges that arise from the differences that are vital.

Celia Davies, Professor of Healthcare, writing in the BMJ 2000.

PAEDIATRIC REFERRALS

The paediatrician and his or her team receives referrals from various sources, including primary care workers such as general practitioners (GPs) and health visitors, because of concerns about either a child's overall development or specific aspects of their development, in this case related to feeding. Alternatively, referrals may be made by, for example, a speech therapist or physiotherapist who has seen the child at the request of a primary care worker because of perceived difficulties with speech and language or gross motor skills. The therapist will then refer to the paediatrician for further assessment if it is felt that the child has significant difficulties and/or to exclude a more serious underlying condition. The assessment stage forms the basis for diagnosis, intervention and evaluation thereafter.

ASSESSMENT

When faced with a child with possible feeding problems, it is essential that a full and detailed assessment is taken, ideally from those who have most experience of dealing with the child (Whaley and Wong, 1998). The five key elements to be considered in the evaluation are as follows.

1   How is the feeding problem manifested?
2   Is the child suffering from any underlying disease?
3   Have the child's weight and development been affected?
4   What is the emotional climate like during the child's meals?
5   Are there any great stress factors in the family?

HISTORY

The medical and nursing history should, where possible, be undertaken collaboratively; this will prevent the family from repeating this information twice. Generic information exists for all types of feeding problems and is important to collate. This should include ante-natal and post-natal history, family history (particularly in relation to atopy or feeding problems), previous illnesses, hospitalisations and so on. Manipulation around the oropharynx area must also be considered.

The onset and chronology of the feeding problem is important. The history should therefore include details of the child's feeding since birth, any changes of formula, introduction of solids, current diet, textures and feeding position. It should also include information about quantities eaten, length of meals and associated routines, strategies already used, and environment and behaviour around mealtimes. Any food aversions and allergies need to be carefully outlined. Assessment must also be sensitive to social stressors, family relationship issues and emotional problems.

PREGNANCY, BIRTH AND THE POST-NATAL PERIOD

It is important to obtain as many details as possible about the child, as these can be extremely helpful in building up a picture of his or her background and any contributing factors. This includes details of the pregnancy, including maternal health problems or drugs taken (including those prescribed over the counter and illicit drugs), and length of gestation, which will indicate any prematurity. By implication, if a baby is born pre-term, there must have been a problem, either for the baby, the mother or both. Thus, premature labour began spontaneously or was induced for either the mother or baby's well-being (e.g. severe pregnancy-induced hypertension or foetal distress).

Details of the events surrounding the birth, such as premature rupture of membranes, the method of delivery of the baby and birth weight, can be very helpful. The method of delivery can indicate whether the baby was having problems before birth. For example, a caesarean section is not in itself a problem, but the reason why the baby was delivered by caesarean section may be significant. The condition of the baby immediately after birth and his or her weight are important. If a baby is small for its gestational age, there may have been intrauterine growth retardation.

TABLE 2.1: Apgar score

Score	0	1	2
Heart rate	absent	<100/min	>100/min
Respiratory effort	nil	slow, irregular	regular with cry
Muscle tone	limp	some tone in limbs	active moments
Reflex irritability	nil	grimance only	cry
Colour	pallor or cyanosis	body pink, extremities blue	pink all over

The Apgar score is frequently quoted (Apgar, 1953). This is a practical and quick method of systematically assessing the infant immediately after birth. The Apgar score evaluates five signs (Table 2.1) at 1 and 5 minutes. Each sign is given a score of 0, 1 or 2. Only the first of these five signs is objective, but the Apgar score does ensure that newborn babies are observed and assessed.

THE POST-NATAL PERIOD AND EARLY DEVELOPMENTAL HISTORY

The progress of the baby in the first few post-natal days can give valuable information. For example, a baby who has been taken home within a couple of days of birth has clearly not had significant perinatal problems. Conversely, babies who suffer from severe birth asphyxia or significant intracranial haemorrhage can have a very stormy time in the post-natal period, during which time they may have seizures and require ventilation and/or prolonged nasogastric feeding.

A baby who has birth asphyxia sufficient to cause brain damage is almost always extremely ill with hypoxic ischaemic encephalopathy; he or she requires neonatal intensive care, ventilation and non-oral feeding, and has seizures. A baby whose oesophagus did not form properly (oesophageal atresia) did not have a functioning oesophagus in utero and therefore is likely to present with feeding problems.

Details of the child's medical history, since the neonatal period, may reveal the need for hospital admissions or surgery. Information about the child's developmental progress will help to indicate whether developmental milestones have been reached within the appropriate time frame. Infants may be described by health professionals or parents as being 'slow' or 'late' to reach a milestone, such as walking. However, this is often in comparison to the 'average' age at which children reach that milestone. By definition, if that is the mean average, then 50% of children would have achieved that particular milestone, but 50% would not have.

FAMILY HISTORY

A family history extending beyond the members of the immediate family can be informative, as it may show that other members of the family had experienced feeding or eating difficulties or were simply 'picky eaters'. Alternatively, it may reveal serious medical conditions in other members of the family. The family history may also reveal numerous miscarriages, stillbirths or early infant deaths, and this has to be of consideration, as it may indicate an underlying genetic problem. In some cases where families have a particular cultural background that permits intra-familial marriage, parents should be asked specifically whether they are 'blood relatives', as consanguinity increases the risk of children having genetic disorders.

The medical history will indicate whether the child has had any significant illnesses, surgery or other admissions to hospital requiring interventions or investigations. Parents need to be specifically asked about whether the child has ever had a nasogastric tube inserted.

THE NURSING ASSESSMENT COMPONENT

Nursing assessment produces information that is used to identify the child and family's need for and response to nursing care. Observation, care, data collection and feedback contribute an ongoing perspective to the assessment process. Additionally, nurses invest in building therapeutic relationships with the family, making further observations (and often gaining further information) and supporting both the family and medical systems. In non-acute situations, family support is probably best undertaken in the home environment where the family is subject to the usual routines. However, in many geographical areas, community nursing support is not widely available, the result of which is that the child is admitted to an acute children's ward for a period so that a full assessment can take place.

Nursing assessments are based on 'models of care' (Roper *et al.*, 1983) and on more family-centred models (Casey, 1998). These models guide the children's nurse towards a holistic view of both child and family. Such models of assessment are used by the nurse when assessing the child and family where there is a potential feeding problem. In particular, parent–child interactions during feeding are often best observed by nurses, as they spend a greater amount of time on the ward with the family than most other practitioners. Positive interactions between parent and child, such as eye contact, reciprocal vocalisations, praise and touch, and negative interactions, such as force-feeding, coaxing and threatening, are important to record, as are the child's non-compliant behaviours (e.g. turning the head away from the spoon and throwing food). It is also helpful for an assessment to include details of behaviour occurring before and after the food is presented, as this can help inform any behavioural hypotheses (Babbit, 1994).

Following the assessment, care plans are formed using the nursing process. First, the nurse collects subjective and objective data, and then organises the data into a systematic pattern, for example:

- What is the current height and weight for this child?
- What is the child total calorie intake per day and in what form are they taken?

- Are family members generally under/overweight?
- Do they eat together as a family?

This step helps identify the areas in which the child and family needs nursing care, advice or support during the child's stay in the paediatric ward.

Based on this, the nurse makes a nursing diagnosis. This may be as simple as the child is receiving too few calories per day; however, it is rarely so simple as by the time they have been referred to the paediatric team, there are usually a number of other elements present and the problem has become complex.

After determining the nursing diagnosis, the nurse must state the expected outcomes, or goals. A common method of formulating the expected outcomes is to reverse the nursing diagnosis, stating what evidence should be present in the absence of the problem (e.g. ingestion of certain calorific intake daily, introduction of new foods/textures). The expected outcomes must also contain a goal date.

After the goal is set, the nursing interventions must be established. This is the plan of nursing care to be followed to assist the child and family in recovery. The interventions must be specific, noting how often it is to be performed, so that any nurse or appropriate health professional can read and understand the care plan easily and follow the directions exactly.

Reassessment after action is expressed as an evaluation. The evaluation is made on the goal date set. It is stated whether or not the child and family has met the goal, the evidence of whether or not the goal was met, and if the care plan is to be continued, discontinued or modified. If the care plan is problem-based and the child has recovered, the plan would be discontinued. If the child has not recovered, or if the care plan was written for a chronic illness or ongoing problem, it may be continued. If certain interventions are not helping or other interventions are to be added, the care plan is modified and continued.

Overall, collaborative assessment should help establish shared perceptions of the onset of the problem, how it has changed, what measures have been tried so far and with what degree of success, if any.

GENETICS

A number of conditions in which feeding difficulties may be one component have a genetic basis. A careful family history may reveal that other members of the family have had similar problems. However, recessive conditions, which require both parents to carry the responsible gene, may go undetected for several generations in a family until someone marries another unsuspecting carrier. Alternatively, the child with the condition may have a new mutation; in other words, he or she may be the first person in that family to have developed an inheritable condition and is thus at risk of passing on the condition to his or her children. Cystic fibrosis is one such chronic, inherited condition and is discussed in Chapter 12.

Genetic counselling may be undertaken by the paediatrician or the family can be referred to a geneticist. The family can be given an estimated risk of any future children having a similar condition. At the same time, they may also be given information about the likelihood of the affected child's offspring having a similar condition. If the condition can be recognised as a syndrome (i.e. a collection of symptoms and signs that constitute a known disorder), then some idea of the prognosis and likely development for the child can be given.

PHYSICAL EXAMINATION

The child needs a thorough physical examination. This will include looking at the overall appearance of the child, including any unusual facial features (referred to as dysmorphic features), which may be characteristic of a particular syndrome, or alternatively may alert the paediatrician to a possible underlying chromosomal abnormality or undefined non-specific congenital abnormality. The skin should be examined for any birth marks or unusual patterns of hyper- or hypopigmentation, as well as the structure of the hair and its patterns of growth (Smith and Gong, 1973) and teeth. The child's height, weight and head circumference should be measured and compared with any previous measurements, if available, to get an estimate of the rate of growth. As well as a general physical examination of the child, muscle bulk should be assessed as an indication of possible malnutrition or wasting.

A careful neurological examination of muscle tone and strength, reflexes and any tremor should be done. The child should be observed walking, if appropriate, as this may reveal abnormalities, such as mild cerebral palsy, which may otherwise not have been picked up. Drooling at an inappropriate age may indicate poor swallowing or poor control of muscles of the lips and mouth or neck. Abnormal eye movements, either as a squint or uncoordinated roving eye movements (nystagmus), may indicate an underlying neurological disorder.

Much information can be gained from observing the child play, and from his or her interaction with parents and strangers such as the doctor. The child's gestures, behaviour with adults and general interest in surroundings help build up an informal picture of the child's developmental abilities and developmental level.

It can be very helpful to observe how the child handles objects, whether he or she puts them to his or her mouth or not, if this is an appropriate developmental stage, or if an older child plays with toys in an imaginative way. It can be helpful to watch the child feed, which may be either breast or bottle feeding, or similarly, if the child is given solids such as biscuits or crisps, this will also provide useful information both in terms of how they are offered to the child as well as how they are received. Careful observation must take account of evidence of any neurological problems, indications of learning disabilities, or any impairment of social, communication or imaginative play skills and repetitive non-constructive actions, which might suggest a disorder along the autism spectrum.

Blood and urine tests may be arranged, as well as imaging techniques such as scans, although most oftenfrequently these are done to exclude conditions rather than to confirm that a specific condition exists. Investigations in both neuro-developmental delay and failure to thrive (FTT) are frequently unrewarding (Berwick *et al.*, 1982; Newton and Wraith, 1995).

GROWTH CHARTS

Growth charts, also known as centile charts, are often used by both health professionals and parents as an indicator of a child's nutritional status and general well being. However, it is important that they are used appropriately, and their limitations are recognised. Growth charts are compiled from serial measurements of a group of children, who are presumed to be normal over a period of time. Growth charts most commonly used are those for weight, height and head circumference, although centile charts are available for chest circumference, hand measurements, foot length, eye measurements, ear length, penile and testicular growth. Growth charts are also available for children with syndromes such as Down's syndrome, Cornelia de Lange syndrome and Turner's syndrome.

Traditionally, the growth charts have been drawn with the 97th, 90th, 75th, 50th, 25th, 10th and 3rd centiles. Recently, growth charts have been produced, which range from the 99.6th centile to the 0.4 centile. However, to get the maximum benefit from growth charts, measurements must be made correctly, plotted correctly and interpreted correctly. It is important to take into account familial growth patterns. Short parents tend to produce short children and vice versa; a significant number of children seen in growth clinics because of short stature are only following their familial trend (*see* Chapter 5).

It is generally accepted that allowance must be made for prematurity when plotting measurements on the growth chart. In other words, if the child was born, say, 8 weeks prematurely, then 8 weeks should be deducted from the child's chronological age. What is less clear is how long this allowance for prematurity should be made. Many paediatricians continue to allow for prematurity for the duration of the first growth chart (e.g. 0–2 years of age). If prematurity is ignored at some stage during the duration of a particular growth chart, for example, at the child's first birthday, then a measurement at approximately 12 months would be plotted and interpreted as if the child were 10 months old. The measurement taken the next day would be virtually the same and would be plotted at 12 months of age (the child's chronological age). It would appear as if the child had had a period of arrested growth.

DEVELOPMENTAL ASSESSMENT

Children with feeding difficulties need a careful developmental assessment. This may be one of the first indicators that the child has a serious underlying problem.

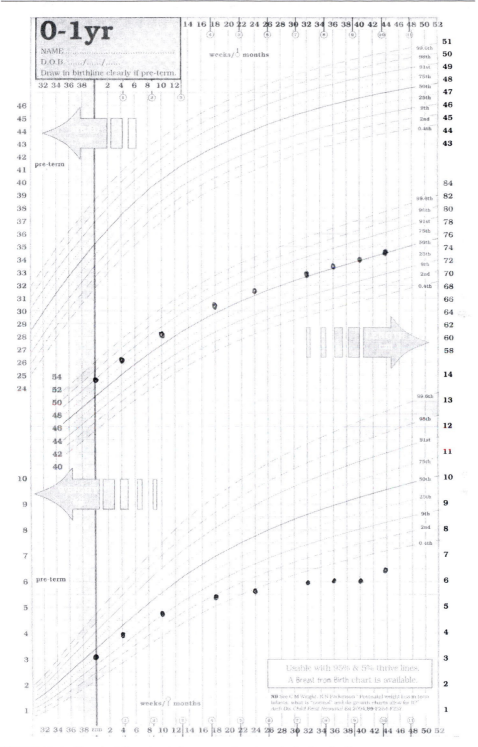

FIGURE 2.1: Classic failure to thrive secondary to caloric deprivation.

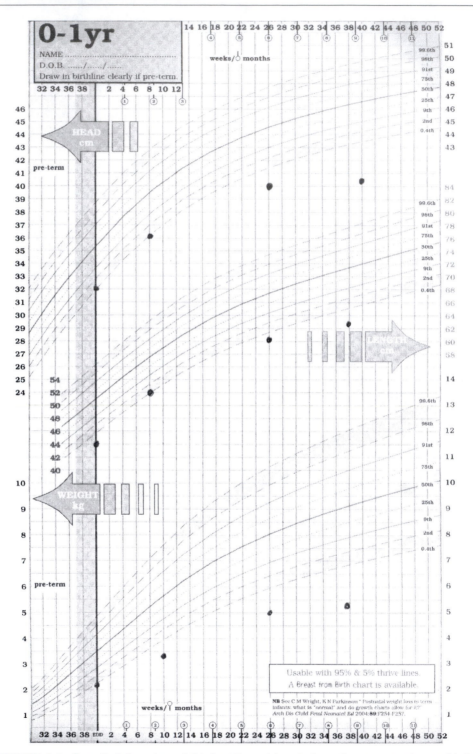

FIGURE 2.2: Growth failure in weight, length and head circumference starting at birth, suggesting a pre-birth organic aetiology.

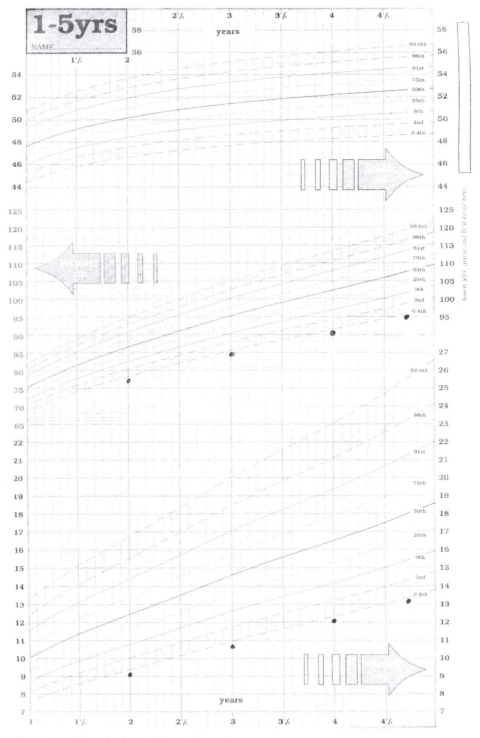

FIGURE 2.3: Constitutional delay of growth.

It will also give an indication of the child's feeding abilities, particularly the ability to communicate needs, wishes and preferences and the ability to self-feed.

The form of multi-disciplinary developmental assessment a child receives vary widely. In some districts, any child referred to the local Child Developmental Centre (CDC) because of suspected developmental delay is automatically accepted for assessment. The child may be seen over a consecutive number of days by a variety of therapists and health professionals, including the speech and language therapist, occupational therapist and physiotherapist. A number of further investigations may be made, such as hearing, vision, play and dental assessments, as well as a medical examination. Sometimes both an educational psychologist and a social worker are involved. In other districts, the child may be seen for a half-day assessment weekly for a number of weeks.

Some districts do not have a CDC, and the child will be seen by the appropriate professionals either at home, at the local clinic or in the child's nursery setting. In other areas, the community paediatrician undertakes an initial developmental assessment. If the child shows a developmental delay affecting one or possibly two areas of development, then referrals can be made to the appropriate therapists (e.g. for speech therapy and for a hearing test). However, if the child is showing delay in more than two areas of development, then a multi-disciplinary assessment is undertaken at the CDC.

From this, a comprehensive assessment of the child's abilities can be made and appropriate services put in place or recommendations made. This may include physical therapies, such as physiotherapy or speech therapy, psychological therapies for the child and family, educational services, such as special nursery placements, and the involvement of the educational and/or developmental psychologist.

INVESTIGATIONS

No laboratory investigations are indicated for infants with normal results of physical examinations, normal growth curves and normal results of developmental assessments. When infants are growing and developing according to the normally established parameters, practitioners should reassure parents in a consistent way and explain why no further investigations are indicated at this point. If a child's growth appears to be faltering, caloric intake should be assessed and, if needed, increased for a period prior to medical investigation. A detailed dietary history must be taken with the help of a dietician, if possible. Quality and quantity of food ingested must be assessed to document deficits in calories, vitamins, trace elements and food aversions. Most foods can be fortified to increase calorific value under the guidance of a paediatric dietician (Castiglia, 2005).

Where there is no improvement with these interventions, there is a need for further medical investigation. First-line laboratory investigations should include a complete blood count and assessment of sedimentation rate, serum albumin and protein, serum iron, iron-binding capacity and serum ferritin to detect specific nutrient deficits and to assess hepatic and renal function, as well as a sweat test to screen for systemic diseases. Antitransglutaminase antibodies for celiac disease are now widely available.

Coexisting medical problems should be addressed. Good medical and nursing management does not always alleviate feeding problems adequately. For instance, young children with cystic fibrosis often have a pattern of eating slowly, having difficulty chewing, preferring liquids, refusing to eat solids and having an aversion to new food (Mitchell, 2004); the families of these children will need support and education in order to be able to understand and accept this.

Despite nursing and other practitioners intervention, neurologically disabled children often need nasogastric or gastrostomy feedings when they are unable to ingest adequate calories safely and when the time required to provide adequate nutrition by mouth consumes parents' and children's lives, leaving little time for nurturing activities (Arvedson, 2002). For more discussion of neurological aspects of children's problems, refer to Chapter 10.

The number of children in United Kingdom who are being fed enterally at home is increasing (Hunt, 2007). While feeding by naso-gastric or gastrostomy tube may not seem particularly unusual to doctors and nurses who care for sick children, it can have a significant impact on both the child and his or her family. Research related to children with disabilities who have feeding problems is focused around the views of their mothers because they are often the main carers of these children. However, eating is a social activity in our society, and tube feeding will have an effect on other members of the family. In order to provide adequate support, nurses need to understand the nature and scale of the impact that continuing with oral feeding or changing to gastrostomy feeding has on the whole family (Hunt, 2007).

TREATMENT

If the child has a feeding problem, the fundamental aim of treatment is to ensure that sufficient calories are consumed for energy requirement and growth. Depending on the complexity of the feeding difficulty, a number of other professionals may be involved. The dietician is frequently involved in providing dietary advice and information about the use of high-calorie feeds and thickeners. His or her input is essential where any proposed changes to a feeding regime are required. Similarly, behavioural management advice may be important in order to promote changes in feeding behaviour (*see* Chapter 3). Practical measures such as positioning may be helpful; for example, in young infants with severe gastro-oesophageal reflux (GERD), placing the infant in a 30° reclined sitting position will help (Larnert and Ekberg, 1995).

PROFESSIONALS WHO MIGHT SEE A CHILD WITH FEEDING DIFFICULTIES

- *Paediatric gastroenterologist*: paediatrician with expertise in disorders of the gastrointestinal system.
- *Paediatric endocrinologist*: paediatrician with expertise in disorders of the glands.
- *Maxillofacial, craniofacial or plastic surgeon*: surgeon with expertise in operating in the area of the head and neck.
- *Geneticist*: doctor specialising in inherited or congenital disorders.
- *Physiotherapist*: examines physical performance, gross motor skills and body organisation.
- *Occupational therapist*: deals with fine motor skills, hand function, activities of daily living, perception and graphic skills.
- *Speech and language therapist*: specialises in the development of a child's communication skills and examines issues relating to oral and pharyngeal functioning.
- *Clinical child psychologist*: specialises in issues relating to functioning in the areas of emotional, behavioural and social development at individual family and group levels.
- *Educational psychologist*: psychologist with expertise in the educational needs of children with chronic or severe disorders which may interfere with access to the National Curriculum in the normal way.

LIAISON WITH EDUCATION SERVICES

Most children with feeding problems are identified in the pre-school years. However, if the feeding difficulty is part of a wider developmental, learning or medical problem, then the child will have difficulties, which will probably impinge on his or her ability to access the educational curriculum in the usual way.

The special needs department of the local education authority therefore needs to be alerted to these children well before the age of school entry. The community paediatrician who has the remit for children with special needs or neurodevelopmental problems will usually liaise with the appropriate education officer. Although it may vary between geographical areas, this is usually the educational psychologist.

DRUG TREATMENT

Many children who have GERD or repeated vomiting are often prescribed alginate combinations (e.g. Gaviscon). These work by forming a viscous layer on top of the gastric contents. Thus, if the child refluxes or vomits, the surface layer, which also contains antacids, will offer some protection to the oesophageal mucosa. The adult formulation of Gaviscon contains relatively high amounts of sodium, and therefore, Infant Gaviscon should be used in children under two years of age.

Prokinetic drugs are useful in that they have an effect throughout the gastro-intestinal tract. These increase tightening of the oesophageal sphincter and promote gastric emptying. Cisapride is the most commonly used prokinetic drug. It can cause colic and diarrhoea as a secondary effect, although as children with feeding difficulties often can have severe neurological impairment and also constipationand this effect on the bowels may be welcome.

Drugs to reduce gastric acid secretion are used in more severe cases. These include H2 antagonists such as cimetidine. Gastric acid secretion can also be reduced by drugs such as omeprazole, which is a proton pump inhibitor that blocks the final step in the pathway of gastric acid production. Many children whose feeding problems are related to severe neurological impairment or to significant neurological immaturity have significant drooling. Although this is not usually distressing for the child, it can be embarrassing for parents and siblings and can also create a lot of washing for the parents as the child may require a change of clothes several times a day. Hyoscine patches can be very effective at reducing drooling. These are slow-release patches that are stuck on the skin, rather like plasters. They are impregnated with hyoscine, which is then absorbed transdermally, and are effective for up to three days.

Other more invasive treatments are sometimes used. The most frequent is a nasogastric tube. These can be used either on an intermittent basis or inserted and removed on a daily basis. They may also be left *in situ* long-term.

SURGICAL AND INVASIVE TREATMENTS
Nasogastric tube

Although nasogastric tubes are normally a hospital-based intervention, they are sometimes used in the community. Briefly, the advantages of nasogastric tubes are as follows:
- they can be inserted rapidly
- parents can be taught to insert them
- they allow food and medicines to be given directly into the stomach
- they can be removed easily and quickly.

Nasogastric tubes also have disadvantages. These are summarised as follows:
- frequent development of sensitivity around the mouth and nasopharynx

This can be a particular problem for children who are taking some food or drink by mouth; this oral feeding, however limited, may be lost if the child becomes sensitive or develops an aversion to things in or around his or her mouth.
- the discomfort of having a foreign body in place; increased saliva production
- the visual impact of the nasogastric tube if it is left in place and strapped to the face
- skin reactions from the strapping and soreness to the nose
- they do not prevent GERD.

Gastrostomy

Gastrostomies are being used increasingly for children who have prolonged periods of significant feeding difficulties in preference to continued or prolonged nasogastric feeding. In consultation with both the parents and other health professionals caring for the child, the child may be referred to a paediatric surgeon for insertion of a gastrostomy. The indications for gastrostomy are given below.

Indications for gastrostomy

- Severe oral and/or pharyngeal dysphagia.
- Unsafe oral feeding.
- Prolonged oral feeding times.
- Inadequate oral intake.
- Failed oral supplementation.
- Chronic food refusal.
- Prolonged nasogastric tube feeding.
- Increased energy needs.

Gastrostomies have several advantages. These include improved nutritional access, improved growth, reduced feeding times, reduced feeding-related choking and reduced incidence of chest infections (Elthami and Sullivan, 1997; Tawfik *et al.*, 1997).

However, they also have disadvantages, both physical and psychological. The physical disadvantages include early complications, such as bleeding from the site of the wound, wound infections, abdominal distension, vomiting and gastroenteritis. Late complications include vomiting, retching, granulation around the wound, late infection, GOR (which can be particularly severe) and 'dumping'. 'Dumping' takes place when there is distortion of the anatomy of the stomach and interference of the normal peristaltic movements of the stomach musculature. A bolus of semi-digested food can be 'dumped' in the upper part of the small intestine and lead to abdominal discomfort, with sweating and pallor.

The disadvantages of gastrostomy feeding also include the surgical nature of the insertion of the tube, the anaesthetic and the fact that it is an 'unnatural' method of feeding – the inability of the parents to provide for the child's nutritional needs in a 'normal' way.

Children must be carefully selected for gastrostomy. This includes:
- careful assessment of the child's nutritional needs and whether or not these are being met by other means
- the views of the family on having a gastrostomy inserted
- the presence of any GERD.

If the child has GERD, this is almost always made worse by the insertion of a gastrostomy. Children will therefore need specialised barium X-rays of the oesophagus and stomach before surgery.

Most paediatric surgeons would correct any GERD or perform a fundoplication (an operation in which part of the stomach is wrapped around the lower end of the oesophagus) to prevent any subsequent GERD (Heine *et al.*, 1995). Many children with feeding difficulties also have bowel problems, of which constipation is by far the most common. It is outside the remit of this chapter to discuss this issue, although a comprehensive review can be found elsewhere (Clayden, 1992).

Excessive drooling

Many children with feeding problems also have problems with drooling. There are a variety of reasons for this, such as difficulty with swallowing, oromotor difficulties or nasogastric feeding. Advice on treatment for drooling should be readily available. Whereas some parents and children may not find this a problem, others will. If required, the community paediatrician can make a referral to the oral surgeon who can perform a relocation of the salivary glands as necessary, which can direct the flow of saliva backwards into the pharynx. Alternatively, the community paediatrician can prescribe hyoscine patches to help to dry up oral secretions, as described above.

Failure to thrive (FTT)

The term FTT refers to the state of inadequate growth from inability to obtain and/ or use calories required for growth. It is a symptom, not a disease, but regardless of the aetiology, all children failing to thrive have malnutrition (Hoare, 2009). FTT has no universal definition, although one of the most common parameters is weight and sometimes height. Percentile charts are routinely used for all children accessing healthcare and constitute an efficient opportunity to identify children who may be failing to thrive. Although definitions vary, most authors use this term only when growth has been noted to be low or to have decreased over time. For instance, some authors define FTT as a height or weight of less than the third to fifth percentiles for age on more than one occasion. Other authors cite height or weight measurements falling 2 major percentile lines using the standard growth charts of the National Center for Health Statistics (NCHS). Still others state that true malnutrition (weight <80% of ideal body weight for age) should be present to state a child is failing to thrive.

All authorities agree that only by comparing height and weight on a growth chart over time can FTT be accurately assessed. Although measurements of head circumference are important in the evaluation of infants and toddlers, failure of the head to grow by itself is not part of the FTT entity (Hoare, 2009).

Two general categories of FTT have been defined (Genero, 1996). In both instances the nurse is ideally positioned to provide parent education and provision of necessary support (financial or psychosocial) which will successfully correct the reasons for the malnutrition.

Organic FTT

This category of FTT is a result of a physical cause, such as congenital heart defect, neurological problems, chronic infection, gastro-oesophageal reflux, malabsorption or cystic fibrosis. However, this category accounts for less than half of all FTT (Levy *et al.*, 2009).

Non-organic FTT

This category of children also has a definable cause but it is unrelated to disease. Non-organic FTT is most commonly the result of psychosocial factors, such as inadequate nutrition information by the parent, deficiency in care or a disturbance in the carer–child attachment (Briggs and Priddis, Chapter 4). However, many other factors can contribute to the inadequate feeding of children, such as poverty, inadequate knowledge, health beliefs, family stress or feeding resistance.

Diagnosis is initially made on anthropomorphic findings documented growth retardation. If FTT is recent, the weight but not the height will be below the accepted standard. If FTT is long standing, both weight and height will be depressed, indicating chronic malnutrition.

Additional diagnostic procedures including a dietary history will be needed. Other investigations are selected by the paediatrician only as indicated to eliminate organic problems. Unfortunately, many children undergo exhausting, traumatic, expensive diagnostic procedures that are often not necessary. To prevent the overuse of diagnostic procedures, non-organic FTT should be considered early in the differential diagnosis and the children's nurse given the opportunity to assess the child and family in order to aid the diagnosis prior to investigation.

This assessment requires the nurse to have knowledge regarding the general characteristics of children (and their families) in whom non-organic FTT is probable. These skills are essential in helping identify these children and hastening the confirmation of a correct diagnosis without the need for invasive investigations. The general characteristics for this group of children include (Klein, 2004):

* growth failure – in weight only or both weight and height
* developmental delay – social, motor and language
* apathy
* poor hygiene
* withdrawn behaviour
* feeding or eating disorders, such as vomiting, rumination and anorexia
* avoidance of eye-to-eye contact
* minimum smiling.

Accurate measurement and documentation of weight and height, as well as a recording of all oral intakes, is essential. The nurse should ensure that there is an agreed process in place that enables the behaviour of the child and family to be directly observed, this would include parent–child interaction generally but be particularly focused on feeding.

In particular, the nurse will be observing for signs of parental maladaptive behaviour toward the child, these may include:

- handling the child only when necessary
- asking few or no questions regarding care of child
- annoyed at nappy changing
- holding child away from body when feeding
- develops inappropriate responses to the child's needs, e.g. over or under feeding
- cannot discriminate between the child's signals for hunger, comfort, rest or contact
- is convinced there is an organic cause for the FTT
- makes negative statements regarding the child.

Implications for nursing

Regardless of the cause of FTT, the role of the nurse is centred on supporting the family to reverse the malnutrition. The general goal is to provide sufficient calories to support 'catch up' growth, which is a rate of growth greater than the expected rate for age. Often in cases of non-organic FTT, there needs to be a team approach to care including, nurse, doctor, health visitor/school nurse, psychologist, social worker and mental health practitioner.

The prognosis of non-organic FTT is very much dependent on the cause and is often dependent on the ability of the parents/carer to engage in partnership working. If the parents/carer has simply been ignorant of the child's needs, education and support may be all that is needed from the nursing staff. However, when the family dysfunction is extensive the role of the nurse is difficult and will always require a team approach to achieve the best outcome for the child and family. This should focus on the following principles: (Whaley and Wong, 1998)

- structuring a feeding environment that encourages the child to consume adequate calories and provide age appropriate foods
- providing appropriate developmental stimulation for the child
- teaching parents/carer feeding techniques and general care-giving activities such as suitable play
- providing a supportive environment for parents/carers, develop partnerships that encourage the parents to develop new skills
- making appropriate referrals to other agencies, e.g. social services, psychologists and speech and language therapists.

The effectiveness of nursing intervention is determined by continuous ongoing support; reassessment and evaluation based on observational guidelines and expected outcomes. Once these outcomes are met, a discharge planning meeting must be undertaken prior to the child and family being transferred to the care of the GP to ensure ongoing support in the community from appropriate practitioners.

OTHER COMMON FEEDING RELATED PROBLEMS SEEN ON THE PAEDIATRIC WARD

Among the commonest causes of admission to the children's ward are children and infants with problems related to possetting and colic.

Possetting

Possetting in young infants is the term used to describe the repeated, effortless regurgitation of small quantities of milk and stomach acid into the mouth after feeding, often when being winded (Plarre, 2007) and can occasionally continue until the next feed (Weldon, 2002). This problem affects a large proportion of infants under the age of 3 months and often continues into early childhood. Some infants are particularly susceptible to possetting, especially if they are very hungry prior to a feed or swallow more air than normal as they feed. In some babies, it is merely the appropriate response to overfeeding.

Possetting causes no significant degree of pain or discomfort, and is no cause for concern if the baby is happy, feeds well and gains weight. The serious underlying pathology is present in only a small minority of cases. It occurs when abdominal pressure overcomes an infant's immature or weak lower oesophageal sphincter (LOS) – the muscular valve between the oesophagus and the stomach, which usually prevents regurgitation. Milk easily bypasses this muscle. Almost all babies posset to some extent in the early months. Some bring back milk at every feed and sometimes more than once.

In most babies, posseting is at its worst between 1 and 4 months of age. It generally resolves naturally by 18 months as the muscle strengthens, the infant eats more solid food and spends more time in the upright position.

Fortunately, in the majority of infants, possetting is self-limiting, resolving spontaneously within the first year of life as the infant starts to eat solids and spends more time in an upright position.

Nevertheless, it is often confused with actual vomiting and causes anxiety and feelings of inadequacy and guilt in the parents. These infants are often admitted to hospital as a result of parental concern. Most posseting can be managed without the need for medical intervention or investigation.

Following a full and detailed nursing assessment, simple management techniques may be encouraged. These are listed below.

Feeding and handling advice for possetting
- Handle the baby extra gently, especially when winding.
- Raise the head of the cot slightly.
- Give smaller feeds more frequently.
- Keep their baby upright during feeding and for at least 45 minutes afterwards.
- Angling the bottle correctly.
- Burping/winding every 5 minutes.
- Avoid nappy changing when the baby's stomach is full.

It is of the utmost importance that the family are clear as to the diagnosis, prognosis and are given practical advice on how to manage this very common condition.

Colic

Colic is generally described as paroxysmal abdominal pain or cramping that is manifested by loud and persistent crying and drawing up of the legs to the abdomen. Other definitions include variables such as crying for more than 3 hours a day and parental dissatisfaction with the child's behaviour. It is more common in young infants under the age of three months and infants with 'difficult' temperaments (Barr *et al.*, 1999). Despite the obvious behavioural indication of pain, the child tolerates the feed well, gains weight and thrives. Despite this, the level of parental anxiety and stress is high.

Many theories have been investigated as to the potential causative factors, but currently no one theory is supported universally. In fact, much controversy exists about the aetiology the condition and many health professionals question if colic merely represents a maturational stage. This in turn can increase the stress levels of parents, as they do not feel listened to or taken seriously (Gilles, 2006).

Therefore, while colic is considered a 'minor' ailment, the presence of a colicky, crying, irritable infant can have an intense emotional impact on parent–child attachment and family relationships. Parents, especially mothers, often relate histories of daily routine that is laden with feelings of guilt, frustration, anger and despair. A vicious cycle ensues in which the parent's own anxiety may be transferred to the infant, further increasing the tension, irritability and crying.

IMPLICATIONS FOR NURSING

The initial step by the nurse is to undertake a detailed history of the usual daily routine of events as follows (Sampson, 2005):

1   diet of the breastfeeding mother
2   time of day when attacks occur
3   relationship of attacks to feeding times
4   presence of specific family members and habits, such as smoking during attacks
5   activity of the mother or usual care giver before, during and after the crying episode
6   characteristics of the cry (duration and intensity)
7   measures used to relieve crying and their effectiveness.

Of special emphasis is a careful assessment of the feeding process via demonstration and direct observation of the parent by the nurse. A common cause of feeding problems is improper feeding technique. Children's nurses are well placed to support families with difficulties in this area.

In order to feed satisfactorily, a number of mechanical skills can be suggested, such as placing the infant to the breast or bottle at the correct angle allowing milk and not air to enter the baby's mouth, reading the babies cues for burping or satiation and holding the baby in the arms rather that propping the bottle against something while the baby is laying flat. A number of other problems can occur singly or in combination, such as feeding too much or too little, selecting incorrect foods for the baby's physical or motor development and incorrectly preparing the milk formula.

While such feeding problems are more common in inexperienced parents, they can also occur with seasoned parents who are unprepared for an infant with different needs or less clear cues of hunger or satiation. Most of these problems are easily corrected with guidance and demonstration. Early assessment and intervention is essential to prevent complex problems from developing between parent and child at mealtimes.

More often than not, little or no change is required in feeding practice. When no cause can be found, it is preferable to determine the time of the onset of crying and attempt to manipulate the circumstances associated with it. For example, there is evidence to suggest that infants have episodes of colic around the family meal time (Hartsell, 2006) when all family members are home and the mother is pre-occupied with cooking. The over-stimulating, tense atmosphere may upset the infant. Often encouraging another family member to prepare the dinner or for the mother to prepare dinner earlier in the day and feed the infant in a quiet area of the house may help to reverse the environmental conditions that may be provoking the attack of colic.

One of the most important areas of nursing concern is the support of parents during the colic period. It should be stressed that despite the crying and obvious pain, the infant is in no danger and in fact is doing well. Colic disappears usually by 3 months, but guarantee should not be given as it can continue much longer.

Most important, it should be stressed by the nurse that colic does not indicate poor or inadequate parenting. Parents need to be reassured that negative feelings toward the infant and insecurities regarding their parenting abilities are normal. Parents should be encouraged to talk about such feelings since active listening may do more to relieve the colic syndrome than offering stereotyped advice and remedies that have very little evidence to underpin their effectiveness.

SUMMARY

A basic definition of feeding is that it is, of course, fundamental to children's growth. If there is a feeding problem, of whatever cause, it is necessary to ensure that the child is getting adequate nutrition, that feeding is safe, efficient, comfortable and enjoyable. Feeding is also a core parenting and nurturing task, which, if it is not going well, can cause parents to feel undermined in their most basic of human roles, namely loving their child. One of the tasks of the paediatric team is to ensure that the appropriate services are offered and put in place, not only to maximise the child's nutrition and growth but also to support the parents in this most fundamental and important of tasks.

REFERENCES

Apgar V. A proposal for a new method of evaluation of the newborn infant. *Curr Res Anaesthesiol.* 1953; **32**: 360.

Arvedson JC. Management of pediatric dysphagia. *Otolaryngol Clin North Am.* 2002; **31**: 453–75.

Babbitt RA, Hoch TA, Coe DA, *et al.* Behavioral assessment and treatment of pediatric feeding disorders. *J Dev Behav Pediatr.* 1994; **15**: 278–91.

Barr, *et al. Child Abuse and Neglect.* London: Elseiner; 1999.

Berwick DM, Levy JC, Kleinerman R. Failure to thrive: diagnostic yield of hospitalisation. *Arch Dis Child.* 1982; **57**: 347–51.

Casey A. A partnership with child and family. *Senior Nurse.* 1998; **8**(4): 8.

Castiglia P. Failure to thrive. *J Paediatr Health Car.* 2005; **B**(1): 50.

Clayden GS. Management of chronic constipation. *Arch Dis Child.* 1992; **67**: 340–4.

Elthami M, Sullivan PB. Nutritional management of the disabled child: the role of percutaneous endoscopic gastrostomy. *Dev Med Child Neurol.* 1997; **39**: 66–8.

Genero A, Moretti C, Fait P. Non-organic failure to thrive: retrospective study in hospitalized children. *Pediatr Med Chir.* 1996 Sep–Oct; **18**(5): 501–6.

Gillies C. Is there anything new? *J Paediatr Health Car.* 2006; **2**(6): 305.

Hartsell M. Babies crying spells. *J Paediatr Nurs.* 2006; **2**(6): 438.

Heine RG, Reddihough DS, Catto-Smith AG. Gastroesophageal reflux and feeding problems after gastrostomy in children with severe neurological impairment. *Dev Med and Child Neurol.* 1995; **37**: 320–9.

Hoare KJ. A baby presenting with failure to thrive in primary care: a case report. *Cases J.* 2009; **2**(1):137.

Hunt F. Changing from oral to enteral feeding: impact on families of children with disabilities. *Paediatr Nurs.* 2007 Sep; **19**(7): 30–2.

Klein M. The nurse's role in the prevention of nonorganic failure to thrive. *J Paediatr Nurs.* 2004; **5**(2): 129.

Larnert G, Ekberg O. Positioning improves the oral and pharyngeal swallowing function in children with cerebral palsy. *Acta Paediatr.* 1995; **84**: 689–92.

Levy Y, Levy A, Zangen T, *et al.* Diagnostic clues for identification of nonorganic vs organic causes of food refusal and poor feeding. *J Pediatr Gastroenterol Nutr.* 2009 Mar; **48**(3): 355–62.

Mitchell MJ, Powers SW, Byars KC, *et al.* Family functioning in young children with cystic fibrosis: observations on interactions at mealtime. *J Dev Behav Pediatr.* 2004; **25**: 335–46.

Newton RW, Wraith JE. Investigation of developmental delay. *Arch Dis Child.* 1995; **72**: 460–5.

Plarre FE. Babies who cry. *J Adv Nurs.* 2007; **36**(4): 27–30.

Reau NR, Senturia YD, Lebailly SA, *et al.* The Pediatric Practice Research Group. Infant and toddler feeding patterns and problems: normative data and a new direction. *J Dev Behav Pediatr.* 2006; **17**: 149–53.

Roper N, *et al.* The meaning of models of nursing. *Nursing Times.* 1983; **21**: 36–9.

Sampson H. Infantile colic, fact or fiction. *J Paediatr Nurs.* 2005; **115**(4): 538.

Smith DW, Gong DT. Scalp hair patterning as a clue to early fetal brain development. *J Pediatr.* 1973; **83**: 374–80.

Tawfik R, Dickson A, Clarke M, *et al.* Caregivers' perceptions following gastrostomy in severely disabled children with feeding problems. *Dev Med Child Neurol.* 1997; **39**: 746–51.

Weldon AP. Vomiting or not? *J Paediatr Nurs.* 2002; **117**(4): 538.

Whaley D, Wong DL. *Children's Nursing.* London: Mosby; 1998.

CHAPTER 3

Behavioural approaches to the management of paediatric feeding disorders

Petula CM Vaz and Cathleen C Piazza

INTRODUCTION

Children with paediatric feeding disorders fail to consume a sufficient quantity and variety of solids or liquids to maintain nutritional status, which may result in weight loss, malnutrition, dehydration, frequent illness, failure to thrive and, if left untreated, death. They may also develop learning and behaviour problems. Therefore, their early identification and timely management are extremely important.

As discussed in Chapters 1 and 2, paediatric feeding disorders are a heterogeneous group of problems that usually result from a combination of multiple factors such as medical conditions (e.g. gastro-oesophageal reflux disease (GERD)), oral motor disorders (e.g. inability to lateralise the tongue), physiological factors (e.g. disorders of appetite regulation or hunger) and behavioural factors (e.g. caregivers terminating the meal following inappropriate mealtime behaviour). For example, a child with GERD may learn to pair eating with pain. So, the child may refuse to eat to avoid these unpleasant consequences. This refusal behaviour may limit the child's ability to master the oral motor skills essential for eating, impede the development of age-appropriate oral motor skills and prevent the child from advancing to age-appropriate textures.

An interdisciplinary team approach is most appropriate for assessing the multiple aetiologies of paediatric feeding disorders. A comprehensive feeding evaluation typically includes:

- medical assessment
- oral motor assessment
- nutritional assessment
- behavioural assessment.

The members of the interdisciplinary team meet following the evaluation to formulate recommendations for the child and consider possible outcomes of the interdisciplinary evaluation (e.g. further medical testing, additional evaluation or intervention). Individualised, structured behavioural approaches have proven to be essential in the management of paediatric feeding disorders, and their effectiveness has good empirical support in the scientific literature. Favourable outcomes have been reported following intensive interdisciplinary paediatric feeding disorders treatment programs (Byars *et al.*, 2003; Irwin *et al.*, 2003; Piazza and Carroll-Hernandez, 2004; Williams *et al.*, 2007).

THE CHILD'S LEARNING HISTORY

From a behavioural perspective, it is important to consider the impact of the child's medical history and the child's and family's learning history on child and parent behaviour. The routes by which a child's feeding behaviour may develop are outlined in Box 3.1.

Box 3.1: Potential routes of learning for the child in the development of a feeding disorder

Aversive conditioning may occur when the child experiences repeated pairing of physically unpleasant sensations (e.g. nausea) with feeding and the stimuli associated with feeding (e.g. bottle and spoon). Following this repeated pairing, the future presentation of the feeding stimuli may begin to elicit behaviours such as crying, nausea, retching, vomiting and gagging. The child also may begin to engage in refusal behaviour such as batting at the spoon and head turning following the presentation of the feeding stimuli. These refusal behaviours may increase if the parent removes the spoon or cup (negative reinforcement) or provides attention, preferred food or toys (positive reinforcement) following the child's refusal behaviour (Girolami and Scotti, 2001; Najdowski *et al.*, 2008; Piazza *et al.*, 2003a).

In addition, oral motor dysfunction may occur due to physical deficits (e.g. cleft lip) or lack of opportunity to eat, such as when the parent ends the meal because of the child's refusal behaviour or when the child has a feeding tube and the parent does not feed the child orally. Children with oral motor deficits may lack the skills to be effective feeders. These skill deficits may also impact the child's motivation to eat (i.e. 'eating is hard, so I don't want to do it'). Finally, early or late introduction of solid foods can contribute to the child's difficulty in managing age-appropriate textures.

Just as the parent's behaviour may affect the child's behaviour during meal-time, the child's responses to the parent may affect the parent's behaviour (*see* Box 3.2).

Box 3.2: Potential routes of learning for the parent in the development of the child's feeding disorder

Repeated pairing of the child's inappropriate behaviour during feeding (e.g. cry-ing) and the stimuli associated with feeding (e.g. spoon and food) may cause mealtime to become aversive for the parent. Parents may try a number of strat-egies to stop the child from engaging in inappropriate mealtime behaviour. Strategies that parents may use to 'calm the child down' include ending the meal, providing attention and offering the child preferred food or toys (Piazza *et al.*, 2003a). If parent behaviour (e.g. ending the meal) results in the cessation of the child's inappropriate behaviour, even momentarily, the parent is likely to engage in that behaviour again in the future. For example, parents may feed only preferred food to their selective child if the child eats when the parents present only the preferred food and the child engages in inappropriate behav-iour and does not eat when offered non-preferred food. When attempting to change parental behaviour patterns, the therapist needs to be aware of how difficult it is to change when parental behaviour is reinforced by not having a crying, oppositional child at the table and by having a child who also eats food that is placed in front of him or her.

Many parents benefit from nutritional counselling with a focus on offering the child a diet that is both calorically and nutritionally appropriate. Parents of children who struggle with weight gain may tend towards providing only high-calorie foods and ignore the need to provide the child with a diet that is nutritionally balanced as well, which may result in the child receiving primarily 'empty' calories. Other par-ents may not realise that the caloric and nutritional needs of a child are different from those of an adult, which may result in the child receiving insufficient calories (e.g. the parent provides the child with only 'low fat' foods). Finally, the parent may need guidance on the textures or consistencies of food that are appropriate based on the child's oral motor skills.

BEHAVIOURAL ASSESSMENT

Before proceeding with a behavioural approach to a paediatric feeding disorder, it is critical that the child has been cleared as a safe oral feeder by a qualified professional and that the child's medical problems (if any) have been resolved to the extent possible, with the medical team recommending oral feeding therapy. After this, it is vital that the professional applying the behavioural treatment has sufficient training and experience in working with children with paediatric feeding disorders. Direct observation of the parents and child at a mealtime enables existing patterns of eating to be assessed and provides a wealth of information about existing maintaining factors (Piazza *et al.*, 2003a).

The main purpose of the behavioural assessment is:

1 to identify the behaviours that characterise the feeding problem
2 to define these behaviours operationally such that they can be observed and measured
3 to identify the antecedents and consequences of appropriate and inappropriate feeding behaviours.

Identification of behaviours

The first step in problem identification is to 'sort through' the various behaviours that may be contributing to the child's feeding disorder. There are a number of common problems, and these are summarised in Box 3.3.

Box 3.3: Commonly occurring problems in a feeding disorder
- Total food refusal (the child does not accept any solid food or liquids).
- Food selectivity by type (the child only eats certain foods of a specific type).
- Food selectivity by texture (the child only eats a certain texture of food).
- Liquid dependence (the child consumes only liquids as the sole source of nutrition).
- Bottle dependence (age-inappropriate dependence on the bottle as a sole source of nutrition).
- Inappropriate mealtime behaviours (e.g. crying, throwing food and batting at the spoon).
- Expulsion (spitting out food).
- 'Packing' or 'pocketing' food (i.e. holding food in the mouth).
- Idiosyncratic eating behaviour (e.g. only accepting the bottle during sleep).
- Excessive meal length (Field *et al.*, 2003; Kerwin, 1999; Munk and Repp, 1994).

Defining behaviours

A useful strategy in evaluating the severity of the child's feeding problem is to compare the child's feeding behaviour with developmental norms (*see* Chapter 1).

Excessive meal length is one of the most commonly identified characteristics of children with a feeding disorder, with meal lengths in excess of 30–40 minutes considered inappropriate (Powers *et al.*, 2002, 2005; Reau *et al.*, 1996; Stark *et al.*, 1997; Young and Drewett, 2000).

Recognising antecedents and consequences

Antecedents might include among others:
- how the caregiver structures the meal (e.g. Does the caregiver serve meals at the same time every day? Does the caregiver serve the meal in the same setting?)
- the child's seating arrangements (e.g. high chair and booster seat)
- the caregiver's style of presentation (e.g. 'Will you please eat this?').

  Possible consequences following inappropriate behaviour might include:
- coaxing and reprimanding (e.g. 'Don't hit the spoon')
- allowing escape or breaks from bite or drink presentations or meal termination
- providing access to tangible items in the form of toys or activities (e.g. turning on the television) or preferred food (giving the child a peanut butter sandwich when he refuses to eat his peas).

Although much of the information during the evaluation may be obtained via records and caregivers' interview, there is no substitute for a direct observation of the caregiver and child at mealtime, as the data-based approach is a hallmark of behaviour analysis, and direct observation is the gold standard.

PRE-ASSESSMENT SPECIFIC CONSIDERATIONS

At the time of the behavioural assessment, specific considerations are given to some of the following contextual aspects:
1 identification of bottles, teats ('nipples'), cup selection and feeding utensils.
2 bolus size
3 texture
4 optimal seating and positioning for feeding.

Identification of bottle, teat, cup selection and feeding utensils

The age of the child, the size of the child's mouth and the child's experience with bottle feeding are important to consider when choosing a teat for bottle feeding. Our most common tools for cup drinking are pink (29.6 mL) and blue (59 mL) cut-out cups (*see* Figure 3.1), which allow a child to drink without moving his or her head backwards.

Feeding utensils (e.g. spoons and forks) should be identified for each child. Common utensils that we use are shown in Figure 3.1. Although many therapists use oral simulator brushes such as the Nuk® brush for non-nutritive stimulation, there is no empirical evidence that non-nutritive stimulation with a Nuk® brush promotes effective feeding skills in children. By contrast, we use the Nuk® brush for

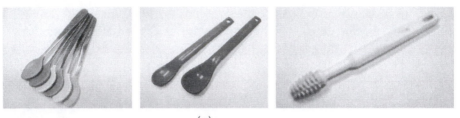

(a)

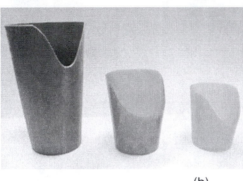

(b)

FIGURE 3.1: Commonly used feeding utensils such as (a) rubber-coated baby spoons, small and large maroon spoons, a Nuk® brush and (b) cut-out or nosey cups.

children who have difficulty in swallowing, as it allows the feeder to place the bolus of food directly on the child's tongue (Gulotta *et al.*, 2005).

Bolus size

Kerwin *et al.* (1995) demonstrated how bolus size can influence the consumption of food or liquid. The general approach is to set the child up for success by making eating and drinking as easy as possible, which typically translates into using a 'small' bolus size. The general guidelines that we use for liquid and solid bolus sizes are outlined in Table 3.1.

Texture

The texture or consistency of food or liquid may need to be modified to promote safe swallowing in children at risk for aspiration, to facilitate consumption in children with food or liquid refusal or to prevent gagging and emesis. It is important to present the texture at which the child is most likely to be successful (*see* Table 3.2).

Optimal seating and positioning for feeding

A primary concern is to provide appropriate seating that will maximise the child's ability to feed and identify seating that will maintain the child's safety while feeding.

In summary, the general approach we follow when treating children with paediatric feeding disorders is to set the child up for success by carefully studying how to make eating and drinking as easy as possible.

TABLE 3.1: Bolus size and cup or utensil type by age of child for use in initial treatment for liquids and solids

Age	Cup type	Bolus
8 months to 4 years	Pink cut-out cup	2 mL
4–8 years	Blue cut-out cup	4 mL
8–12 years	Regular open cup	8 mL

Age	Spoon type	Bolus
4–8 months	Coated baby spoon	¼ level
9–12 months	Coated baby spoon	½ level
12–18 months	Coated baby spoon	Full level
18–30 months	Small maroon spoon	½ level
2.5–6 years	Small maroon spoon	Full level
6 years plus	Large maroon spoon	Full level

TABLE 3.2: Texture and food type by age of child for use in initial treatment for solids

Texture	Food type	Preparation method
Stage 1: jarred baby foods	Fruits and vegetables	Store bought
Stage 2: jarred baby foods	Fruits, vegetables and proteins	Store bought
'Magic bullet' table purees	Table foods	Blend in Magic Bullet® until smooth (add liquid if needed)
Strained table purees	Table foods	Blend in chopper or blender until smooth and then strain (add liquid if needed)
Puree table foods	Table foods	Blend in chopper or blender until smooth (add liquid if needed)
Wet ground	Table foods	Blend in chopper or blender until the mix is pureed foods with small (0.32×0.32 cm^2) pieces within the puree
Ground	Table food	Blend in chopper or blender with no added liquid until the mix is 0.32×0.32 cm^2 pieces in a relatively dry medium
Chopped	Table food	Use knife to cut into 0.46×0.46 cm^2 pieces
Cut	Table food	Use knife to cut into 1.27×1.27 cm^2 pieces

BEHAVIOURAL ASSESSMENTS

The first step should be to identify the target behaviours specific to the child's identified feeding problem(s) that will serve as the focus of intervention. The target behaviours should be observable and measurable. We observe this behaviour within the conditions in which it normally occurs (*home baseline*). We also observe the child's and caregiver's behaviour, interacting with a variety of different foods, textures, liquids and feeding methods to measure and compare the child's progress over time (*standard outcome baseline*).

Some examples of target child behaviour might include:

- *acceptance* (all of the food or liquid in the child's mouth within 5 seconds of presentation)
- *mouth clean* (no food or liquid larger than the size of a pea visible in the child's mouth 30 seconds after acceptance)
- *expels* (solid or liquid greater than the size of a pea visible outside the plane of the lips after the child has accepted the bite)
- *inappropriate behaviour* (e.g. head turning, hitting the spoon, cup or feeder's hand or arm).
- *negative vocalisations* (e.g. crying and saying 'no')
- *grams consumed* (the difference between the pre- and post-weight of food and liquids minus the spill).

Some examples of target parent behaviour might include:

- *escape* (caregiver removes the spoon or cup more than 4 cm away from the child's mouth before the child has consumed all of the presented food or drink)
- *incorrect attention* (caregiver directs comments to or touches the child within 5 seconds of the child's inappropriate behaviour)
- *correct praise* (caregiver delivers a positive remark after the child demonstrates targeted behaviour).

Caregivers should be asked to identify 16 foods (four from each of the food groups of protein, starch, vegetable and fruit) that will be the targets of intervention.

Home baseline

Data collected from the observation of the caregiver feeding the child as he or she normally would do at home are used to generate hypotheses about the environmental variables that may be maintaining the child's inappropriate and appropriate mealtime behaviour.

The results of a study by Piazza *et al.* (2003a) showed that the consequences used by caregivers (providing escape from solid or liquid presentations, terminating the meal, coaxing and reprimanding and giving the child an item or preferred food) were associated with a worsening of inappropriate mealtime behaviour for 67% of the children.

Standard outcome baseline

We observe:

- the caregiver feeding the child pureed foods
- the child self-feeding pureed foods
- the child self-feeding regular-textured foods
- the caregiver feeding the child an age-appropriate and nutritionally appropriate beverage (e.g. whole milk)
- the child self-feeding that same beverage.

The caregiver presents the same type of foods in each solid-food condition, prompts the child to take a bite or drink (depending on the condition) once every 30 seconds, but otherwise responds to the child, as he or she would during meals at home.

Food-type or texture-preference assessment

A preference assessment by food type or texture is appropriate for children who demonstrate inappropriate mealtime behaviours with certain types or textures of food (Munk and Repp, 1994; Patel *et al.*, 2002, 2005). In this assessment, a feeder presents pairs of the 16 foods selected by the caregiver at a single texture (e.g. puree) for the food-type assessment or 16 foods at different textures (e.g. ground and puree) for the texture assessment. The child's preference hierarchy can be established based on the number of times the child selects a particular type or texture of food.

Paired-choice item preference assessment

During the paired-choice preference assessment (Fisher *et al.*, 1992), the child's caregivers select 16 items or activities that the child appears to prefer. The therapist then presents the items in pairs to the child. The results produce a preference hierarchy to identify preferred items or activities to be used as reinforcement for appropriate feeding behaviour.

FUNCTIONAL ANALYSIS

The term functional analysis refers to a specific clinical assessment used to identify environmental contingencies that maintain a child's inappropriate mealtime behaviour. This assessment involves analogue conditions to test the effects of reinforcers, antecedents and consequences on the child's inappropriate feeding behaviour. The results of a functional analysis can be used to develop the treatment for the child's feeding problems.

For example, Piazza *et al.* (2003a) conducted functional analyses with 15 children diagnosed with a paediatric feeding disorder. The assessment consisted of four conditions, namely, escape, attention, tangible and control. In these conditions, the feeder presented bites or drinks to the child once every 30 seconds and the specific response to the child's inappropriate mealtime behaviour are described in Table 3.3.

TABLE 3.3: Experimental conditions and consequences.

Name of the condition	What the feeder does when the child has an inappropriate behaviour
Escape	Removes the spoon/cup for 20 seconds (escape)
Attention	Provides 20 seconds of attention (e.g. reprimands) and holds the spoon/cup stationary
Tangible	Provides 20 seconds access to a tangible item and holds the spoon/cup stationary
Control	Ignores inappropriate behaviour and holds the spoon/cup stationary

Results of this study indicated that one purpose of inappropriate mealtime behaviour was to get a break from eating. These results suggested that negative reinforcement plays a primary role in the maintenance of feeding problems. However, many children also engaged in inappropriate mealtime behaviour to gain adult attention or to receive a tangible item (e.g. a preferred toy or food). Therefore, a significant number of children with feeding disorders may be sensitive to other sources of reinforcement like attention and access to tangible items.

Corey

Corey, a 17-month-old child with a medical history of GERD, was referred for food and liquid refusal. A functional analysis, using the escape, attention and control conditions described earlier, was completed. The results (*see* Figure 3.2) showed that Corey's rates of inappropriate mealtime behaviour were higher in the escape condition in comparison with the control condition, suggesting that his inappropriate mealtime behaviour was maintained by escape from eating (i.e. he engaged in inappropriate mealtime behaviour to receive breaks from presentations of food).

BEHAVIOURAL INTERVENTION PROCEDURES

Treatments and interventions based on theories of operant conditioning (often referred to as 'behavioural' treatments) have been reported to be effective in the management of paediatric feeding disorders (Benoit *et al.*, 2000; Byars *et al.*, 2003; Irwin *et al.*, 2003; Kerwin, 1999; Linscheid, 2006; Piazza, 2008; Piazza and Carroll-Hernandez, 2004; Volkert and Piazza, in press; Williams *et al.*, 2007). Kerwin and Volkert and Piazza reviewed the treatment literature on paediatric feeding disorders and concluded that the only treatments that had empirical support in the

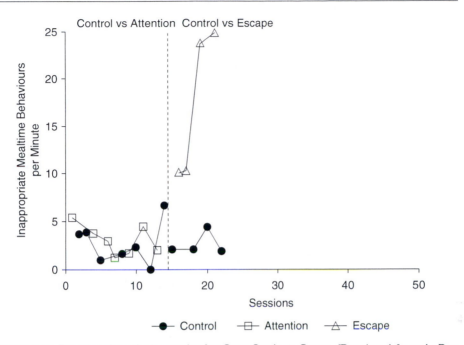

FIGURE 3.2: Functional analysis results for Case Study 1: Corey. (Reprinted from LaRue *et al.*, in press.)

literature were based on behaviour-analytic principles and employed single-subject designs.

Escape extinction

Research data show that children engage in inappropriate mealtime behaviour to escape from presentations of solids or liquids (Girolami and Scotti, 2001; Najdowski *et al.*, 2008; Piazza *et al.*, 2003a). Escape extinction (EE) involves no longer providing escape from the bite or drink presentation when the child engages in inappropriate mealtime behaviour (i.e. the inappropriate mealtime behaviour no longer 'works' to make the spoon or cup go away). Data from a number of studies have shown that these procedures are effective as treatment for children with feeding disorders (Ahearn *et al.*, 1996; Cooper *et al.*, 1995; Hoch *et al.*, 1994; Patel *et al.*, 2002; Piazza *et al.*, 2003a,b; Reed *et al.*, 2004).

The two frequently used EE procedures are outlined below.

* *Non-removal of the spoon*: the feeder presents the spoon or cup at the child's lips until the child opens his or her mouth to accept the solid or liquid presentation (Ahearn *et al.*, 1996; Hoch *et al.*, 1994; Piazza *et al.*, 2003b; Reed *et al.*, 2004).
* *Physical guidance*: if the child does not accept the bite within a specified time period (e.g. 5 seconds), the feeder applies gentle pressure to the child's mandibular joint to physically guide the child to open his or her mouth. The feeder then deposits the solid or liquid into the child's mouth (Ahearn *et al.*, 1996).

Corey: what happened next?

We previously described a case study of Corey, a 17-month-old child with GERD, who engaged in higher levels of inappropriate mealtime behaviour during the escape condition of the functional analysis, which suggested that escape extinction (EE) would be effective as treatment.

During baseline, we assessed two conditions:
1 The feeder removed the spoon and waited 30 seconds until presenting the next bite when Corey had a mouth clean (escape for mouth clean).
2 Corey's mouth clean resulted in no differential consequence.
  In both conditions, the feeder removed the spoon for 30 seconds if Corey engaged in inappropriate mealtime behaviour.

The data in Figure 3.3 show that Corey's inappropriate mealtime behaviour remained high, and the acceptance of food was low in these baseline conditions.

The treatment was the same as baseline for mouth clean (either the feeder removed the spoon for 30 seconds or the feeder did not respond to mouth clean). In both conditions, the feeder held the spoon at Corey's lips until he opened his mouth to accept the bite (i.e. EE). Inappropriate mealtime behaviour decreased to low levels, and acceptance increased to high levels in both conditions.

Positive reinforcement-based treatments

Some earlier studies in paediatric feeding disorders reported that positive reinforcement alone may be effective for increasing food acceptance (Riordan et al., 1980, 1984). However, the results of these studies were difficult to interpret because of procedural limitations. Further research addressed these limitations by evaluating the effects of positive reinforcement alone, positive reinforcement with EE and EE alone (Patel et al., 2002; Piazza et al., 2003b; Reed et al., 2004). Results from these studies suggested that EE may be necessary for increasing acceptance and decreasing inappropriate mealtime behaviour for children with paediatric feeding disorders, and the addition of positive reinforcement may be beneficial, but not necessary, for some children.

Function-based treatment

Bachmeyer et al. (2009) extended the work on function-based treatment of paediatric disorders by identifying four children whose inappropriate mealtime behaviour was maintained by adult attention and escape. Feeders implemented function-based extinction procedures. The EE procedure consisted of non-removal of the spoon, and the attention extinction procedure consisted of the therapist providing no differential consequence for inappropriate mealtime behaviour. Attention extinction alone did not result in increased acceptance or decreased inappropriate mealtime behaviour.

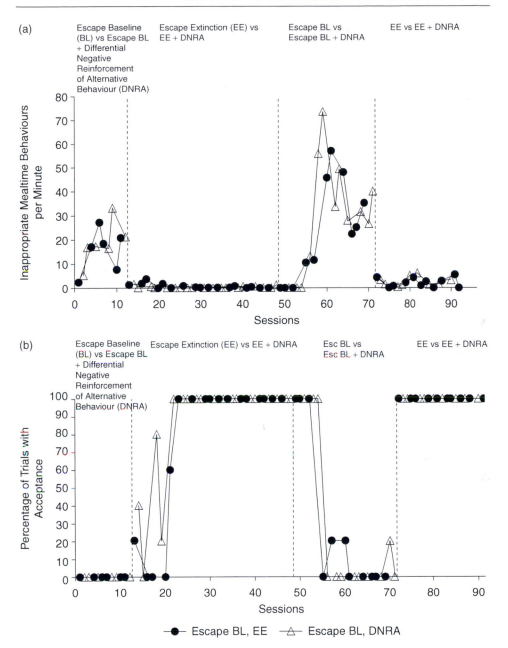

FIGURE 3.3: (a) Inappropriate mealtime behaviour per minute (top panel) and (b) percentage of trials with acceptance (bottom panel) for Case Study 2: 'Corey: what happened next'. (Reprinted from LaRue *et al.*, in press.)

By contrast, EE alone resulted in an increase in acceptance and a decrease in inappropriate mealtime behaviour. However, declines in inappropriate mealtime behaviour did not reach clinically acceptable levels, and acceptance did not increase to high and stable levels until the feeder implemented a combined extinction technique (i.e. escape and attention extinction). The results of the Bachmeyer *et al.* (2009) study suggested that a functional analysis of inappropriate mealtime behaviour may be useful for prescribing treatment for children with paediatric feeding disorders.

EE combined with other treatment procedures

Although EE is effective as treatment for many children, some children may not respond to this procedure alone and may need the application of EE in combination with other procedures:

1 *Blending*: mixing preferred and non-preferred foods when combined with EE was an effective method of increasing consumption of non-preferred foods for two children who did not respond to EE alone (Mueller *et al.*, 2004). Similarly, Patel *et al.* (2001) treated a child diagnosed with autism who would consume water, but no other beverage. Because the goal of treatment was to increase the child's consumption of a calorically dense beverage, we gradually blended water with a calorie-dense and nutritionally complete powdered supplement (Carnation Instant Breakfast (CIB)). Initially, we added 10% of the 35.8-g packet of CIB to 237 mL of water. Once the child consumed this mixture, we increased the amount of CIB added to the 237-mL glass of water in small increments (e.g. 20%, 30%). Once the child was drinking 100% of the 237-mL glass of water with the entire 35.8-g packet of CIB, we added milk to the water and CIB mixture in small increments (e.g. 10%, 20%). This blending procedure, in conjunction with EE, was effective in increasing the child's consumption of milk with CIB.

2 *High probability (high-p) sequence*: the high-p sequence procedure (Dawson *et al.*, 2003; Patel *et al.*, 2005) involves the feeder delivering a series of commands for which the child has demonstrated high levels of compliance (e.g. acceptance of an empty cup). The feeder then follows the high-p demands with a demand for which the child had demonstrated low levels of compliance (e.g. acceptance of a cup containing liquids). For example, the sequence for one child could be: 'take a drink' (presentation of the empty cup), 'take a drink' (presentation of the empty cup), 'take a drink' (presentation of the empty cup) 'take a drink' (presentation of the cup with liquids).

3 *Response effort*: the amount of effort or difficulty associated with eating has been demonstrated to affect food consumption. Kerwin *et al.* (1995) varied the amount of food presented on a spoon, with and without EE. Smaller amounts of food on the spoon were associated with higher levels of acceptance. These results suggested that altering response effort may be effective in the treatment of feeding disorders.

4 *Treatment for expulsion*: treatment of refusal behaviour may be associated with increases in expulsion (spitting out food or liquid) for some children (Sevin *et al.*, 2002). Re-presentation, in which the feeder places the expelled food back into the child's mouth, is one method of treatment for expulsions (Coe *et al.*, 1997; Girolami *et al.*, 2007; Sevin *et al.*, 2002). Patel *et al.* (2002) showed that the type and texture of food could influence expulsions. Decreasing the texture of meat resulted in decreased expulsions.

Ann

Ann, a 2-year 8-month-old child, was born prematurely at 24 weeks and had a medical diagnosis of short-gut syndrome secondary to necrotising entero-colitis. Ann was referred for food and liquid refusal and G-tube dependence. On the basis of functional analysis results, the feeder implemented a treatment package consisting of EE (non-removal of the spoon) and attention extinction (the feeder ignored inappropriate mealtime behaviour). Although the treatment package was effective for increasing bite acceptance, a high rate of expulsions continued to be a problem with liquids. The feeder then implemented a chin-prompt procedure in conjunction with the treatment package. This procedure consisted of the feeder counting aloud to five while applying gentle upward pressure on Ann's chin to prompt Ann to close her mouth after acceptance and after the feeder re-presented the drink following an expulsion. Expels decreased when the feeder added the chin-prompt procedure to the treatment package (*see* Figure 3.4). When the feeder discontinued the use of the chin-prompt procedure, expels increased. When the feeder re-introduced the chin-prompt procedure, expels decreased again.

5   *Treatment of packing:* another problematic mealtime behaviour commonly seen in children with paediatric feeding disorders is packing (pocketing or hold-ing food or liquid in the mouth). Gulotta *et al.* (2005) used a re-distribution procedure to treat packing successfully. During re-distribution, the feeder used a Nuk® brush to remove packed food from the child's mouth. The feeder then placed the food back on the child's tongue. Re-distribution was effective for reducing packing.

John

John, a 6-month-old infant with a medical diagnosis of short-gut syndrome sec-ondary to gastroschisis (a congenital disorder in which the small bowel develops outside of the abdominal cavity), was referred for food and liquid refusal, G-tube dependence and total parenteral nutrition dependence. He engaged in high lev-els of crying (negative vocalisations) during the baseline condition (*see* Figure 3.5, top panel). In the first intervention, the feeder presented a pacifier to John immediately after each bite presentation to decrease negative vocalisations. Using a pacifier was effective in decreasing negative vocalisations; however, John continued to demonstrate low levels of acceptance during the baseline and pacifier intervention (*see* Figure 3.5, middle panel). The feeder used EE in the form of non-removal of the spoon (NRS) to increase acceptance and re-presented expelled bites. Bite acceptance increased during the NRS procedure. However, John also demonstrated low levels of mouth clean (*see* Figure 3.5, bottom panel). The feeder then used a flipped-spoon procedure, which involved the feeder placing the bite with the upright spoon into John's mouth and then flipping the spoon over 180° in the mouth to deposit the bite. Flipping the spoon enabled the feeder to place the food directly onto John's tongue. Using the flipped-spoon procedure resulted in increased mouth cleans for John. This procedure may be helpful when children are not able to or do not use their lips to remove food from the spoon and manoeuvre the bolus with their tongue to swallow.

6   *Texture fading*: texture selectivity or problems with age-appropriate advancement of textures is commonly encountered in paediatric feeding disorders. Shore *et al.* (1998) showed that texture fading, which involved gradually advancing a child's texture from pureed to chopped, was an effective treatment for texture advancement. However, clinical experience suggests that not all children with feeding disorders respond to texture fading and that maintaining children on

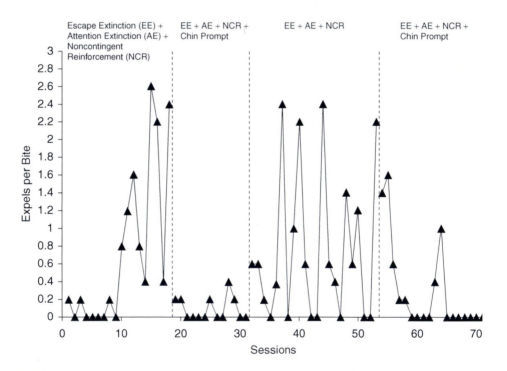

FIGURE 3.4: Number of expels per bite with and without the chin-prompt procedure for Case Study 3: Ann. (Reprinted from Wilkens, Piazza, Groff, and Vaz. (in press). Chin Prompt plus Representation as Treatment for Expulsion in Children with Pediatric Feeding Disorders. *Journal of Applied Behavior Analysis.*)

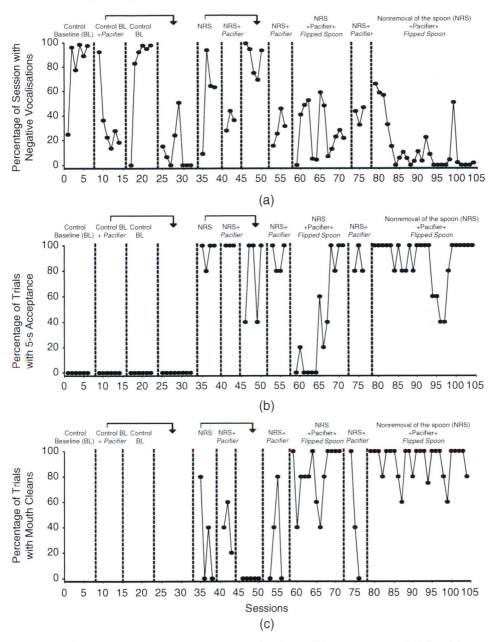

FIGURE 3.5: (a) Percentage of negative vocalisations, (b) percentage of trials with 5-s acceptance and (c) percentage of trials with mouth cleans, in the control baseline (BL), BL and pacifier, NRS, NRS and pacifier, NRS, pacifier and flipped-spoon conditions for Case Study 4: John. (Reprinted from Rivas *et al.*, in press.)

pureed textures while simultaneously teaching them to chew can prove a more effective strategy. This approach allows for the child to be transitioned from puree to table food once his or her chewing skills and stamina have improved to the extent that sufficient table food can be consumed in a timely manner to maintain growth.

7   *Self-feeding*: Piazza *et al.* (1993) used a three-step prompting procedure to teach five girls with Rett syndrome to self-feed. The three-step procedure involved sequential verbal, modelled and physical prompts along with verbal praise for bite acceptance following the verbal or modelled prompt. The results of this study suggested that the modelled prompt, which provides demonstration of the requested response, is helpful for children who are unable to follow verbal instructions. With physical prompting, children who are unable to follow verbal instructions or imitate a model may be physically assisted in completing the required task.

8   *Caregiver training*: Long-term successful feeding program outcomes depend to a large extent on the ability of caregivers to efficiently implement treatment procedures. Therefore, caregiver training, to ensure that treatment protocols are implemented with a high degree of integrity, is a crucial component of treatment. A number of studies on the treatment of paediatric feeding disorders have demonstrated that caregivers can be trained successfully to implement treatment protocols (Anderson and McMillan, 2001; Mueller *et al.*, 2003; Najdowski *et al.*, 2003; Werle *et al.*, 1993). Mueller *et al.* (2003) showed that multiple components were necessary to train parents to implement paediatric feeding disorders protocols. A combination of written and verbal instructions, modelling and rehearsal; written and verbal instructions and modelling; written and verbal instructions and rehearsal; or written and verbal instructions were all effective for increasing parental integrity with the treatment protocols.

SUMMARY

Feeding disorders can seriously compromise nutrition, growth and development in children and can have a huge impact on the quality of life for the child and family. Because multiple factors contribute to feeding disorders, the interdisciplinary team approach to assessment and treatment is essential. Functional analysis procedures are useful in determining the function of inappropriate mealtime behaviours and prescribing treatment. Strategies based on the principles of operant conditioning have been found to be effective in the treatment of paediatric feeding disorders. Negative reinforcement has been identified as a significant contributing factor to feeding disorders in children. The efficacy of EE treatment procedures in isolation or in combination with other procedures is well established. There are a variety of empirical studies that have evaluated the effectiveness of procedures in conjunction with EE, such as blending, the high-p sequence and modifying the response effort associated with eating. Re-presentation and re-distribution appear to be effective as treatment for expulsion and packing, respectively. Finally, caregiver training is a primary determinant of the long-term success of treatment and, therefore, an essential component of the program.

REFERENCES

Ahearn WH, Kerwin ME, Eicher PS, *et al*. An alternating treatments comparison of two intensive interventions for food refusal. *J Appl* Behav *Anal*. 1996; **29**: 321–32.

Anderson CM, McMillan K. Parental use of escape extinction and differential reinforcement to treat food selectivity. *J Appl Behav Anal*. 2001; **34**(4): 511–15.

Bachmeyer MH, Piazza CC, Fredrick LD, *et al*. Functional analysis and treatment of multiply controlled inappropriate mealtime behavior. *J Appl Behav Anal*. 2009; **42**(3): 641–58.

Benoit D, Wang EE, Zlotkin SH. Discontinuation of enterostomy tube feeding by behavioral treatment in early childhood: a randomized controlled trial. *J Pediatr*. 2000; **137**: 498–503.

Byars, KC, Burklow KA, Ferguson K, *et al*. A multicomponent behavioral program for oral aversion in children dependent on gastrostomy feeding. *J Pediatr Gastroenterol Nutrit*. 2003; **37**(4): 473–80.

Coe DA, Babbitt RL, Williams KE, *et al*. Use of extinction and reinforcement to increase food consumption and reduce expulsion. *J Appl Behav Anal*. 1997; **30**: 581–3.

Cooper LJ, Wacker DP, McComas JJ, *et al*. Use of component analyses to identify active variables in treatment packages for children with feeding disorders. *J Appl Behav Anal*. 1995; **28**(2): 139–53.

Dawson JE, Piazza CC, Sevin BM, *et al*. Use of the high-probability instructional sequence and escape extinction in a child with food refusal. *J Appl Behav Anal*. 2003; **36**: 105–8.

Field D, Garland M, Williams K. Correlates of specific childhood feeding problems. *J Pediatr Child Health*. 2003; **39**: 299–304.

Fisher W, Piazza CC, Bowman LG, *et al*. A comparison of two approaches for identifying reinforcers for persons with severe to profound disabilities. *J Appl Behav Anal*. 1992; **25**: 491–8.

Girolami PA, Boscoe JH, Roscoe N. Decreasing expulsions by a child with a feeding disorder: using a brush to present and re-present food. *J Appl Behav Anal*. 2007; **40**: 749–53.

Girolami PA, Scotti JR. Use of analog functional analysis in assessing the function of mealtime behavior problems. *Educ Treat Mental Retard Develop Disabil*. 2001; **36**: 207–23.

Gulotta CS, Piazza CC, Patel MR, *et al*. Using food redistribution to reduce packing in children with severe food refusal. *J Appl Behav Anal*. 2005; **38**: 39–50.

Hoch TA, Babbitt RL, Coe DA, *et al*. Contingency contacting: combining positive reinforcement and escape extinction procedures to treat persistent food refusal. *Behav Modif*. 1994; **18**: 106–28.

Irwin MC, Clawson EP, Monasterio E, *et al*. Outcomes of a day feeding program for children with cerebral palsy. *Arch Phys Med Rehabil*. 2003; **84**: A2.

Kerwin ME. Empirically supported treatments in pediatric psychology: severe feeding problems. *J Pediatr Psychol*. 1999; **24**: 193–214.

Kerwin ME, Ahearn WH, Eicher PS, *et al*. The costs of eating: a behavioral economic analysis of food refusal. *J Appl Behav Anal*. 1995; **28**: 245–60.

LaRue RH, Stewart V, Piazza CC, *et al*. Escape as reinforcement and escape extinction in the treatment of feeding problems. *J Appl Behav Anal*. In press.

Linscheid TR. Behavioral treatments for pediatric feeding disorders. *Behav Modif*. 2006; **30**(1): 6–23.

Mueller MM, Piazza CC, Moore JW, *et al*. Training parents to implement pediatric feeding protocols. *J Appl Behav Anal*. 2003; **36**: 545–62.

Mueller MM, Piazza CC, Patel MR, *et al*. Increasing variety of foods consumed by blending nonpreferred foods into preferred foods. *J Appl Behav Anal*. 2004; **37**: 159–70.

Munk DD, Repp AC. Behavioral assessment of feeding problems of individuals with severe disabilities. *J Appl Behav Anal*. 1994; **27**: 241–50.

Najdowski AC, Wallace MD, Doney JK, *et al*. Parental assessment and treatment of food selectivity in natural settings. *J Appl Behav Anal*. 2003; **36**: 383–6.

Najdowski AC, Wallace MD, Penrod B, *et al*. Caregiver-conducted experimental functional analyses of inappropriate mealtime behavior. *J Appl Behav Anal*. 2008; **41**: 459–65.

Patel MR, Piazza CC, Kelly ML, *et al*. Using a fading procedure to increase fluid consumption in a child with feeding problems. *J Appl Behav Anal*. 2001; **34**: 357–60.

Patel MR, Piazza CC, Layer S, *et al*. A systematic evaluation of food textures to decrease packing and increase oral intake in children with pediatric feeding disorders. *J Appl Behav Anal*. 2005; **38**: 89–100.

Patel MR, Piazza CC, Martinez CJ, *et al*. An evaluation of two differential reinforcement procedures with escape extinction to treat food refusal. *J Appl Behav Anal*. 2002; **35**: 363–74.

Patel MR, Piazza CC, Santana CM, *et al*. An evaluation of food type and texture in the treatment of a feeding problem. *J Appl Behav Anal*. 2002; **35**: 183–6.

Patel MR, Reed GK, Piazza CC, *et al*. An evaluation of a high-probability instructional sequence to increase acceptance of food and decrease inappropriate behavior in children with pediatric feeding disorders. *Res Develop Disabil*. 2005; **27**: 430–42.

Piazza CC. Feeding disorders and behavior: what have we learned? *Develop Disabil Res Rev*. 2008; **14**: 174–81.

Piazza CC, Anderson C, Fisher W. Teaching self-feeding skills to patients with Rett's syndrome. *Develop Med Child Neurol*. 1993; **35**: 991–6.

Piazza CC, Carroll-Hernandez TA. Assessment and treatment of pediatric feeding disorders. In: Trembly RE, Barr RG, Peters RDeV, editors. *Centre of Excellence for Early Childhood Development* (online). 2004. Available at: www.childencyclopedia.com/Pages/PDF/Piazza-Carroll-HernandezANGxp.pdf (accessed 29 June 2009).

Piazza CC, Fisher WF, Brown KA, *et al*. Functional analysis of inappropriate mealtime behaviors. *J Appl Behav Anal*. 2003a; **36**: 187–204.

Piazza CC, Patel MR, Gulotta CS, *et al*. On the relative contributions of positive reinforcement and escape extinction in the treatment of food refusal. *J Appl Behav Anal*. 2003b; **36**: 309–24.

Powers SW, Byars KC, Mitchell MJ, *et al*. Parent report of mealtime behavior and parenting stress in young children with type 1 diabetes and in healthy control subjects. *Diabetes Care*. 2002; **25**(2): 313–18.

Powers SW, Mitchell MJ, Patton SR, *et al*. Mealtime behaviors in families of infants and toddlers with cystic fibrosis. *J Cyst Fibrosis*. 2005; **4**(3): 175–82.

Reau NR, Senturia YD, Lebailly SA, *et al.* Infant and toddler feeding patterns and problems: normative data and a new direction. *J Develop Behav Pediatr.* 1996; **17**: 140–53.

Reed GK, Piazza CC, Patel MR, *et al.* On the relative contributions of noncontingent reinforcement and escape extinction in the treatment of food refusal. *J Appl Behav Anal.* 2004; **37**: 27–41.

Riordan MM, Iwata BA, Finney JW, *et al.* Behavioral assessment and treatment of chronic food refusal in handicapped children. *J Appl Behav Anal.* 1984; **17**: 327–41.

Riordan MM, Iwata BA, Wohl MK, *et al.* Behavioral treatment of food refusal and selectivity in developmentally disabled children. *Appl Res Mental Retard.* 1980; **1**: 95–112.

Rivas KD, Piazza CC, Kadey HJ, *et al.* Sequential treatment of a feeding problem using a pacifier and flipped spoon. *J Appl Behav Anal.* In press.

Sevin BM, Gulotta CS, Sierp BJ, *et al.* Analysis of response covariation among multiple topographies of food refusal. *J Appl Behav.* 2002; **35**: 65–8.

Shore BA, Babbitt RL, Williams KE, *et al.* Use of texture fading in the treatment of food selectivity. *J Appl Behav Anal.* 1998; **31**: 621–33.

Stark LJ, Mulvihill MM, Jelalian E, *et al.* Descriptive analysis of eating behavior in school-age children with cystic fibrosis and healthy control children. *Pediatrics.* 1997; **99**(5): 665–71.

Volkert VM, Piazza CC. Empirically supported treatments for pediatric feeding disorders. In: Sturmey P, Herson M, editors. *Handbook of Evidence Based Practice in Clinical Psychology.* USA: Wiley. In press.

Werle MA, Murphy TB, Budd KS. Treating chronic food refusal in young children: home-based parent training. *J Appl Behav Anal.* 1993; **26**: 421–33.

Wilkens JW, Piazza CC, Groff RA, and Vaz PCM. (in press). Chin prompt plus re-presentation as treatment for expulsion in children with pediatric feeding disorders. *Journal of Applied Behavior Analysis.*

Williams KE, Riegel K, Gibbons B, *et al.* Intensive behavioral treatment for severe feeding problems: a cost-effective alternative to tube feeding? *J Develop Phys Disabil.* 2007; **19**: 227–35.

Young B, Drewett R. Eating behavior and its variability in 1-year-old children. *Appetite.* 2000; **35**(2): 171–7.

CHAPTER 4

Feeding difficulties in infancy and childhood: psychoanalytic perspectives

Stephen Briggs and Lynn Priddis

INTRODUCTION

This chapter applies psychoanalytic perspectives to understanding the dynamics of feeding difficulties in childhood. Concentrating primarily on the early feeding relationship in infancy, we will explore the role of psychoanalytic thinking and practice in understanding and providing ways of intervening. In a field in which there has been rapid change and innovation, psychoanalytic thinking and practice now forms a key aspect of an integrated approach to understanding infant development and problems. There has emerged a primary focus on the infant–parent relationship, a new emphasis that has changed the ways in which infant development is considered and also how professional interventions are delivered. In particular, there have been significant developments in infant–parent psychotherapy and an emphasis on observationally led methods.

We apply the relational approach to discuss the distinctive dynamics of feeding difficulties within the infant–parent relationship, paying particular attention to the 'container-contained' relationship and thus to how the infant–parent relationship regulates emotions, particularly anxiety, and provides opportunities for intimacy and companionship. We explore the connection between feeding difficulties and problems in experiencing intimacy and separateness, illustrating this discussion with some examples from clinical practice and observational research. The chapter then highlights the implications of feeding difficulties for the infant's future development, especially in the arenas of thinking, relating and symbolising. We conclude with a discussion of some issues arising in interventions exploring ways that the turn towards a relational approach to infant development has led to the development of new and innovative ways of working, especially in infant–parent psychotherapy, and has provided also a focus for the application of psychoanalytic understanding for a wide range of professionals working with infants and parents.

PARENT–INFANT RELATIONSHIPS IN EARLY INFANCY

The distinctive quality of psychodynamic approaches to feeding difficulties in infancy and childhood lies in the emphasis that is placed on understanding the emotional qualities of the feeding relationship. From the beginning of life, the infant and the mother are engaged in a relationship that is emotionally significant for both. Winnicott (1964) suggested that:

> "If you set out to describe a baby, you will find that you are describing a baby and someone else. A baby cannot exist alone, but is essentially part of a relationship."

This can be said to be the point at which psychoanalytic theory of infant development began to concentrate, within the object relations tradition, on a two-person rather than a one-person psychology. The psychoanalytic emphasis on the link between the physical and emotional aspects of feeding within the infant–mother relationship foreshadowed recent developments in thinking about infancy, particularly from the perspective of infant mental health (Barlow and Svanberg, 2009). There is now a fruitful focus on the parent–infant relationship, one that reflects a successful integration of psychoanalytic thinking about the dynamics or early relatedness, developmental research revealing the qualities of relatedness, understanding of the development of attachment patterns in childhood and neuroscientific studies. The emphasis that emerges from these studies is that the relationship between infants and parents is concerned, in overarching terms, with two themes; the need to regulate emotions, especially anxiety, and the need for companionship.

Thus, there is now a considerable body of empirical evidence to support the focus on the relationship for it is now well recognised that the infant is oriented towards relationships from birth and it is in the context of this emotional environment in primary relationships that the infant develops. Where Winnicott wrote of the 'holding environment', Stern (1995, 2002) described how the dance between a mother and her child introduces the child to the inter-subjective world of others through 'vitality affects'. Tronick (2007) has identified subtle processes that unfold in mother–infant interactions to conceptualise how mutual emotional regulation occurs, and how disruptions or mis-attunements are repaired through interactions. Malloch and Trevarthen (2009) identify that the musical rhythms of communication between a mother and her child in the first few months guide the child into the world of meanings, of intentions and of knowing. Together mothers and infants are understood to make sense of each other through the rhythm and synchronicity of their exchanges. The idea of attunement first observed by psychoanalytic practitioners is now thought to be established in neuronal circuits in the brain, in particular those of the mirror neuron system and temporal cortex (Siegal, 2007).

Recognition of the importance of the need for companionship has led to an emphasis on keeping the baby 'in mind' (Barlow and Svanberg, 2009), an approach that owes much to the concept of mentalisation (Fonagy *et al.*, 2008). The developing dominance of this conceptualisation of mother–infant relationships (Barlow, 2009) indicates a remarkable shift from the time, barely two decades ago, when the emphasis on the physical aspects of feeding predominated. Now, the predominance of mentalisation requires a restatement of the importance of the bodily, physical aspects of the infant–mother relationship, including the feeding relationship (Downing, 2005).

Alongside the mentalisation of the infant–parent relationship, there is a strong emphasis in recent studies on the agency of the infant, who is an active participant in the relationship, bringing to it the capacity to develop patterns of timing and rhythm in relationships (Alvarez, 1992; Tronick, 1989), and distinct and individual ways of communicating (Trevarthen and Aitken, 2001). Recognition of the baby's need for emotional regulation is linked with the idea that the mother's role is to attend to and transform the infant's emotional experiences, a focus that follows or parallels Bion's (1962) formulation of the container and contained relationship. The infant's anxiety not only spills over when experiencing intense emotional experiences, but he seeks to communicate non-verbally by making the mother feel what he is feeling. The parent then has the task of taking in, making sense of and detoxifying these intense emotions and putting back to the baby an experience which is manageable, and digested by the (adult) mother's capacity to think. In developmental terms, the mother positions herself to manage the infant's need for emotional regulation through her physical and mental responses to such moments.

ESTABLISHING THE FEEDING RELATIONSHIP

Establishing a feeding relationship is a momentous experience for both mother and infant. Of course, the infant brings to the relationship capacities which enhance the process, notably the sucking reflex and the capacity to indicate, through a range of communications, which are both observed and emotionally experienced, the desire to be fed and the wish for companionship. The mother too brings both the desire to feed her infant, to establish a relationship with him or her, and also anxieties which reflect both the newness of the experience – even if this is not the first baby – and the responsibilities of the role. As Daws (1995) describes it:

> "Parents who have just had a baby are normally in a heightened state of emotion. Life and death feelings are part of the ordinary stuff of [infancy]."

This 'heightened' state of emotion was thought by Winnicott (1965) to be a means whereby the mother, through 'primary maternal preoccupation', made a space in her mind for the arrival of her new baby and prepared herself for a kind of communication which of necessity depends upon pre- or non-verbal modes. Empirical studies have demonstrated just how normative maternal preoccupation is in the immediate period preceding delivery and in the first 3–6 months post-delivery for both mothers and fathers. Studies on post-partum depression inform us that the state of preoccupation is beneficial for the infant–parent relationship; too little maternal preoccupation may be problematic, and too much preoccupation as in obsessive–compulsive states can also present problems (Swain *et al.*, 2008).

Bion (1962) described the mother's state of readiness to relate to and receive infant communications as 'reverie'. Reverie is a state of mind in the mother in which she allows herself a space within herself to receive the baby's experiences; to allow them to enter her mind, so that she can think about and gather a sense of their meaning. From this she formulates, consciously and unconsciously, responses to the infant's communications and needs. The parental capacity for reverie and primary maternal preoccupation depends upon the experience and internalisation of a similarly receptive mother in the mother's own infancy and childhood.

The intensity of the infant's earliest experiences almost defies words, psychoanalysis has tried to encapsulate this in descriptions of the generic term 'primitive anxieties'. Winnicott wrote of 'primitive agonies' (Winnicott, 1974), and Bion of 'nameless dread', appropriately conjuring the idea that, for the infant, these feelings and experiences do not yet have names. Bick, like Winnicott, thought of the experiences of falling, of falling apart, as if 'liquefying' or 'falling for ever' (Bick, 1986). The vulnerability of the infant in these moments is such that he or she is unable to hold within himself or herself the emotional experiences to which he is subjected to. He turns, therefore, using primitive methods of communication, particularly projective identification (Bion, 1967; Klein, 1946), to a parent who can undertake, on his or her behalf through reverie, the emotional work of first allowing the infant's experiences to permeate her, making sense within herself of the infant's communications before responding to her baby, through her words, gestures and deeds. The infant then experiences the parental function to be one that holds or contains his/her emotional experiences as well as one that integrates these so that the infant is not overwhelmed. Rather than feeling he or she is falling apart, held together by the mother's containing function, the infant has the experience of remaining within his or her own 'psychic skin'. The 'good enough' (Winnicott, 1974) and 'balanced' (Bion, 1967) mother, who is able to make sense of her own experiences of heightened emotion and communicate in this way with her infant, provides names for emotional experiences, which through repetition, enables the infant to build within an internal world in which he or she has felt understood and can understand his or her own emotional experiences. This is the 'container-contained' relationship, a concept which has had a tremendous influence on the psychoanalytic thinking and practice.

Alongside the intensity of these emotionally intense experiences, dominated by the need to regulate anxieties, there are moments of integration, when the infant is held or feeding, and these moments also need a distinctive description. What is at stake now is not simply the amelioration of anxious moments, but the origins of the capacity to develop intimate relationships. Through a sense of timing and developing rhythms of interaction with her baby, through her reverie and understanding, the mother has the responsibility of making available to the infant a subjective world of shared meaning (Stern, 2002). The feeding aspect of the relationship thus takes on the significance of being one of the most important dimensions through which the infant develops a notion and experience of intimacy. Feeding is not just about the passing of physical nurture from one person to another, but rather about the communication of elemental aspects of intimacy, love, hate and truth. The link between body (food) and mind (intimacy) is a crucial one to maintain when thinking about the feeding relationship.

Difficulties in feeding have to be understood through identifying problems within the infant–mother relationship and thus identified through assessing the individual infant–parent relationship. According to Stern (2002) the feeding experience becomes a 'we' experience, not only a 'me' experience, with long-lasting effects that influence the later development of the child, the nature of the parent–child relationship as well as the other intimate relationship. In a significant compilation that reflects on the work of the Eating Disorders Workshop in the Tavistock Clinic's Adolescent Department, Williams et al. (2004) identify that a key aspect of the internal dynamics for both feeding difficulties in infancy and early childhood and eating disorders in later childhood and adolescence[1] is a failure in some aspects of the early relationships. That is, there is an identifiable disturbance of the relationship between the container and the contained, persistent enough to generate a lack of 'fit' between the parent and infant and characterised by a reciprocal problem in giving and taking. In Tronick's (2007) terms there is (or has been) a failure to effect interactive repair in the relationship.

Williams et al. (2004) explore the nature of the problem thus experienced in the container-contained relationship. This can include: first, the parent being unable to process the infant's experiences, through a lack of reverie, leaving the infant unable to effectively communicate with the parent through projective identification; and second, a reversal of the container-contained relationship, in which the infant becomes the receptacle for the parent's projections. The container-contained relationship is thus replaced by a 'receptacle–foreign body' relationship (Williams et al., 2004, p. xiv). This is a serious situation in which crucial developmental processes

---

[1] The striking similarity of internal relatedness patterns in feeding difficulties and eating disorders, including what Williams (1997) refers to as a 'no-entry system of defences' is particularly apparent in the therapeutic relationship with adolescents with eating disorders. These patterns are, of course, expressed through different fears and preoccupations in later childhood .and adolescence.

are endangered. The main consequences are disturbance to the infant's capacity for dependence and – as an inevitable corollary – an inability to develop a capacity to be separate. Both dependence and separation become dreaded experiences, and in the face of feeling overwhelmed by these experiences, the infant develops defences which aim to protect him from overwhelming experiences but which tend to reinforce the developmental difficulties, through, for example, avoiding or obliterating experiences of separateness and through omnipotent attempts to make do without needing parents. We will discuss, below, some particular examples in which disturbance of the infant–parent relationships and the development of defences are illustrated.

AN OBSERVATION-LED APPROACH

Increasingly, particularly in the field of child psychotherapy, psychoanalytic thinking is influenced by direct observation. A method of observation, where an infant and a young child are observed weekly in the home for 1 hour for a period of 1 or 2 years, is now an essential training experience for therapists and a wide range of professionals in health and social care (Bick, 1964; Miller *et al.*, 1989). The extensive applications of the method and the knowledge generated thus are reported in *The International Journal of Infant Observation*. Increasingly, this method of observation is used as a research methodology generating a distinctive 'experience near' approach (Briggs, 1997, 2005; Rustin, 1989, 1997, 2002, 2006; Urwin, 2007). It underpins clinical practice and provides a flexible basis for practice interventions. Health visitors, for example, find it invaluable for their practice (Benihoud, 2004).

Closely detailed accounts of interaction between infant and mother, and other family members and the behaviour and communications of the infant are encouraged in this essentially naturalistic method of observation. Open, unstructured descriptive accounts of mother–infant relationships are produced for discussion in seminar groups, and the observer develops qualities of reflectiveness based on openness to the emotionality in the setting. This reflective capacity is a precondition for the therapist developing 'reverie', mirroring the function of the mother and thus a willingness to remain in a state of 'not knowing' long enough to develop a sense of the impact of the emotionality in the relationship between mother and infant. The observer thus becomes equipped to make use of the feelings he or she has in the course of therapeutic work, the countertransference. Experienced practitioners use such observation training alongside their own experiences of analysis and therapy to develop the capacity to use feelings and reactions within themselves economically and creatively.

Daws (2005, 2008) demonstrates the capacity the skilled therapist has to apply the observational approach, and the facility this provides for moving, in her mind, through thinking about interactions between parent and infant, the internal experiences of both, and what happens inside himself or herself, the therapist. The therapist applies the open, reflective, observational approach to notice and make use of her own reactions. Often, working thus, the therapist can make connections between the dynamics in the families and the impact of these families on her, the therapist. A range of emotions impacts on the worker, 'from voracious greed to an inability to take in what is offered' (Daws, 1993, p. 75), and these feelings make sense of a particular part of the experiences within the family.

Applying the observational approach, and linking it with the theoretical background discussed above, we can now discuss and illustrate some key aspects of feeding difficulties in infancy.

FEEDING DIFFICULTIES AND DISTURBANCES IN THE INFANT–PARENT RELATIONSHIP

We have suggested that disturbance in the infant–parent relationship should be the focus for working with feeding difficulties. To discuss this further, we can illustrate through exploring some thinking and practice. Daws' work (1993, 1997, 2005, 2008) focuses on psychotherapy with parents and infants particularly where there are problems in eating, or sleeping. Frequently, these difficulties are connected in some way with anxieties about separation, so that overcoming these anxieties is the key to resolution. 'Daring to be different' means believing 'individuation need not be the end of intimacy' (Daws, 2008, p. 253).

Daws distinguishes between two kinds of feeding difficulty. On one hand, there are situations where the infant is underfed, leading to failure to thrive; on the other hand, there is a pattern where the infant is fed little and often, but both mother and infant become exhausted by the constant feeding cycle. While she does pay attention during the consultations with the families to the individual qualities of the infant, the emphasis in her work is on the different ways in which the parent is influenced by the impact of her baby, what is stirred up in the mother from the past, and the way this becomes patterned into her relationships with the infant and others. The two categories of feeding difficulty are best considered separately.

The infant who 'feeds too much' is a snack feeder. Here the mother may be responding to infant communications more at a physical level than an emotional one, and 'there is no shape to the meal as an emotional encounter' (Daws, 1993, p. 73). Daws shows that the repeated snack feeding masks a deep-seated fear in the parent of separation, which often takes the form that the infant will die if separate (a response therefore to the problem of heightened emotion about life and death). Also, in these circumstances, the mother's own infantile feeding experiences have been stirred up by the experience of feeding her baby. Here, as Daws (1993, p. 73) puts it, 'mothers who endlessly feed their babies may also be expressing unending hunger in themselves and are not able to feel reciprocally fed and satisfied by their babies' satisfaction'.

A particular manifestation of this dynamic can be the mother's preference for interpreting communications at a physical level – as a need for food – rather than as emotional needs. This creates a sense that the mother is missing her infant's communications. This may be the consequences of depression in the mother (Murray *et al.*, 2003) or of a mother's other troubling or difficult preoccupations, or other stressful circumstances. A combination of these factors, and a lack of confidence within the mother in being able to be guided by the qualities of the actual relationship she has with her baby (her reverie) can lead to the mother turning away from the intimacy of direct communication with the baby. Harris (1975) gave an example from an observation of a mother who, in contrast, though feeling herself to be limited in some respects and aware of her own childhood difficulties, allowed herself to learn from experience with her baby, to be taught by her baby, so to speak. An example from a study undertaken by one of us (Briggs, 1997) shows a mother, Anne, appearing to lack confidence and having difficulty in establishing interactions with her baby.

Samantha feeding

Samantha, at 13 days, was asleep in her mother's arms, then Anne moved a little and Samantha, still asleep, moved with her so that her head was lying back, almost out of Anne's arms in a slightly unsupported way. Anne told me she felt a lot of pain after the caesarean and this was the first day she had not thought about having a painkiller. Samantha stirred, opening her eyes slowly, quietly. She looked towards Anne's face. Anne said she was awake at last and said 'I'm just going to feed her'. She offered the right breast to Samantha and made a grimace as she took the nipple. She readjusted and Samantha lost the nipple, then took it again and sucked steadily. Anne sat cross-legged on the sofa, holding Samantha quite low down so that her face seemed to be hidden in Anne's top.

In this piece of interaction, Samantha is seeking mother with her eyes, demonstrating her wish to relate to her; mother took this to mean she wanted feeding. Samantha sucked steadily, making a good grip on the nipple. She was not perturbed by needing to start the feed twice. On the other hand, for mother Anne, the feed was preceded by her reporting pain from the childbirth and the process of making contact with Samantha was also painful; that is to say, she grimaced. As the feed progressed, Anne's conversation followed a wide range of subjects all of which seemed to reflect on her lack of confidence. She then returned to the subject of breastfeeding:

Samantha's feed and mother's anxieties

Anne said she had found she was running out of milk by the evening, and her first child, Donald, had always been hungry. She said that when Donald had been a baby she had not closed the curtains of the room which led to his waking at 4:00 a.m. Samantha stopped sucking, holding the nipple in her mouth and Anne looked down at her and then lifted her away from the breast and held her over her shoulder. Anne looked at her again and said 'you're hungry, that's what you are'. She said she thought she would go and make a bottle for Samantha.

Her lack of confidence in herself, in the face of her many preoccupations, is graphically illustrated in her turning to a bottle – as though she feels unable to feed Samantha from within herself. Feeding difficulties emerged later when, perhaps following this script, Samantha was not satisfied by breastfeeding, and she regurgitated bottle feeds. Anne herself had a background in which she had experienced her mother as not able to feed her adequately. The presence in any combination of lack of confidence, depression, anxiety about meeting the baby's needs and preoccupation with troubling issues – in Anne's case her older child's development was causing considerable anxiety – can lead a mother to miss her baby's cues and to withdraw from relating to the baby. In an unusual observational example provided by Reid (1997), a glimpse is obtained of the way a mother's own infantile feeding experiences can influence her feeding of her own baby. In these observations there is seen repeatedly a difficulty stemming from mother's apparent need to control the feeding situation:

The observer noted feed after feed the way that mother firmly held on to the bowl and the spoon. The infant was never allowed to hold the spoon or touch her food, certainly not to play with it and explore its qualities. This made the observation of feeds tense and difficult. The mother returned to work when the infant was 6 months old and the observations continued in the maternal grandmother's home. To the observer's amazement, she found that the grandmother fed in an identical way to the infant's mother. Reid (1997, p. 10) comments

"Of course the infant's mother had no conscious memory of this, but perhaps an unconscious blueprint had been made of the experience. It seemed to have survived totally unmodified."

'GHOSTS IN THE NURSERY' AND FAILURE TO THRIVE

The impact on parents of early but consciously not remembered experiences, which, as Reid notes, have somehow remained unmodified by time and experience, can in some circumstances form 'ghosts in the nursery', to use Fraiberg's (1980) term.

Fraiberg's work has had a significant impact on therapeutic work with parents and infants (Hopkins, 2008) highlighting the way in which undigested past experiences resurface in the heightened anxieties after the arrival of a new baby. Often, these 'ghost-like' experiences are of the impact of an actual, retrievable event, either from the recent or more distant past, which impacts on the parent and interferes with parenting. For example, a mother, Yvonne, who appeared to be affected by a distant 'ghost' who was both known and unknown to her repeatedly talked about an event from her own childhood:

A 'ghost in the nursery'

Yvonne made repeated references to the cot death of her younger brother when she was a small child. These references seemed unconnected in the way she told me about them from the current situation, in which she found herself in an often aggressive and sometimes quite cruel relationship with her infant daughter, Hester, her second child. Her fear of damaging her baby, of strangling her, or of hurting her in other ways suggested Yvonne's identification with a mother who could not keep babies alive and a murderous older sibling. Breastfeeding was ended prematurely so that neither she nor her older child should know these feelings of jealousy of the new baby, Hester, who was repeatedly sick after feeds (Briggs, 1997).

In this case the 'ghost in the nursery' is dimly remembered but creates a painful and difficult scenario for all the family. At times, the presence of a 'ghost' can be 'detected' with dramatic outcome. Brazelton and Cramer (1991, p. 139) give a number of illustrations of how these events lead to the parent relating 'to the ghost who is interposed - like a screen - between themselves and the child'. They give as an example the experiences of one mother who sought help for her baby boy, who had vomited feeds from birth. In the course of clinical consultation, the mother described the recent death of her brother, who also regurgitated (he had intestinal cancer). The connection made by the clinician ('he regurgitates like your brother') enabled the mother to separate her grief for her brother from her anxiety about her (boy) child. The clear and striking example of this 'ghost in the nursery' provides dramatic clinical possibilities. However, it also simplifies a complex configuration, in which it is as important to ask, as Reid implies in the example above, how the events remain so unmodified, despite time and experience.

Infants who fail to thrive present a painful and distressing picture in which the identification of the presence of a 'ghost in the nursery' helps to elucidate the emotional predicament. In one example (Daws, 1997) describes a 3-week-old baby who was removed from home by workers after gaining no weight from birth. On reflection, it appeared that the older sister's jealousy was placated in that way, so that she, the sister, did not have to know that she had been displaced as the baby in the family. This is a similar and probably more extreme example of the problems faced by Hester, whom I have described above. Some very powerful emotions were mobilised in the workers so that they too did not think about the new baby's needs. There was thus withholding of food supported by a parental rationalisation, in this case that the baby was not putting on weight, and fears of the infant's death were projected rather than thought about.

The painful sense of parental cruelty stems from the inability of parents (and workers) to notice and recognise the infant's needs, because of their own unmet needs, their inability to respond to the infant's needs, or feeling that they do not wish to share what they have with the infant. Daws (1997, p. 197) concludes that:

> "The major cause of the kind of feeding that leads to a withholding of food from the infant is undoubtedly the experience by the parent of neglect, deprivation and hunger in all its meanings, in their own childhood."

The withholding of food should be seen as an emotional issue played out on a physical level. Unmet needs, 'ghosts in the nursery' and the legacy of deprived and disturbing experiences all form the material for experiences which are projected into the infant or child, reversing the container-contained relationship. It is in this way that the child becomes a receptacle for these projections (Williams *et al.*, 2004). These can be primarily emotional intrusions of the parent's own uncontained, distressing or disturbing experiences, or they can be physical intrusions. They impact on the infant in a way which precipitates an 'at risk' situation for the infant, and, through repetition, affect a range of aspects of development.

POOR FEEDERS

Parental deprivation, unmediated by past or current supportive relationships, has a central part to play in the development of feeding difficulties in infancy. However, it is also important within the parent–infant relationship to take into account the particular qualities the infant brings to the development of such difficulties or, alternatively, a capacity to overcome these difficulties. In the 'fit' between a mother and her infant the infant is also an active participant. The degree of 'fit' depends not only on the mother's capacity in general, but also her particular capacity to deal with and respond to the constellation of feelings that are aroused in her by her baby. Some infants arouse in the mother a sense of her ability to understand and meet their needs; feeding, is thus experienced as rewarding at a physical and emotional level. On the other hand, some infants seem to push the mother beyond her own limitations or to arouse in her emotional experiences which are difficult for her.

Williams (1997, p. 91) gives a striking example of a 'poor feeder'. This infant, whom she calls Robert, is from the beginning almost impossible to feed. He does not demand to be fed, and when he is fed he regurgitates then sucks his thumb, his tongue and his lip. At 2 days old, she described him as making 'little stretching movements and his forehead was creased in a deep frown, a deep cleft on the lower lip was pulled up towards his mouth as though he was sucking in the flesh. Then he started to cry hard. His tongue was a little crescent raised inside his mouth.

The refusal of this infant to feed almost from the start of life aroused in the mother a very disheartened state of mind. The more disheartened the mother became, the less she felt she could meet his needs. This 'fit' between them led quickly to the development of a pattern in which the infant used parts of the body, his hand, lip and tongue, began to substitute for, or defend against, relying on another person to provide him with what he needs. Eventually, he had to be tube-fed.

Some groups of infants are known to be poor feeders, including premature babies (McFadyen, 1994). Skuse (1993) emphasises the 'subtle interaction between infant characteristics and parental response'. He distinguishes between the two groups of poor feeders: those who are restless, cry excessively and do not complete feeds, and the others who do not demand to be fed and go long periods between feeds. The development of these difficulties can be related to the qualities of the parent–infant relationship and, in particular, the qualities of containment in the relation-ship. Problems in the capacity of the parent to feed and of the infant to internalise the feed, at a physical and emotional level, lead to infants relating in ways which express a lack of internalisation of good experiences or which defend against the difficulties of depending on another person.

The two patterns of infant feeding characteristics described by Skuse relate closely to the relationship patterns demonstrated by infants when infants begin to develop defences arising through problems in the container-contained relationship. The first of these is a vigorously muscular kind of development (Bick, 1968), in which infants attempt to use their bodies to achieve mastery over distress. These are the distressed, restless feeders. One example (Briggs, 1997) is an infant, Timothy, whose mother felt she did not have enough to offer him, and they become involved in a cycle of distress, in which the mother felt she could not understand or 'know what he wants'. Problems of dependency and separation loomed large. For example (Briggs, 1997), at 5 months Timothy did not allow mother to be separate from him. During one observation, he continued crying and mother said she was sewing. She went to him and gave him a mirror and a rattle. He looked round, continued to cry and then lifted himself up, leaning towards his mother. He went right forward almost on to all fours and cried again.

Timothy's movements show that he wished to be with his mother and that as she did not come towards him, he must move towards her. He did reach physical milestones early, almost precociously. The mother seemed to feel that he should be able to allow this degree of separation from her. This is perhaps understandable at his age (5 months), but the experiences of lack of containment did not equip him, internally, to co-operate with this maternal wish.

The second pattern of defensive relatedness was that infants withdrew from relationships in the face of either parental projections or unresponsiveness. These infants showed a lack of emotional contact with others, lack of curiosity and a lack of evidence of physical development. Withdrawal from the world of relationships is accompanied by a closing down of attempts to make demands for attention and feeds. These infants also succeed in arousing considerable anxiety in others, particularly of a life and death dimension. Michael was one such infant (Briggs, 1997).

Michael withdrawing

In the early weeks of life Michael demonstrated through his sucking gestures and his crying a wish to relate, feed and make demands. His withdrawal was dramatically worrying to observe. At times he lay quietly with only the faintest signs of life and liveliness. For example, at 3 months: Michael was lying on his back with his eyes open the slightest amount. His mouth was open making some sucking movements. He lay still and moved his feet, turned his head slowly, still with his eyes open the merest crack.

He was sick in almost every feed I observed and at times he regurgitated almost the entire feed. His mother fed him irregularly and reluctantly. When she did feed him, she was intrusive and mechanical, Similarly, she was intrusive, and hostile, when wiping his mouth On occasions, even as he appeared most withdrawn, he could find it in him to respond to others, to become alert for a time and, almost covertly, to make developmental progress. There was a 'fit' between a mother who, through her antagonism towards him, wished her baby not to be there and a baby who made himself invisible. Failure to thrive physically was matched by difficulties in emotional development. Infants like Michael demonstrate capacities and wishes to make contact, to feed and to demand feeding at birth and soon after. The pattern of withdrawal clearly emerged within the early relationship.

FEEDING DIFFICULTIES AND DEVELOPMENT

We have emphasised that feeding difficulties have to be understood within the infant–mother relationship, and thus they arise when there is a disturbance within this relationship. Feeding difficulties may thus draw attention to and be an indicator of, particularly, problems in the container-contained dynamics. However, we have also pointed out that feeding difficulties can also be a sign that there are underlying problems with issues of dependency and separation. The example of Timothy shows, for example, an infant contending with such problems. Weaning in particular may well be experienced as an unbearable loss or as a broken link with the mother (Briggs, 1998; Williams *et al.*, 2004). Thus, infants may develop difficulties in maintaining a relationship in which there is a trusting reliance or dependency on the parent. In these circumstances, food itself can be rejected and/or felt to be contaminating. At an emotional level there is a parallel process in which learning can become impaired (Briggs, 1995). In Williams' case of Robert, discussed above, she makes an analogy between taking in food and taking in knowledge. There is strong clinical evidence from work with children to suggest that feeding, internalising physical nourishment and love, is akin to internalising knowledge through thinking. Food for thought is a common expression which underscores this link. Daws (1997) points out that there is a connection between feeding difficulties and speech delays. The way these learning difficulties are seen in observational study is through difficulties in developing symbolic forms of communication.

Both Timothy and Michael, the infants described above, had difficulties with language development and symbolising in their play. Michael, in his play, demonstrated a close similarity between the quality of contact he had with his mouth on the teat and the difficulty he had in maintaining contact with an object when playing. His mouth became slack, loose and open; he had difficulty maintaining a grip on an object with his mouth. In his play, he also showed a difficulty in making a firm contact. For example, he played with a football when he was 14 months old:

> "He held it, pushed it, and he followed it; every contact pushing it away. He seemed to slip against it, with movements that were indecisive, neither trying to hold it nor move it."

His contact with the ball was very like his loose, open-mouthed contact with the bottle. Learning is difficult when there is such a loose grip on objects and relationships. Timothy developed a mild food faddishness, which could be seen at 20 months to be clearly related to his feelings about father

---

Timothy's distaste

Mother passed him his plate and said it was daddy's courgettes and tomatoes. Timothy took one mouthful and then made a face of distaste and spat out the food. Sally used a spoon to give him a mouthful. He took a fork and took a mouthful from this. Sally tried to sort out what he liked and what he did not, and then she said 'you really don't like it', adding to me that he usually ate most things. She gave him an apple and he began to eat it. Then he started to choke. Disgust about father's 'courgettes and tomatoes' was probably connected with his reaction to recent events in the family, in which a second baby was conceived and miscarried.

The attitude of disgust shows also a disturbance of trust and a problem in symbolising, in which the food is experienced concretely as parts of daddy's body. It is the concreteness of experience and the disturbance to the dependent relationship which forms the indigestible experience.

APPLICATIONS IN PRACTICE

We have noted that in recent years there has been a significant growth in methods designed to help parents and infants, and we have emphasised that the basis for these interventions is a reliance on detailed observation linked with the integration of theoretical perspectives to form a relationally oriented approach. The new methods of intervention include infant–parent psychotherapy and the application of infant observation to professional work roles. The context for these interventions, in many countries, is an emphasis on early intervention to combat social exclusion; national and international Associations of Infant Mental Health provide a coordinating network for professionals engaged in early intervention.

We identify that methods of intervention tend to form one of two genres: firstly, there are those that apply understanding of the transference–countertransference dynamics to the understanding of parent–infant relatedness. In this model, the professional or therapist does not introduce any techniques but makes use of reflections on the emotional relationship between herself and the infant–parent couple. Daws (2008) suggests that the role of the therapist is to assist the parent–infant attempts to make interactive repair when they have not been able to achieve this alone (Tronick, 1989, 2007). She gives an example of a health visitor, Helen, who worked with a mother and her infant where there were difficulties in getting the breastfeeding relationship going.

Helen experienced that the mother 'seemed to approach me with intense feelings of need but little hope of them being met'. Helen worked to build trust with mother who told her of her childhood difficulties and traumas. Helen then commented, 'I hope that having opened up a little more to me having let her story out, she might be more able to let the milk flow'. This is indeed what happened; Daws (2008, p. 244) comments:

> "We see how naturally the body–mind connection is made by Helen. The imagery is compelling. The work did continue to 'flow' and the breastfeeding became much easier".

In a similar way of working, Benihoud (2004, p. 21) observes an infant–mother relationship.

> "The manner in which the baby was feeding seemed to mirror the way the mother was feeling … overwhelmed by her experiences".

So the baby's feed spilled out of her mouth and over her face. Again, attention to mother's troubled state of mind brought greater containment for mother and a more contained feeding experience for the baby.

Williams *et al.* (2004) show how more severe difficulties in the relationship, where the lack of 'fit' between mother and infant can also be treated through attention to the transference and counter transference relationship. Pinheiro (2004) discusses two infants with feeding difficulties, one who refused all food – and thus generated heightened anxiety – and one who refused solids and who seemed to communicate a refusal to 'taste' new experiences. Anxieties about separation filled the infant–parent relationship. Pinheiro describes how she undertook a patient process of understanding in lengthy interventions, which focused on the quality of liveliness in the relationship.

The second distinct method of intervention within infant–parent psychotherapy introduces specific techniques including the therapist and parent viewing together a video recording of mother–infant interaction. This aims to provide a 'third eye' that helps the parent become more thoughtful about the way she interacts with her baby (Baradon *et al.*, 2009, p. 151). An example of the application of this technique is the following Australian psychotherapy undertaken by Priddis. Video feedback in infant–parent psychotherapy was used in conjunction with individual psychoanalytic psychotherapy for the mother, Belle who was expecting twins, and her 14-month-old daughter, Mandy. Belle herself had been one of twins, but her twin was stillborn and she grew up with a favoured older brother and a younger sister. Belle's story is one of feeling she never got enough. Even as a baby she reported of her older brother, 'when I was a baby he stole my bottles and took them away and sucked them'. Belle thus appears to have been a receptacle for strong projections in her childhood.

Belle described how she was 'not getting on well with Mandy' whom she viewed as 'strong willed' adding 'I don't feel anything for her much…' Feeding difficulties took the form of a battle between mother and daughter at mealtimes. Mother controlled this battleground by restricting the foods Mandy was allowed since she felt she was a very messy eater.

Mandy and Belle: "I wanted someone to play with me"

In the first video play back session Mandy presented as a dour looking, beautifully dressed, unresponsive infant who sat quietly with a fixed expression on her face. Belle unstrapped Mandy, lifted her free of the stroller and sat her on the floor by some toys. Mandy made no protest and nor did she look interested in anything in the room either me, or the toys or her mother. Belle appeared nervous and unsure of where to start. She sat herself behind Mandy and both stared at the toys. Mandy moved towards a soft toy and almost simultaneously

Belle moved towards a bucket of blocks. Mandy drew the toy to her mouth. Belle turned away from Mandy taking the blocks with her and huddled over them fingering them absently. While Mandy moved about a little finding other things to touch and rarely referencing her mother, Belle remained huddled over her blocks, manipulating them quietly. My sense was of two young children in the room engaged in separate play. Belle's reaction to seeing the video was that she felt really strongly 'I wanted someone to play with me.'

In a subsequent session Belle and Mandy sat either side of a tea set that Belle had pulled from the shelf. Belle set out four cups and four saucers, a milk jug and a teapot. She took her time and arranged them carefully while Mandy watched, again with a soft toy in her mouth and a dour expression on her face. Belle placed a doll at each tea cup and carefully poured the play tea. Again Mandy looked on following her mother's moves. Belle smiled at Mandy and said 'They are taking tea.' Mandy turned to the toy cupboard. Belle kept her attention on the tea set…. Later in the session Belle showed Mandy the blocks from the previous session. Mandy didn't appear interested…. Mandy turned to Belle and held up a large mug. Belle said 'Oh are you thirsty', and gave Mandy a bottle of water from out of her bag Mandy knocked it away and held up the mug again. Belle lifted Mandy onto her lap and tried to give her the bottle of water …. I said, speaking for Mandy, 'Mum, I just wanted to take tea' Belle continued to hand Mandy the bottle again as though she didn't hear me.

The video session thus demonstrated the total preoccupation that Belle had with her own needs, her grievance from childhood and her competitiveness with her daughter; there was a significant gap between the roles she took up, and that required being a parent. Through containment in her individual therapy and in the parent–child relationship therapy Belle become more able to see Mandy's needs, wishes and intentions, to have space for these and to differentiate Mandy's needs from her own. As she said, 'at least I know now what Mandy is trying to tell me and if I don't respond I usually know I'm not'.

CONCLUSION

In this chapter we have discussed recent theoretical and practice developments that have created a rich milieu for understanding the infant–parent relationship. Underpinned by psychoanalysis, the theoretical framework for understanding this relationship is an integration of different approaches, strongly supported by both empirical studies and clinical experiences. Feeding difficulties are thought of as indicating difficulties in the infant–parent relationship especially difficulties relating to dependency and separation. Through looking at these difficulties from the perspective of container-contained, we have discussed ways in which a lack of 'fit' between infant and mother describes different patterns of difficulty within the infant–mother relationship, and how disturbances within the container-contained relationship constitute a failure of reciprocity, of giving and taking. There is, a 'generosity of acceptance' (Williams *et al.*, 2004) in feeding which becomes possible with sufficient containment for both infant and mother and an absence of generosity when this is lacking. Difficulties in the feeding aspect of the infant–mother relationship, if persistent, can impact adversely on development, particularly in the areas of thinking, learning and symbolising.

With the new orientation to a relational approach, new methods of intervention have been developed, treating the relationship as the focus. Some psychoanalytic approaches have received support from these changes, including the observation-based approach that focuses on the quality of emotionality between infants and parents, and, in the transference relationship, with therapists. We have highlighted approaches that concentrate on the sensitive understanding of the transference–counter-transference dynamics, and which can be used either in formal psychotherapy or in professional practice that adapts the observational stance. Alongside this, more structured practice settings make use of distinctive techniques, including reflective video feedback, and we have illustrated the application of these to a case with feeding difficulties.

REFERENCES

Alvarez A. *Live Company: psychoanalytic psychotherapy with autistic, borderline, deprived and abused children*. London: Routledge; 1992.

Baradon T, Gerhardt S, Tucker JS. Working with the hidden obstacles in parent–infant relating. In: Barlow J, Svanberg PO, editors. *Keeping the Baby in Mind: infant mental health in practice*. New York, NY: Routledge; 2009. pp. 141–54.

Barlow J, Svanberg P. *Keeping the Baby in Mind: infant mental health in practice*. Hove: Routledge; 2009.

Benihoud E. *How can Informed Observation Contribute Towards Understanding Infant Feeding Difficulties?* MA Thesis in Tavistock/University of East London Library Collection; 2004.

Bick E. Notes on infant observation in psychoanalytic training. *Int J Psychoanal.* 1964; 45: 484–8.

Bick E. The experience of the skin in early object relations. *Int J Psychoanal.* 1968; 49: 484–6.

Bick E. Further consideration of the function of the skin in early object relations: findings from infant observation integrated into child and adult analysis. *Br J Psychother.* 1986; 2(4): 292–301.

Bion W. *Learning from Experience*. London: Heinemann; 1962.

Bion W. *Second Thoughts*. London: Maresfield; 1967.

Brazelton T, Cramer B. *The Earliest Relationship*. London: Karnac; 1991.

Briggs S. Parallel process: emotional and physical digestion in adolescents with eating disorders. *J Soc Work Pract*. 1995; 9(2): 155–68.

Briggs S. *Growth and Risk in Infancy*. London: Jessica Kingsley; 1997.

Briggs S. The contribution of infant observation to an understanding of feeding difficulties in infancy. *Int J Infant Obs*. 1998; 1(3): 44–60.

Briggs S. Psychoanalytic research in the era of evidence-based practice. In: Bower M, editor. *Psychoanalytic Theory for Social Work Practice*. London: Routledge; 2005. pp. 15–29.

Daws D. Feeding problems and relationship difficulties: therapeutic work with parents and infants. *J Child Psychother*. 1993; 19(2): 69–84.

Daws D. Consultation in general practice. In: Trowell J, Bower M, editors. *The Emotional Needs of Young Children and Their Families*. London: Routledge; 1995.

Daws D. The perils of intimacy: closeness and distance in feeding and weaning. *J Child Psychother*. 1997; 23(2): 179–93.

Daws D. A child therapist in the baby clinic of a general practice: standing by the scales 30 years on. In: Launer J, Blake S, Daws D, editors. *Reflecting on Reality: psychotherapists at work in primary care*. London: Karnac, Tavistock Clinic Series; 2005.

Daws D. Sleeping and feeding problems: attunement and daring to be different. In: Emanuel L, Bradley E, editors. *What Can the Matter Be? Therapeutic Interventions with Parents, Infants and Young Children*. London: Karnac; 2008.

Downing G. Emotion, body and parent–infant interaction. In: Nadal J, Muir D, editors. *Emotional Development*. Oxford: Oxford University Press; 2005.

Fonagy P, Gergely G, Target M. Psychoanalytic constructs and attachment theory and research. In: Cassidy J, Shaver P, editors. *Handbook of Attachment: theory, research and clinical applications*. New York, NY: Guilford; 2008. pp. 783–810.

Fraiberg S. *Clinical Studies in Infant Mental Health*. London: Tavistock; 1980.

Harris M. Notes on maternal containment in good enough mothering [Reprinted]. In: Harris Williams M, editor. *The Collected Papers of Martha Harris and Esther Bick*. Perthshire: Clunie Press; 1975.

Hopkins J. Infant–parent psychotherapy: Selma Fraiberg's contribution to understanding the past in the present. In: Emanuel L, Bradley E, editors. *What Can the Matter Be? Therapeutic Interventions with Parents, Infants and Young Children*. London: Karnac; 2008.

Klein M. Notes on some schizoid mechanisms (1946) [Reprinted]. In: Klein M, editor. *Envy and Gratitude and Other Works 1946–63*. London: Virago; 1988.

Malloch S, Trevarthen C, editors. *Communicative Musicality: exploring the basis of human companionship*. Oxford: Oxford University Press; 2009.

McFadyen A. *Special Care Babies and their Developing Relationships*. London: Routledge; 1994.

Miller L, Rustin ME, Rustin MJ, *et al.*, editors. *Closely Observed Infants*. London: Duckworths; 1989.

Murray L, Cooper P, Hipwell A, *et al*. Mental health of parents caring for infants. *Arch Women's Ment Hlth*. 2003; 6(Suppl. 2): 571–7.

Pinheiro M. Feeding difficulties in infancy: Faruk and Shereen. In: Williams G, Williams P, Desmarais J, *et al.*, editors. *Exploring Feeding Difficulties in Children: the generosity of acceptance*. Vol 1. London: Karnac; 2004. pp. 21–42.

Reid S, editor. *Developments in Infant Observation: the tavistock model*. London: Routledge; 1997.

Rustin M. Reflections on method. In: Miller L, *et al.*, editors. *Closely Observed Infants*. London: Duckworths; 1989. pp. 52–75.

Rustin M. What do we see in the nursery? Infant observation as laboratory work. *Int J Infant Obs Appl*. 1997; **1**(1): 93–110.

Rustin M. Looking in the right place: complexity theory, psychoanalysis and infant observation. *Int J Infant Obs*. 2002; **5**(1): 122–44.

Rustin M. Infant observation research. What have we learned so far? *Int J Infant Obs Appl*. 2006; **9**(1): 35–52.

Siegal D. *The Mindful Brain*. New York, NY: WW Norton & Co; 2007.

Skuse D. Identification and management of problem eaters. *Arch Dis Child*. 1993b; 604–8.

Stern D. *The Motherhood Constellation: a unified view of parent–infant psychotherapy*. New York, NY: Basic Books, Inc; 1995.

Stern D. *The First Relationship: infant and mother*. Cambridge, MA: Harvard University Press; 2002.

Swain JE, Thomas P, Leckman JF, *et al.* Parent-infant attachment systems. In: Jurist EL, Slough NM, Bergner S, editors. *Mind to Mind: infant research, neuroscience, and psychoanalysis*. New York: Other Press; 2008. pp. 264–303.

Trevarthen C, Aitken K. Infant intersubjectivity: research, theory, and clinical applications. *J Child Psychol Psychiatr*. 2001; **42**(1): 3–48.

Tronick E. Emotions and emotional communications in infants. *Am Psychol*. 1989; **44**(2): 113–19.

Tronick E. *The Neurobehavioral and Social-emotional Development of Infants and Children*. New York, NY: WW Norton & Co; 2007.

Urwin C. Doing infant observation differently? Researching the formation of mothering identities in an inner London borough. *Int J Infant Obs Appl*. 2007; **10**(3 Special Issue): 239–51.

Williams G. *Internal Landscapes and Foreign Bodies*. London: Duckworths/Tavistock Clinic Series; 1997.

Williams G, Williams P, Desmarais J, *et al.*, editors. *Exploring Feeding Difficulties in Children: the generosity of acceptance*. Vol 1. London: Karnac; 2004.

Winnicott D. *The Child, the Family and the Outside World*. Harmondsworth: Penguin; 1964.

Winnicott D. *The Maturational Processes and the Facilitating Environment*. London: Hogarth Press; 1965.

Winnicott D. Fear of breakdown. *Int Rev Psychoanal*. 1974; **1**(1): 103–7.

CHAPTER 5

Developmental, cognitive and regulatory aspects of feeding disorders

Terence M Dovey and Clarissa Martin

INTRODUCTION

There is little published data within the literature on the development of a child with feeding disorders. As such, we are almost totally reliant on explaining feeding disorders by characterising children in terms of their deviation from 'normal' eaters. There is one obvious and unsubstantiated assumption within this approach that must be challenged. This is that there is such a thing as 'normal' development, cognition and appetite regulation. If the title of this chapter were read literally, then the assumption would be that one of two things has happened to the child in order for them to become 'disordered': either the feeding disorder has occurred as a consequence of some biological infirmity or it has emerged as a result of significant developmental disruption, causing inappropriate food-related cognitions that are also inappropriate for the child's chronological age. These basic beliefs about the underlying cause(s) of the development of feeding disorders are predicated on the assumption that all feeding disorders are homologous, that is, their development from 'normal' into 'disordered' behaviour is both linear and predictable. However, recent tentative research from different authors would strongly refute this and suggests that such simplistic interpretations seriously underestimate the complexity of feeding problems and disorders in children, while also failing to reflect the experience of clinical practice. A more accurate interpretation would be that the term 'feeding disordered' should be considered as an umbrella term for the many children who present with an inability and/or lack of desire to consume food. Each presentation is unique, requiring a tailor-made management strategy to overcome it, though there are some distinct groups whose underlying causes may have significant similarity. This chapter will offer an explanation of what constitutes an appropriate development of feeding, as well as at which points a feeding disorder may manifest.

DIFFERENTIATING NORMAL FROM DISORDERED FEEDING

To understand what constitutes normal feeding, it is important to briefly review children's developmental milestones and feeding and to discuss what we define as a functionally viable diet.

Developmental milestones and feeding

Theory and research on child development emphasises the notion of 'achieving milestones' (*see* Table 5.1). However, it is important to consider that the timeframes suggested in the literature are representative of an average. Developmental changes run parallel to chronological age, but it is accepted that some children may achieve various developmental milestones earlier or later than this average while still being within the normal range (*see* Chapter 2).

Within the first few months of life, children will require feeding on demand until they reach the weaning stage. At weaning, the consumption of foods with increased energy density will give the child energy security and lessen their requirement for constant access to food, which, in turn, allows exploration of their world. This explorative stage is essential to learning and is arguably integral to overcoming food neophobia and sensory sensitivity. The child's engagement and frequency of exploration depend primarily on the quality of the attachment to the primary caregiver. The more predictable the caregiver's behaviour, the more confident the child will be to explore their environment, experience new things and develop.

Expanding our understanding of the concept of a normal diet

In the non-clinical population the emphasis is on having a healthy diet, as determined by the consumption of a wide range of nutritious foods. This diet is not 'normal': it is an aspiration. Normality should be defined by the 'average' diet within the wider population, which often shows variation to this 'ideal'. In an environment where it is easy to gain weight and to over-consume (in terms of total calories per day), it is highly incongruent to find children who do not have any known biological problem (having either totally recovered from a medical ailment or have never had one) and yet are rapidly losing weight. Within this context, children who present with feeding disorders seem particularly unusual, difficult to understand and somewhat difficult to treat.

Rapid weight loss is invariably determined by the consumption of too few calories compared to the child's energy and growth requirements. Growth is usually determined by a comparison to a peer group, although it could also be

TABLE 5.1: Developmental milestones and feeding

	Cues of hunger	Motor skills	Feeding and eating skills	Textures and types of food	🥄
From 0 to 2 months	Cries, show irritability and/or fussiness when hungry. Opens mouth looking for nipple. Stops sucking and spits out nipple when full.	Strong reflexes movements. Can move head from side to side. No head support. Uncoordinated arms movements.	Suckle swallow pattern. Suckle reflex. Tongue thrust reflex.	Breast milk or bottle infant formulas.	Stiffening body when feeding. High frequency of irritability and crying when feeding. Coughing/choking.
From 2 to 4 months	Cries, show irritability and/or fussiness when hungry. Open mouth looking for nipple. Stops sucking and spits out nipple when full.	Developing head control. Can smile and track objects with eyes.	Better coordination of suck/swallow/breath pattern. Tongue moves forward and backwards to suck.	Breast milk or bottle infant formulas.	Prolonged feeding times. Frequent vomiting and spitting. Recurrent respiratory infections. Difficulties in gaining weight/height.
From 4 to 6 months	Moves head forward to reach spoon. May scream when hungry. Turns head away from spoon and is distracted by surroundings when full.	Holds the head at 90° when in prone position. Can sit with support. Can maintain their weight on both legs with help. Laugh and smile. Pay attention to objects and try to reach for them.	Loss of sucking reflex. Uses primitive phasic bite-release pattern. May suck a biscuit instead of biting. May use intermittent up–down chewing movements.	Breast milk or bottle infant formulas. From 5 months can start tasting baby cereals and some puree foods.	Recurrent respiratory infections. Observation of problems in relation with aspiration risks, swallowing or oro-motors problems. Difficulties in gaining weight/height.
From 6 to 8 months	Reaches for food or spoon, leans towards spoon and/or points to food when hungry. Can close the mouth, turn head and/or push food away when full. Eats slowly when full.	Sits independently. Pick up small objects and hold onto them.	Long sequences of sucking/swallowing and breathing. Open mouth and relax tongue to accept food. Improving tongue movements. Self-feeding skills. Keeps food in mouth. Uses upper lip to reach food. Drink from a cup with help.	Bottle infant formulas. Thin and thicker puree baby foods. Junior foods. Soft mashed food without lumps.	To monitor when eating and drinking as the child. May have continuous sucking followed by uncoordinated swallowing (losing liquid). Larger mouthfuls through drinking by cup may result in choking. Aversive reaction to the introduction of foods. Difficulties in gaining weight/height.

Age					
From 8 to 12 months	Show excitement in the presence of food. Can point to food and will reach out to food when hungry. Pushes food away when full.	Learning to crawl. Pull self to stand. More coordinate hand movement (i.e. pass objects from one hand to another, waves hands to say goodbye, claps etc.). Use thumb and finger to grasp things. Identify themselves in the mirror.	Show graded bite. Diagonal rotary and lateral tongue movements. At 10 months, move lips to remove food from spoon. Use jaw and tongue to mash food. Play with spoon at meal times. Hold cup. Independently pick and hold food with thumb and first finger.	Puree food. Mashed table foods with some soft lumps. Feed self finger foods and/or crunchy food that dissolve (i.e. crackers).	Difficulties in accepting new textures. Sensitive to be touched around mouth. High frequency of coughing, gagging and vomiting before/during/after meals. Difficulties in gaining weight/height.
From 12 to 18 months	Indicate needs with gestures and own style. Shows temper when hungry. Ask for foods with words or sounds. Shake the head to express 'no' when full.	Pulls self to stand and stand alone. Takes early steps.	Active lips during chewing. Uses upper gums or teeth. Uses controlled bite on soft biscuits. Can chew with closed lips. Diagonal rotary chewing movements. Feeds self with fingers. Can hold cup with two hands. Dips spoon on food.	Express desire for specific foods. Toddler foods, ground mashed or chopped table foods. Easily chewed meats. At 18 months eats most meats and raw vegetables. Familiar food recognition is established.	Difficulties in accepting new textures. High frequency of coughing, gagging and vomiting before/during/after meals. Not showing interest in others eating. Tantrums to avoid eating and/or some foods.
From 18 to 24 months	Can use language to express needs. Leads parent to refrigerator and point or ask for food/drink. Arrived at completion of food when full.	Walks alone. At 24th month: can run alone, kicks ball and climbs up–downstairs.	Uses controlled bite. Opens mouth more than required to accept big pieces. Swallow from a cup without losing liquid. Chewing, mixing vertical and rotary movements. Eats at the family table.	Toddlers drink 100% juice and eat chopped food. Efficient at eating different textures. Takes controlled bites of soft, hard and crunchy solids at 24th month.	Not showing interest in others' eating. Tantrums to avoid eating and/or some foods. Persistent fussiness and irritability associated with eating.

determined through a comparison to the child's previous weight status. Growth is a vector-based anatomical assessment of the child's development and has historically been the basic diagnostic determinant of feeding disorder. Growth and food intake, along with genetic predisposition, are symbiotic: the more the child eats the faster they grow, and the more they grow the more food they need to consume to maintain their weight status and continue to grow. The initial manifestation of a feeding disorder can come at any stage during this process. It may happen from birth resulting in the child's growth faltering (also termed 'failure to thrive') or alternatively can happen at any time during the first 6 years of life, when the child fails to adequately consume sufficient calories to match their current energy needs.

The diet in terms of quantity may end with the child not growing or losing weight; however, it can also be characterised by its quality and significant nutrient deficiency. A feeding disorder may also be attributed to a child that suffers medical consequences because their diet is characterised by poor dietary variety. The child may only accept a very limited repertoire of food items that leads to a variety of medical problems. Clearly, these children require intervention as much as those who have lost weight or have not grown compared to their siblings and peers. The common theme between those children with feeding disorders characterised by consuming a lack of quantity and those who eat a lack of variety is the reliance on the waiting until the food refusal results in serious medical consequences.

Dysfunction or specific medical diagnosis often provides the impetus to intervene in feeding disorders. This has largely been due to the tendency of many professional groups to wait for presentation of growth faltering. While this delay may provide absolute evidence for the necessity of professional intervention, it disregards the importance of the initial deviation from 'normal' development that must have occurred for the child's feeding to 'become disordered'. Intervention at an earlier point will be more successful, as measured by the speed of response to intervention and better short-, medium- and long-term prognoses.

Deviation from 'normal' development can occur within five distinct domains.

1   Biological dysfunction/dysregulation resulting in interruptions in the normal developmental process.
2   Disruption of attachment, resulting in a lack of reciprocity between child and carer; in the child, this may manifest as a lack of responsiveness or not registering innate drives to eat
3   Lack of psychological development of familiarity based on frequency, duration and type of exposure to foods, so that the child formulates appropriate 'trust' in food.
4   Inappropriate reactions to food especially within the sensory domain, developmental delay or autism spectrum disorders (ASDs), resulting in the rejection of food based on inappropriate rationalisation.
5   Anxiety-related refusal, resulting in an inappropriate aversion to food and leading to a phobic-like reaction.

Medical complications/interruptions leading to feeding disorders

This chapter does not cover the problems that these complications can have on normal development. These can be found in other chapters of this book, primarily Chapter 2, which outlines medical and nursing perspectives. Feeding problems in children with neurological problems and chronic illnesses are also covered in Chapters 10 and 12, respectively. However, it is paramount to remember that any form of illness, especially chronic gastrointestinal disorders, can affect feeding and by proxy the required learning process about food. A variety of ailments and medical treatments can also require long periods of hospitalisation or result in increased caregiver anxiety around food intake. In both situations, the child will not have the chance to experience their world as other children would.

DEVELOPMENT OF ATTACHMENT AND APPETITE AWARENESS

Children must develop within an environment where they feel secure. It is only within this context that they can learn to associate their appetite signals with feelings of hunger and fullness. The child is reliant on their parent to offer guidance about 'what', 'where' and 'when' it is appropriate to eat. Problems in caregiver/child attachment may lead directly to problems in eating behaviour (*see* Chapter 4).

Attachment between the parent and the child has been extensively characterised through the term 'styles'. It is a dyadic relationship requiring both parties to 'understand' one another. The parent must accurately empathise, understand and respond to the child's demands and the child must learn to associate the parent's response with the behaviour they initially expressed. It is only once this 'cycle of understanding' has been repeated several times with consistent outcomes that both parties can perceive consistency in the relationship and become attuned to one another. This consistency is frequently termed secure attachment. If the child is securely attached then he or she will be able to learn about their 'inner world' around appetite regulation and their wider environment (Rees, 2008).

The importance of attachment

Secure attachment is the only style of attachment with positive outcomes, where both parent and child feel at ease with one another. Other forms of attachment (anxious attachment, ambivalent attachment, avoidant attachment and disorganised attachment) are characterised as problematic and have multiple repercussions. They can be differentiated from one another through how 'attuned' the child is to the parent. These insecure attachment styles have been linked to eating disorders especially around emotion regulation and cognitive distortions (Tasca *et al.*, 2006, 2009) and to some degree in feeding disorders (Martin *et al.*, 2008).

It is impossible to consider the role of attachment and appetite-awareness in feeding disorders without acknowledging the similar psychiatric diagnosis of 'infantile
anorexia', so-called because of its apparent sharing of similar characteristics with the
other sub-types of adult anorexia nervosa, notably the drive for autonomy (Chatoor
et al., 1998).

Chatoor's (1997) diagnostic criteria for 'infantile anorexia' are given below.
• The behaviour will vary from meal to meal.
• The behaviour will vary depending on the person feeding them.
• The child will have a poor calorie intake for at least 2 months.
• The child's weight status will be below the 5th percentile for age.
• The parent will report that their child has:
  – a poor appetite
  – is overly attention-seeking and curious
  – stubborn during feeding.
• The parent usually responds to the constant and consistent rejection of food by:
  – coaxing the infant to eat more
  – distracting the infant with toys to induce eating
  – feeding the infant at any time of the day or night
  – offering different foods if the infant does not eat
  – force-feeding the infant.

The fact that these criteria fail to distinguish 'infantile anorexia' from 'feeding disorder' emphasises the continuing need for consensus around a shared language and
classificatory system. Until such time as consistency is reached within the literature,
there will be continuing conflict in approaches to management strategies and which
group has clinical responsibility. Furthermore, the field will progress at a slower
rate, as equally conflicting investigatory results will be published due to differential
conceptualisations and rationales offered by different authors. Above all else, this
issue needs resolution.

BIOLOGICAL AND COGNITIVE LINKS

The descent into feeding disorder through poor attachment can occur directly
through psychological dysfunction, but there are also some biological repercussions. Disruption in the mother–child bond has been shown to affect the microflora of the intestinal tract in monkeys presumably through elevated levels of stress.
Similar elevation in stress responses have been observed in children who have been
maltreated (Cicchetti and Rogosch, 2001) or neglected (Gunnar *et al.*, 2001). This
biological repercussion can lead to significantly elevated levels of sickness and poor
digestion (Bailey and Coe, 1999). Manifestations of illness during childhood can
also lead to inappropriate association of the illness with food intake and, without
parental rectification, lead to further food rejection.

Attachment and energy regulation

The primary role of attachment is to allow the child to learn about their environment safe in the knowledge that they have energy security and protection from any potential threat. In effect, the child does not have the experience or cognitive capacity to understand what is, and is not, potentially dangerous, and is reliant on others to rectify or guide their behaviour. Only within this form of relationship can they learn what they should and should not be fearful of. For eating behaviour, this learning refers to physiological and gastric markers of hunger and fullness. Successful associations of hunger and fullness allow the child to learn energy security for themselves and will become less reliant on others to regulate this for them.

How children learn associations between their biology and its energy needs is through flavour-nutrient learning. In flavour-nutrient learning, the child learns to associate a particular taste with the potential energy, satiation and satiety repercussions of consuming it. This information gives the individual the relative comfort of being able to predict the energy content of a particular food and weigh up its intrinsic motivational value. Moreover, it gives the individual energy security so that they can concentrate on other aspects of life than the acquisition of food (Brunstrom, 2007).

The complexity of this learning process also needs to consider energy usage too. Not only must the child learn about the nutrient value of the food but also how much energy will they need on any given day dependent on how much physical activity they engage in. Failure to learn this complex interplay between flavour, energy, nutrient and physical activity will eventually lead to failure to grow adequately. Such children often present with little desire or behavioural motivation to consume food and will not understand the link between food and their well-being. An obvious example of these children is those who are tube-dependent following full recovery of a medical ailment.

Development of taste in infants

- Taste begins to emerge at 7–8 week gestation (Schaal *et al.*, 2005).
- Evidence of foetal swallowing of amniotic fluid flavoured by mother's diet (Schaal *et al.*, 2000).
- Dislike of sour flavours at birth and a preference for sweet tastes (Birch, 1999).
- Experiences of taste and smell through mother's breast milk for breastfed infants.
- Development of a preference for a slightly salty taste (appears between 4 and 6 months, indicating development of taste sensitivity; Birch, 1999).
- Evidence of a 'window of opportunity' between 5 and 6 months, as at this stage, acceptance of new tastes is relatively easily to achieve (Schwartz *et al.*, 2009).
- Establishment of familiar food recognition by around 1 year of age.

DEVELOPMENT OF TRUST AROUND FOOD

For some children, one aspect that could be identified as a contributory factor in feeding disorder is that of appropriate development to overcome age-dependent food neophobia. All children will progress through a developmental stage whereby they will suddenly become highly distrustful of new foods. The beginning of this phase will be observed alongside the child's increased mobility and exploration of his or her environment. Depending on the child, their family and environment, food neophobia will peak between 2 and 6 years of age (Addessi *et al.*, 2005) and should gradually diminish to a relatively stable trait-based level before early adolescence (Nicklaus *et al.*, 2005). Many factors have been identified that affect the progression and magnitude of expression of food neophobia. These include innate and rapidly acquired taste preferences (Visser *et al.*, 2000), cognitive ability or attention span (El-Chaar *et al.*, 1996), cultural norms (Kannan *et al.*, 1999), parenting style/ pressure (Galloway *et al.*, 2005), parental dietary preferences and eating behaviours (Fisher *et al.*, 2002), sensation-seeking (Galloway *et al.*, 2003), trait anxiety (Loewen and Pliner, 1999), openness (McCrae *et al.*, 2002), neuroticism (Steptoe *et al.*, 1995) and emotivity (MacNicol *et al.*, 2003). Despite a plethora of factors affecting the normal child's expression of food neophobia, one factor above all will predict how quickly the child overcomes it. This factor is experience.

The defining feature of food neophobia is that the rejection of the food item presented is based on its novelty. The more experience a child has with a food item, the less novel it is and, therefore, the more likely they are to accept it as a food item and try it. Within the literature, it has been reported that 8–15 different exposure episodes are required to overcome food neophobia-based rejection in a 'normal' child (Birch *et al.*, 1987; Wardle *et al.*, 2005). It must also be inferred from this data that this 'mean' number of exposures also has a natural standard deviation and any child considered resistant will require significantly more exposures to overcome their food neophobia. These problematic children are referred to by many different names; however, 'picky' or 'fussy' eaters appear more frequently than any others. These children are often defined as those that refuse a large number of familiar foods in addition to having higher levels of food neophobia (Dovey *et al.*, 2008). Picky eaters, if based solely upon a food neophobia argument, may appear to be of clinical significance; however, not all will be. The households of families in developed countries typically contain functional and energy dense foods and, therefore, it is possible for a child to survive and even thrive on a relatively low dietary quantity and variety. Through the consumption of a comparatively low number of food items, a child may be able to meet both their nutritional and energy requirements. It is only when the dietary-related factors are undermined that the child's feeding may come to be understood as disordered.

Development of a feeding disorder may occur as a result of the child's inability to progress beyond their food neophobic stage. Although the parent may control each food exposure, including both quality and quantity, it is important to not under-estimate the role the child has in this dyadic relationship. It is unarguable that the parent controls the exposure episode in terms of frequency, environment, approach, pressure to conform and type of foods offered; however, the child will express his or her own desires, preferences and personality characteristics too. The child's preferences during this developmental stage will reflect innate hedonistic food choices and they will employ strategies to gain these choices in preference to any new food offered. Therefore to blame the parents for the development of a feeding disorder derived from insufficient experience with a food item alienates them from any possible interventions and assumes parental fault. Instead, focus must be on the presentation of the problems and how to effectively overcome them; early assumptions about 'blame' will undermine intervention strategies and thus effective outcome.

DEVELOPMENT OF FOOD ACCEPTABILITY

Concurrent to the increase and eventual decrease in expression of food neophobia, the child also progresses through a sensory exploration stage. Indeed, learning to process sensory information and not derive insult or aversion from it could be argued to be the underlying factor to overcoming food neophobia (Dovey *et al.*, 2008). Each child will have a pre-determined set level of sensory defensiveness that will eventually constitute part of their overall trait-based interpersonal interaction (especially in the case of tactile defensiveness). However, this initial level will decrease based on the child's ability to learn and their experiences within early life. For example, once the child has stable and functional categorisation criteria for various objects, it will allow them a certain amount of expectation around it (Aldridge *et al.*, 2009). They then will not view the item as a threat and will not react and interact with it accordingly.

Heightened sensory processing ability (Dovey *et al.*, 2010b) and/or clinical levels of sensory defensiveness (Smith *et al.*, 2005) will lead to food rejection based on its visual, olfactory or texture properties rather than its utility as a food item. Sensory defensiveness is characterised as an overreaction, or offence, resulting in withdrawal from the sensation of being touched, either by another person, or by something in their environment, which most would consider inoffensive (Wilbarger, 2000). Heightened sensory ability would be defined as those individuals that have the ability to tell the difference between items based solely on their sensory properties that others, including expert categorisers, would find difficult or impossible. Both the sensory sensitive and heightened ability children may have a higher propensity to develop a feeding disorder. Such disorders are likely to be characterised by diets that are extremely limited and contain foods of a similar colour, taste and/or texture. In short, food is rejected due to inappropriate assumptions about it rather than its actual properties (e.g. children may say they 'don't like green food' or 'it smells funny' or 'it's too crunchy').

All children will express some degree of sensory defensiveness, especially towards items they have limited experience with. The child must learn that the item poses no threat to them and so will naturally progress through a sensory processing hierarchy based on distance required in order to process the object. Therefore, a new item will be investigated through a set sensory process of sight, then smell/touch and then taste. Taste exposure is believed to be the strongest method of forming trust (Kalat and Rozin, 1973), acceptance and preference towards consuming any food item (Arvola *et al.*, 1999). Some theorists have also proposed that exposure effects are modality specific (Birch *et al.*, 1987). Therefore, a child that has any form of sensory defensive characteristics will not cycle through the appropriate hierarchy of exposure episodes. Thus they will not learn to trust the food presented and will not have the opportunity to create learned food preferences. Without intervention, the child will always rely upon their innate neurobiological hedonic preferences to formulate what food is acceptable.

It is possible that sensory defensive children have no other pathologies beyond their feeding disorder; however, there are obvious links with ASD. Children who have ASD are often referred to feeding disorder specialists in order to effectively intervene in their poor or low dietary variety (not all children with autism develop problems around food acceptance). It is possible to differentiate children with sensory sensitivity from ASD relatively easily. Although anecdotal clinical evidence suggests that some children with ASD can respond reasonable well to desensitisation intervention, research suggests that, in comparison to children with sensory sensitivity, they do not (Dovey *et al.*, 2010b). The reason behind the differential response is probably due to the total profile of the child. ASD children have additional social pathologies that may prohibit effective desensitisation learning. Similarly, selective food rejection in ASD is hard to effectively treat (Matson and Fodstad, 2009). Some research concludes that management strategies for feeding problems in ASD cannot be offered until the individual reaches adolescence (Ahearn, 2003) or at least late childhood (Piazza *et al.*, 2002). An exception to this would be if the child with autism was willing to taste the foods offered; for these children, it appears that increasing dietary variety is an easier process (Williams *et al.*, 2007). In all cases, ASD is beyond the scope of this chapter and cannot be considered a 'true' feeding disorder despite the presentation of medical symptoms and behavioural responses to foods. This is due to the simple fact that their food rejection is resulting from their ASD profile. Interested readers for feeding interventions with ASD are referred initially to Matson and Fodstad (2009).

Max: a case of sensory sensitivity

Max, a 6-year-old Caucasian boy, was referred to the feeding specialist due to his extremely limited diet. During the clinical interview, it came to the light that the child could not tolerate certain smells. The presence of these smells made him vomit. He had become reluctant to attend school as he could not cope with the smells without feeling sick. This was interpreted by his parents and teachers as an excuse for his school avoidance.

The feeding specialist decided to conduct several 'experiments' with Max to establish his smell sensitivity in comparison with that of other members of his family. It transpired that Max was able to identify the clothes of his brothers and his parents through their smell while the rest of the family could not. This gave the family a more objective perspective of his sensitivity and allowed a helpful re-frame of the problem. With Max's sensitivity viewed as 'special', his rejection of specific smells could be viewed as a challenge that they could help him overcome.

As Max did not present with any co-morbid features, a desensitisation program was designed for him and his parents to work through at home. For example, Max was encouraged to find ingredients that his mother was using when cooking or in the food presented through smell. His parents also made a chart monitoring his progress with tolerating smells, including those associated with school. This systematic desensitisation approach was supported by a cognitive-behavioural strategy to help Max to extinguish his vomiting behaviour. The desensitisation treatment worked well and Max was able to return to the school where a similar approach was followed by his class teacher. Once the smell sensitivity difficulties were resolved, Max and his parents embarked on a taste exposition treatment to expand his acceptance of a greater variety of food.

Developmental delay

Feeding problems may also occur as concomitants of developmental delay. Learning in all its forms precedes any aspect of behaviour including eating (Dovey, 2010). If the child does not learn appropriate behaviour then he or she will not have an appropriate understanding of their environment, themselves or the potential repercussions they may encounter. Therefore, any factor that interferes with the learning process irrespective of any other factor will predispose the child to a variety of problems including feeding disorders. It is conceivable and frequently observed within clinical samples (Dovey *et al.*, 2010a) that a significant proportion of children who present with extremely limited diets will have an additional pathology within their learning ability. This includes both developmental delay and significant learning difficulties. These children can be categorised as lying somewhere between the children with sensory sensitivity and those with ASD in terms of their responsiveness to desensitisation interventions. Responsiveness in these children will depend heavily on the severity of their developmental delay and/or presence of other co-morbidities.

The inclusion of children with developmental delay within this section rather than the learning-dependent-based developmental section is due to the experiences they have been exposed to. Children with learning-dependent food rejection will not accept a food because they have not had sufficient experience with the food item to accept it. Children with developmental delay, in contrast, are likely to have had the necessary amount of experience, they just have not learnt from these experiences. Getting children with developmental delay to accept specific food items will often require a concerted and specialist management strategy. Multiple exposure scenarios tailored to the child's intellectual capabilities will be needed for the child to learn to accept new foods. Sometimes it will be necessary to wait until the child has acquired progress in other areas of the development (i.e. oral motor skills) before supporting the child to develop their diet (i.e. cope with advanced textures).

COGNITIVE DEVELOPMENT AND SIGNIFICANT LIFE EVENTS

A child must learn to cross-categorise foods (i.e. assign multiple meanings to a specific food) (Ross and Murphy, 1999). Early taxonomic arrangements (cognitive organisation based on shared common functions or properties) of food occur quite early in a child's development, but they often are flawed. The categorisation of foods is often undertaken by higher order and more cognitive factors (e.g. fruit is defined by the presence of seeds inside it; rather than its sensory properties). Food can also have meaning beyond its sensory and energy value, which equally require learning. Any given food belongs to taxonomic (dairy, meat, vegetables, etc.), script (snack, substantial meal, dessert, etc.) and thematic (meat and two vegetables equals a substantial meal, etc.) categories. Most adults will reach a level where they can cross-categorise foods on a taxonomic- and script-based level (Ross and Murphy, 1999). It has been shown that children are able to cross-categorise foods by the age of four and are almost as good as adults by the age of seven (Nguyen and Murphy, 2003), which appears to coincide with the diminishing of food neophobia. Errors in this cognitive development can lead to rejection of foods. Large or numerous errors associated with food can lead to a problem with dietary variety and, eventually, to a feeding disorder.

Many feeding disordered children progress through 'normal' development concerning their food intake and then suddenly deviate into a feeding disorder. This deviation into disorder can be described through one of two possible situations. The first situation concerns some form of inappropriate and sudden rationalisation that food constitutes a significant threat. Through inaccurate cross-categorisation processes, the child cognitively conceptualises food as belonging to additional cognitive 'groups' and believes that eating food or particular foods is painful or harmful. Often this form of food rejection is accompanied by other generalised anxiety and behavioural problems (Dovey et al., 2010b). The second situation involves the child suffering from a significant life event that was powerful enough to invoke a fear response strong enough to override all appetite-related motivations. These children will present with much stronger reactions to food compared to other forms of feeding disorders that they are often referred to as 'food phobic' (McNally, 1994).

Fear-based food rejection can occur at anytime (McNally, 1994). It is not specific to childhood and is not always of clinical significance. Like any phobia, there will be a specific cause to the food rejection that once effectively identified will respond to psychological intervention. Clinically significant fear-based food rejection will be determined by the magnitude and pervasiveness of the problem. Many children will be confronted with events that could be perceived as negative enough to elicit food rejection (e.g. a choking episode). Those children who go on to develop a feeding disorder will over-interpret this experience in terms of potential for harm and the likelihood of re-occurrence. Children with a propensity to globalise (expecting the outcome of the specific experience to occur in all future eating episodes) the experience beyond both the situation and specificity to the food are more likely to be of clinical significance than those that do not. Indeed, rejection of a specific food item and even food group may not have dietary repercussions for the child and therefore will not require immediate attention.

CONCLUSION

Specific quantitative or qualitative research into the developmental, cognitive and appetite regulation aspects to feeding disorders is absent within the literature. There are no longitudinal studies that have attempted to explain the propensity for a child to develop a feeding disorder and as such we are reliant on clinical practice and experience to determine the main cause(s) for the manifestation. This experience unarguably derives from an expert understanding and extensive experience of what constitutes 'normal' feeding development and the key markers within it. As such, this field is heavily reliant on information gained from normal, clinically insignificant, children's food refusal and dietary development. Any explanation of the development of a feeding disordered child is hindered by this limitation.

The overarching component to all 'forms' of feeding disorder is that of learning or lack thereof. All children progress through food neophobic and sensory defensive tendencies, which directly impact on their future food choices and preferences. Inappropriate confrontation of these tendencies will invariably end in the development of a feeding disorder. An explanation for some of these weak confrontations within feeding disordered children may come from the role that attachment plays within the exploration phases of childhood and the acquisition of knowledge and expectations around food through experience and exposure. Poor attachment with the caregivers will have a wide variety of potential negative consequences including problems with dietary variety. Another explanation could equally derive from long-term medical problems resulting in similar problems in terms of eating behaviour.

Feeding disorders are a pervasive problem for the child and his or her family resulting in some cases in mortality. The fact that the disorder has the potential to kill the child should provide the impetus for practitioners to uncover the causes, consequences and potential management strategies that are employed to intervene in these children's lives. In most situations, the child will present with a low dietary variety resulting in insufficient weight gain or even weight loss in the more severe cases. Most will have an exaggerated fear-like response to the presentation of novel food items and all will attempt to undermine any exposure-based intervention to gain preferred foods. Any management strategy with these children is likely to require some form of tailoring for their individual needs and is unlikely to be a quick process. Armed with this knowledge, the practitioner should be able to recognise the underlying causes of the child's food rejection and reinitiate/re-engage them with their innate appetite drives and increase their dietary variety.

REFERENCES

Addessi E, Galloway AT, Visalberghi E, *et al*. Specific social influences on the acceptance of novel foods in 2–5-year old children. *Appetite*. 2005; **45**: 264–71.

Ahearn WH. Using simultaneous presentation to increase vegetable consumption in a mildly selective child with autism. *J Appl Behav Anal*. 2003; **36**: 361–5.

Aldridge V, Dovey TM, Halford JCG. The role of familiarity in dietary development. *Dev Rev*. 2009; **29**: 32–44.

Arvola A, Lahteenmaki L, Tuorila H. Predicting the intent to purchase unfamiliar and familiar cheeses: the effects of attitudes, expected liking and food neophobia. *Appetite*. 1999; **32**(1): 113–26.

Bailey MT, Coe CL. Maternal separation disrupts the integrity of the intestinal microflora in infant rhesus monkeys. *Dev Psychobiol*. 1999; **35**: 146–55.

Birch LL. Development of food preferences. *Annu Rev Nutr*. 1999; **19**: 41–62.

Birch LL, McPhee L, Shoba BC, *et al*. What kind of exposure reduces children's food neophobia? Looking vs tasting. *Appetite*. 1987; **9**: 171–8.

Brunstrom JM. Associative learning and the control of human dietary behaviour. *Appetite*. 2007; **49**: 268–71.

Chatoor I, Getson P, Menvielle E, *et al*. A feeding scale for research and clinical practice to assess mother-infant interactions in the first three years of life. *Inf Ment Health J*. 1997; **18**, 76–91.

Chatoor I, Hirsch R, Ganiban J, *et al*. Diagnosing infantile anorexia: the observation of mother-infant interactions. *J Am Acad Child Psychiatr*. 1998; **37**: 959–67.

Cicchetti D, Rogosch FA. Diverse patterns of neuroendocrine activity in maltreated children. *Dev Psychopathol*. 2001; **13**: 677–93.

Dovey TM. *Eating Behaviour*. Maidenhead, UK: Open University Press; 2010.

Dovey TM, Isherwood E, Alridge VK, *et al*. Typologies of feeding disorders based on a single assessment strategy: formulation of a clinical decision-making model. *Inf Child Adoles Nutr*. 2010a; **2**(1): 45–51.

Dovey TM, Isherwood E, Alridge VK, *et al*. Typologies of feeding disorders based on a single assessment strategy: case study evidence. *Inf Child Adoles Nutr*. 2010b; **2**(1): 52–61.

Dovey TM, Staples PA, Gibson EL, *et al.* Food neophobia and picky/fussy eating: a review. *Appetite.* 2008; **50**(2–3): 181–93.

El-Chaar GM, Mardy G, Wehlou K, *et al.* Randomized, double-blind comparison of brand and generic antibiotic suspensions: II. A study of taste compliance in children. *Pediatr Inf Dis J.* 1996; **15**: 18–22.

Fisher JO, Mitchell DC, Smiciklas-Wright H, *et al.* Parental influences on young girls' fruit and vegetable, micronutrient, and fat intakes. *J Am Diet Assoc.* 2002; **102**: 58–64.

Galloway AT, Fiorito LM, Lee Y, *et al.* Parental pressure, dietary patterns and weight status among girls who are 'picky/fussy' eaters. *J Am Diet Assoc.* 2005; **105**: 541–8.

Galloway AT, Lee Y, Birch LL. Predictors and consequences of food neophobia and pickiness in children. *J Am Diet Assoc.* 2003; **103**: 692–8.

Gunnar MR, Morrison SJ, Chisholm K, *et al.* Salivary cortisol levels in children adopted from Romanian orphanages. *Dev Psychopathol.* 2001; **13**: 611–28.

Kalat JW, Rozin P. Learned safety as a mechanism in long delay taste aversion learning in rats. *J Comp Physiol Psychol.* 1973; **83**: 198–207.

Kannan S, Carruth BR, Skinner J. Cultural influences on infant feeding beliefs of mothers. *J Am Diet Assoc.* 1999; **99**: 88–90.

Loewen R, Pliner P. Effects of prior exposure to palatable and unpalatable novel foods on children's willingness to taste other novel foods. *Appetite.* 1999; **32**: 351–66.

MacNicol SA, Murray SM, Austin EJ. Relationships between personality, attitudes and dietary behaviour in a group of Scottish adolescents. *Pers Indiv Differ.* 2003; **35**: 1753–64.

Martin C, Southall A, Shea E, *et al.* The importance of a multifaceted approach in the assessment and treatment of childhood feeding disorders: a two-year-old in-patient case study in the U.K. National Health Service. *Clin Case S.* 2008; **7**: 79–99.

Matson JL, Fodstad JC. The treatment of food selectivity and other feeding problems in children with autism spectrum disorders. *Res Autism Spect Dis.* 2009; **3**: 445–61.

McCrae RR, Costa PT Jr, Terracciano A, *et al.* Personality trait development from age 12 to age 18: Longitudinal, cross-sectional, and cross-cultural analyses. *J Pers Social Psychol.* 2002; **83**: 1456–68.

McNally RJ. Choking phobia: a review of the literature. *Comp Psychiatr.* 1994; **35**: 83–9.

Nguyen SP, Murphy GL. An apple is more than just a fruit: cross-classification in children's concepts. *Child Dev.* 2003; **74**(6): 1783–806.

Nicklaus S, Boggio V, Chababnet C, *et al.* Prospective study of food variety seeking in childhood, adolescence and early adult life. *Appetite.* 2005; **44**: 289–97.

Piazza CC, Patel MR, Santana CM, *et al.* An evaluation of simultaneous and sequential presentation of preferred and nonpreferred food to treat food selectivity. *J Appl Behav Anal.* 2002; **35**: 259–70.

Rees C. Children's attachments. *Pediatr Child Health.* 2008; **18**: 219–26.

Ross BH, Murphy GL. Food for thought: cross-classification and category organization in a complex real-world domain. *Cognitive Psychol.* 1999; **38**: 495–53.

Schaal B, Marlier L, Soussignan R. Human foetuses learn odours from their pregnant mother's diet. *Chem Senses.* 2000; **25**: 729–37.

Schwartz C, Issanchou S, Nicklaus S. Developmental changes in the acceptance of the five basic tastes in the first year of life. *Br J Nutr.* 2009; **102**: 1375–85.

Smith AM, Roux S, Naidoo NTR, *et al.* Food choices of tactile defensive children. *Nutrition.* 2005; **21**: 14–19.

Steptoe A, Pollard TS, Wardle J. Development of a measure of motives underlying the selection of food: the food choice questionnaire. *Appetite.* 1995; **25**: 267–84.

Tasca GA, Kowal J, Balfour L, *et al.* An attachment insecurity model of negative affect among women seeking treatment for an eating disorder. *Eating Behav.* 2006; **7**: 252–7.

Tasca GA, Szadkowski L, Illing V, *et al.* Adult attachment, depression, and eating disorder symptoms: the mediating role of affect regulation strategies. *Pers Indiv Differ.* 2009; **47**: 662–6.

Visser J, Kroeze JHA, Kamps WA, *et al.* Testing taste sensitivity and aversion in very young children: development of a procedure. *Appetite.* 2000; **34**: 169–76.

Wardle J, Carnell S, Cooke L. Parental control over feeding and children's fruit and vegetable intake: How are they related? *J Am Diet Assoc.* 2005; **105**: 227–32.

Wilbarger P. *Sensory Defensiveness and Related Social/Emotional and Neurological Disorders.* Port Elizabeth, South Africa: SAISI; 2000.

Williams PC, Riegal KE, Gibbons B. Combining repeated taste exposure and escape prevention: an intervention for the treatment of extreme food selectivity. *Appetite.* 2007; **49**: 708–11.

CHAPTER 6

Cultural aspects of feeding: some illustrations from Indian and other cultures

Kedar Nath Dwivedi and Jeremy Woodcock

INTRODUCTION

Among the Malays who live in the highlands of the island of Langkawi on the northern coast of Malaysia, there is a belief that breast milk is derived from blood, and that therefore any child who is breastfed becomes family. People in Langkawi say, 'If you drink the same milk you become kin. You become one blood, one flesh' (Carsten, 1995). Furthermore, if one eats rice from the same hearth, one becomes kin. Blood, milk, rice and hearth are of one substance. To be fed milk or rice from the mother creates an emotional bond, but even more substantially, it creates kinship, so that children who have suckled at the same breast or eaten rice cooked on the same hearth may not marry, even if they are not related in any way at a biological level. Such beliefs are a world away from Western ideas of food and kinship and they point up how food, eating practices and beliefs are intricately tied up with each other in all our cultures in ways we almost always take for granted within our own cultural setting. But the lesson from the Malays of Langkawi is that when we come across people from other cultures we cannot assume that their beliefs and habits will be the same as our own, even if when viewed from the outside, their day-to-day practices of food preparation and their eating arrangements appear to fit our norms.

Culture influences virtually all aspects of human behaviour and practices and perhaps none more so than food and feeding habits. Although it would be extremely useful to compile a body of knowledge in this respect from many different cultures, such a compilation would be beyond both the scope of this chapter and the expertise of the authors. It is proposed therefore to exemplify the above with an extended illustration from the Indian culture added to which illustrations will be drawn from the culture and feeding practices found in Africa, the Middle East and the Caribbean. The aim is to offer some news of difference out of which lessons can emerge about how professionals can work alongside cultural differences in feeding.

The chapter looks at food and emotion, cultural rites, religious cosmology relating to food, and the impact of culture on social identity and child-rearing. It also covers the ascribed properties of food and concludes by examining elements pertaining to the professional relationship within a multi-cultural setting. In the past, it was assumed that living for long periods of time in different geographical environments led to different groups developing their characteristic inborn temperaments. Categorisation has moved through several stages, based on the philosophical climate and zeitgeist, culminating in beliefs that have shaped our understanding of different peoples.

In recent years, a 'new culture and personality' approach has emerged that aims to go beyond the 'old culture and personality' movement, which was essentially Eurocentric (Stocking, 1986). The new approach attempts to understand cultures from their own indigenous ideological perspectives in order to conceptualise contrasting human nature. Geertz (1973), therefore, sees culture as a 'web of meaning', and Laungani (1992) emphasises the fact that 'it is these assumptions which often are culture-specific. Not the experience itself as has been mistakenly assumed by the cultural relativists'.

Just like individuals, cultures also grow and mature. In a multi-cultural context, we have people and societies belonging to cultures that may be many millennia old living side by side with those belonging to cultures that are only a few centuries old. For example, in the Indian culture, as early as the 6th century BC, a detailed, coherent and systematic theory of consciousness became available, something that did not begin to happen in the Western science until the 19th century AD (Reat, 1990).

FOOD AND EMOTION IN INDIAN CULTURE

In the Indian culture, one finds a huge variety of paths to salvation (Dwivedi and Prasad, 1999). These range from subjugating feelings and emotions through the rigours of asceticism (such as in Jainism and most schools of Buddhism and Hinduism) to encouraging exuberant emotional and sensuous experiences (such as in the Ajivika and Tantric schools in Hinduism and Buddhism) exemplified by the Kamasutra. For example, Ajivikas (8th century BC) challenged the karmic theory and gave the slogan 'eat, drink and be merry'. Pushti Marg (Bennett, 1990) is an example of exciting the passions as a form of worship.

There can also be cultural differences in the very conceptualisation of emotions. The Western conceptualisation of emotion has had its emphasis on the physiological and irrational aspects of emotions. Recently, however, the social constructivists and cognitivists have begun to point out the fact that emotions are essentially culturally constructed appraisals. For example, Lynch (1990a) shows that:

Contrary to Western devaluation of emotion in the face of reason, India finds emotions, like food, necessary for a reasonable life, and, like taste, cultivable for the fullest understanding of life's meaning and purpose…

In the Indian way of thinking, the mind and body are part of, and continuous with, one another and thus identical. Therefore, emotions are grounded not only in self but also in food, scent, music, play and so on. For example, an offering, such as food, is conceived as the embodiment of an emotional attitude (such as devotion to god): 'In offering the food to god, in its return to his devotee, and in its consumption as prasada, emotions are believed to be exchanged between humanity and divinity' (Lynch, 1990b). Food left over from god is called prasada, and its consumption by the devotee is to experience the self transformed through the act of giving. The proper equivalent of saying grace in the Indian culture is not so much of thanking god for the food, but offering food to god and then eating the leftovers.

In most cultures, life-cycle rites, such as initiations and weddings, are often used for the purposes of transformation. Bennett (1990) describes ritual as:

A culturally constructed system of symbolic communication comprising a structured sequence of words and acts directed towards a 'telic' or 'performative' outcome.

He continues:

Ritual has the capacity to shape and intensify experience by means of patterning, sequencing, repetition, and the controlled arrangement of multiple sensory media.

In the Indian culture, these rites (or Sanskaras in Sanskrit) are meant to have a refining quality (as evident from the meaning of this Sanskrit word), and this refining process has essentially three main phases: physical, mental and spiritual. Marglin's (1990) description of this is reproduced below.

The refining process in Indian culture

The process of refining implies that one starts with a concrete or physical or gross level and by successive processes of refinement extracts from these concrete emotions their essence. The basic processes of refining are cooking, and the most basic cooking is that which takes place in the earth when a seed germinates under the heat of the sun and the moisture of water. The grain or fruit that is eventually produced out of this cooking is the refined product. When the body is refined, out of its physicality several refined products emerge: emotions, thought and, finally, the most refined product of all, corresponding to the fragrance of the food offered to the deities, spiritual experience (pp. 231–2).

THE INDIAN THEORY OF 'RASA'

The Indian theory of emotions known as the 'Rasa (essence, flavour, extract, juice) theory' was established several millennia ago, as evident in Bharat's famous Treatise on Natyashastra (dramatology) of 200 BC, outlining the catalytic purpose of aesthetic forms to activate and refine our already present emotions (de Bary *et al.*, 1958; Dwivedi, 1993b; Dwivedi and Gardner, 1997). In such a cultural context, food is perceived not only as containing nutrients but also emotion and morality, and its purity is as important as (sometimes more important than) its nutrient value. Food is supposed to become easily impure while it is being prepared, as it is imbued with the moral and emotional qualities of those who prepare it. Thus, purity of thoughts, feelings, conduct and actions while preparing food is also very important. A food prepared and offered lovingly, selflessly and solely for the enjoyment of the eater is more likely to be pure. Thus, food is supposed not only to affect the moral and emotional disposition of the eater, but it can also be imbued and invested with the moral and emotional qualities of those who prepare and offer it (Bennett, 1990). In this sense, it is therefore difficult to be sure of purity in ready-to-eat food obtained from supermarkets, restaurants, hospitals and so on.

There is no doubt that such cultural ideologies in their full form may not be operative in many Indians today, living in either India or in the West. However, these are often present at least in diluted forms and influence many practices around food, feeding and eating (e.g. bringing food into hospital). A professional's appreciation of this cultural dynamic is essential for a better sharing of concerns and strategies between the professionals and families.

IMPLICATIONS OF THE INDIAN THEORY OF KARMA ON VEGETARIANISM AND FEEDING

In the Indian culture, the attempt to make sense of the existential issues began as early as during the Indus Valley civilisation and continued through the Vedic period culminating (Reat, 1990). In it all sentient beings understood as being caught up in the cycle of birth and rebirth in different planes of existence until they manage to free themselves through salvation, nirvana or enlightenment. One can be reborn in any plane of existence (e.g. god, human, animal, ghost and so on) depending upon one's actions or karma. Thus, a non-vegetarian food may come from an animal (i.e. a sentient being) that might have been one's parent, partner, sibling or offspring in a previous life. In addition, killing or being intentionally responsible for the killing of any sentient being can also have its negative karmic consequences.

It is understandable that, in such an ideological climate, many Indians are vegetarian. However, they find that the strength of their feeling in this respect, in the Western context, is seldom fully appreciated. Many (at least during their early days of being in the West) also feel shocked by the abhorrent sight of animal carcasses hanging in the butchers' shops (Dwivedi, 1996). The sight of non-vegetarian food can arouse a similar feeling in some. The concept of purity mentioned earlier also

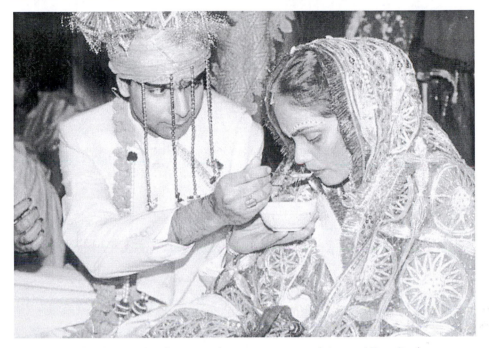

FIGURE 6.1: Feeding each other as an important aspect of the wedding ritual.

influences their feelings towards consuming vegetarian food that may have been in contact with a non-vegetarian food, cooking utensils, equipment, site and so on.

One of the Buddhist and/or Hindu precepts for monks or nuns involves not taking anything unless it is given to them, such as not eating unless it has been served in their bowl. It is also traditional for Indian hosts to serve food on their guest's plate for the same reason. It prevents the guest from performing a negative karma (of taking what is not formally given) and allows the host to gain merits by giving. The same principle is extended to feeding the other with one's own fingers, particularly in a very loving relationship. Parents often do this to their young children as an expression of their love. Similarly, partners feed each other, as an essential part of the wedding ritual (*see* Figure 6.1).

CULTURAL IDEOLOGY, SOCIAL STRUCTURE
AND CHILD-REARING IN INDIA

Child-rearing practices can differ widely across cultures depending upon their socio-cultural and ideological differences. Shweder and Bourne (1982) describe the tendency in the Eastern cultures of not separating or distinguishing the individual from the social context as a 'sociocentric' conception of relationships, in contrast to the 'egocentric' conception in the Western cultures. 'In Western cultures, individuality is the prime value and relatedness is secondary…' (Tamura and Lau, 1992, p. 30). Child-rearing practices are the most important manifestations of such cultural ideologies.

TABLE 6.1: The historical aspect of ideological developments in India

Period	Ideological aspects
Indus Valley civilisation (5000 BC–2500 BC)	Yogic concepts of individual soul; layered consciousness; rebirth and release
Vedic Period (2500 BC–1200 BC	Cosmogonic concept of world soul; rituals; afterlife
Vedantic period (1200 BC–500 BC)	Upanishads linking the world soul with individual soul, layered consciousness, karma and rebirth
Heterodox schools (800 BC–200 AD)	Ajivikism; Jainsim; Buddhism
Revival of Hinduism (200 AD onwards)	Buddhism, having spread abroad, deteriorated in India. Hinduism included revival of Vedic authority, Smrities, Yoga, Sankhya, Mimansa, Nyaya and Vedanta

To make sense of the child-rearing practices in the Indian culture, it is useful to look at its ideological history. In India, between the 8th and 5th century BC, a number of heterodox schools emerged to challenge the well-established authority of the Vedas (Table 6.1). Of these, Buddhism had the greatest impact and it spread not only in India but far and wide abroad. It revealed the illusory nature of self or ego and developed practical (meditative and psychosocial) ways of realising freedom from self (Dwivedi 1992, 1994a,b). Such an ideal became an integral part of the Eastern cultures and even the later revival of Hinduism in India contained this ideal within it. Thus, the development of social structures in India was greatly influenced by such an ideology (Dwivedi 1993a, 1994c).

INDEPENDENCE VERSUS DEPENDABILITY

Independence is one of the most cherished ideals in the Western cultures, and it permeates all aspects of life, including parenting and psychotherapy. Parents are usually at pains to make their children independent as quickly as possible. This is reflected not only in sleeping arrangements for their babies but also in the encouragement of their children to have and express their own opinions, views and voices. The Eastern cultures, on the other hand, have placed more emphasis on 'dependability' as their cherished ideal (Roland, 1980). Parents are often at pains to ensure their child's dependability. This is reflected in indulgence, prolonged babyhood, immediate gratification of physical and emotional needs, continuous physical closeness and common sleeping arrangements. The idea is to create an atmosphere whereby children can model on their parents and cultivate dependability. The process is seen to be successful when they grow up to become model, dependable 'parents' not only for their children but also for their elderly parents. For an elderly person in the

Western culture, the idea of living with their grown-up children is usually associated with the feeling of being a burden on them and can become a source of intense shame and guilt. In the Eastern cultures, it is a source of great joy and pride that one has nurtured one's children in such a way that they have now become truly dependable (Vatuk, 1990; Dwivedi, 1996a,b,c).

PLACE OF EXTENDED FAMILY IN TRANSCENDING NARCISSISM

Another aspect of the social structure that helps in overcoming or transcending self or narcissism is the effort to make the institution of extended family a success. The tendency of love is to flow towards one's own and, therefore, extended families can easily break around nuclear family boundaries unless an extra effort is made so that love begins to flow across such nuclear family boundaries (Kakar, 1981). A mother in such a family would give affection and food to other children before her own, and the children are encouraged to share food and play materials. When they go out they carry each other's children and in conversation 'your' child would mean 'their' child and 'their' child would mean 'yours' (Trawick, 1990).

FOOD AND THE INFLUENCE OF THE AYURVEDIC SYSTEM OF MEDICINE

Food is not just food, it also has medicinal qualities. The medicinal values of a number of traditional Indian foods and herbs are now being studied with very encouraging results (Dwivedi, 1996). Most Indian foods and herbs have already been examined by Ayurveda. Ayurveda (literally translated as the science of life) has been a popular medical system in India since the 8th century BC. It is described as a holistic system. It aims to manage life in such a way as to prevent disease and prolong life. Thus, the Ayurvedic and Unani system of medicine in India has had an enormous impact on food habits. Observance of certain rules regarding food, such as Parhej derived from Ayurvedic medicine, has traditionally been an essential code of practice. These are supposed to be observed in order to maintain good health and to get rid of specific illness (Rai and Dwivedi, 1988). Thus, feeding someone, and in particular a pregnant or lactating mother and her child, needs a great deal of care involving a range of traditional cultural and family specific customs and also the availability of certain foods and their properties.

Let us now go beyond the lessons that can be drawn from Indian culture to consider food and eating practices in Africa, the Middle East and the Caribbean.

FOOD AND FEEDING IN NIGERIA, ETHIOPIA AND IRAQ

Western perceptions of Africa and its food most often focus on famine, food security and nutrition, and while these are of enormous importance, recent commentators have noted that too little attention is paid to the richness and adequacy of African cuisine and the enjoyment and diversity of African food practices (Osseo-Assare, 2009). Beliefs and food practice intermingle, so that food is rarely viewed entirely from the aspect of nutrition, it embodies meaning. This section outlines food in Nigeria and Ethiopia, before moving on to consider food practices in Iraq. Each of these is offered as an example of the diversity of food culture, and children's feeding across the world and with their examples will lead to discussion about how to understand cultural difference in food and feeding practices in the clinical setting.

Nigeria

Trade and food are inextricably bound up with each other, and like many countries in West Africa and across the world, trade played a huge role in changing the ingredients and flavours of Nigerian cuisine. Before trading between Africa and Europe began, the main staple foods in Nigeria were probably rice, millet, and lentils. The Portuguese were the first Europeans to reach Nigeria, and in the 15th century, they established a slave trading centre. British, Dutch, and other European traders later competed for control of the trade, and by the 18th century, the British were the main European traders of slaves on the Nigerian coast. However, it was the Portuguese who traded between West Africa and Latin America who introduced cassava, which they had found probably in Brazil, to western Africa, where it is now one of the most important staples in West Africa. Cassava known in the West as tapioca, and across West Africa as fou-fou, is now the third largest source of carbohydrate in the world. It is rich in starch, calcium, phosphorous and vitamin C, and is eaten across Latin America, the Caribbean, West and Central Africa, India, Vietnam, Cambodia, Laos Indonesia and China. It is the tuberous root of the Manioc shrub, which is prepared in various ways in different countries. In West Africa, it is most often prepared by pounding, followed by fermentation, which breaks down the fibres, and releases the natural occurring cyanide toxins in the root. It is then cooked to a sticky consistency, and is gathered up in the fingers, and depressed by the thumb, so as to form a scoop, with which to gather up stews and soups.

Cassava, however is not eaten everywhere for Nigeria is one of the world's most ethnically and culturally diverse countries, and it is impossible to define national characteristics of Nigerian diet, although food does have some distinctive regional identities. For instance, people of the northern region, most of whom are Muslim, have diets based on beans, brown rice and sorghum, a type of grain. Sorghum, which probably originated in Egypt, is now the fifth largest grain crop in the world and is a very useful staple crop in the arid climate of North Africa because it is extremely drought and heat tolerant.

The Igbo people who live in the eastern part of Nigeria, and the Yoruba people of the southwest and central areas eat dumplings made from gari and flour made from the cassava root. They also eat pumpkins and yams, which are less sweet than Western yams and more similar in taste to potatoes. Yams are eaten as the accompaniment to stews and soups, and Nigerian stews are typically spiced with peppers and chillies, eaten with rice, yams, cassava and corn.

In the coastal areas from Lagos to Port Harcourt and beyond, seafood stews are eaten that are made with the abundance of fish, shrimp, crab and lobster caught off the coast by commercial fisheries and by local fishermen. Seafood is typically fried in peanut oil with yams and other vegetables, cooked in tomato sauce spiced with ginger and pepper and very often served with rice.

Urban centres in Nigeria are well served with street stalls and restaurants, and they teem with hawkers selling snacks. Hawkers are frequently young people who very often regard the work as a stop gap between school and something more established, cannot afford to set up stalls and very often get caught in the precarious returns that only just afford them a living. They congregate wherever there is human traffic and sell foods that can be eaten on the move such as moin-moin, a cake made from steamed black-eye beans or other beans mixed with meat or fish, and other things such as kebabs and fried plantain, which are often served with rice.

Although indigenous animistic beliefs are formally upheld by as little as ten per cent of the population of Nigeria, they also shape customs and beliefs in Muslim and Christian communities. Animism means that people experience the fabric of life as continuous, so that people, animals, trees and plants, rivers and mountains share a single substance and that man's incursions into nature need to be undertaken with reverence, and what is taken needs to be done with respect and with a sense of reciprocity. This means that game, or wild berries, roots and so forth that are hunted or gathered, or shopped for in local markets are never merely food; they have a significance in the natural order of things that transcends there nutritional value. It follows from this that food gathered, prepared, cooked and served serves to create and maintain bonds between families and their neighbours; as such, food always has significant social and cultural meaning and influence. Furthermore, ancestors, particularly the recently departed, maintain an interest in the living and impose an order on Nigerian society. Hence, family ghosts and primordial spirits are honoured, and they reinforce rights to resources and social relations.

The honouring of elders upholds the patriarchy of Nigerian society and privileges men, and men are often given the preferred portions of food at feasts and festivals, and in general run of life. Very often, this means that men will be served first and may eat separately, while the women and children eat later. At festivals, children eat with their elders and participate in the available food, although some may be especially reserved for honoured guests and men, leaving children to feed on less nourishing food. Furthermore, in some regions, because of food taboos, children are not served some foods. For instance, children are forbidden to eat meat or eggs, the belief being that the introduction of such rich foods will encourage them to desire the food and to steal (Onyesom *et al.*, 2008). Earlier studies of food beliefs concluded that such beliefs compromise the nutrition of women, children and the elderly because they tend to forbid them the cheaper animal proteins that are more easily available (Ogbeide, 1974).

Various lines of thinking about food taboos are worth considering; these include the protection of resources, often in favour of men, who at least in Nigerian society suffer the least food taboos; social cohesion and the protection of health (Meyer-Rochow, 2009). However, the combination of poverty, food beliefs and food insufficiency means that Nigeria is among the top ten countries in the world with children suffering from malnutrition, with 38% suffering from moderate-to-severe stunting (UNICEF, 2008). Across Africa, people speak of the 'hungry season', which in Nigeria falls between the time of the rains in March, and the 'season of surplus' that follows the harvest in October. Across Nigeria, food and beliefs intermingle and the high attention paid to the importance of food comes through in various festivals such as the 'New Yam Festival' celebrated by the Igbo people at the end of the harvest in August, and the beginning of the New Year. Prayers of thanks for the yam are offered, and all the mortars and pestles, and calabashes involved in the preparation of yams are washed and a huge feast prepared at which friends and relatives congregate.

Ethiopia

Because of its location in East Africa and its mountainous geography, Ethiopia has remained relatively untouched by powerful outside influences other than the period when it was under Italian military control from 1935 to 46. However, the kingdom lay on trade routes between Europe and the Far East, and exotic spices were introduced to Ethiopian cooking by traders travelling those routes. The influence of these has meant that Ethiopian cooking is very spicy. Spices are used for flavouring the food, and for preserving meat in a country where in the past, and in the countryside today, refrigeration is rare.

One of the fundamental ingredients of Ethiopian cooking is Berbere, which is composed of chilli peppers, ginger, cloves, coriander, allspice and rue, a bitter herb, used throughout North Africa and the Middle East. Berbere is used to preserve and flavour foods such as stews of beef, lamb, chicken and goat and very often, in poorer families and in poorer times, lentils, chickpeas and vegetables. The *wot*, or spicy stew, is mopped up in the hands with anjera. Anjera has the texture of pancakes and is made from dough that has been fermented for several days.

Anjera is usually made from teff or lovegrass, a grain native to the Ethiopian highlands, now grown in India, Australia and the United States, which is high in fibre, iron, calcium and is a good source of protein. It has a slightly sour flavour, which with fermentation gives anjera its distinctive taste.

Food customs

Nearly fifty per cent of Ethiopians are Orthodox Christians. The church claims to date back to the time of the first apostles and follows the Coptic rite. What can be said with certainty is that it has been in unbroken existence since the 4th century. Orthodox Ethiopians follow Biblical food beliefs, similar to those of Muslims and Jews, for instance, they do not eat pork. Similarly, they are strict in their adherence to fasts such as lent, the forty days before Easter, when they do not eat animal products; hence, they consume no meat, cheese, milk or butter, and instead, they eat dishes made from beans, lentils and chick peas, flavoured with berbere. In contrast, Christmas and Easter are celebrated exuberantly with feasts, for those who can afford them, to which family and neighbours may be invited.

It is the custom before eating for Ethiopians to wash their hands under water poured from a pitcher into a basin. Then a prayer or grace is said. Food is served communally and often the meal will not begin until the head of the household or guest of honour has offered bread to each person at the table. The right hand is used to pick up a piece of anjera, wrap some meat and vegetables inside and eat. Children eat with their family, consume the same food and join in with the rituals of meals as soon as they are able. Adults take coffee at the end of important meals in a ceremonious way. Ethiopia is considered the birthplace of coffee; it spread from there into the Arab world, where it was first recorded in the 15th century, and then into Europe. The coffee ceremony consists of the beans being roasted on a small charcoal brazier to release their flavour, and then boiled on the brazier with frankincense. The aroma of coffee and the powerful smell of incense perfume the air.

This rather ideal picture also disguises the fact that a large proportion of Ethiopians survive on the edge of food insufficiency. Outside of the richer urban centres, food poverty is a daily reality, and it is suggested as a more lasting and significant effect on the population than the periodic famines (De Waal *et al.*, 2006). Studies reveal that it is children who are most at risk of malnourishment, and that girls are more likely to experience food insecurity, than do boys, because boys are likely to be buffered against the sharpest effects of food shortage, while by contrast, girls are more likely to experience its sharpest ill effects (Haider *et al.*, 2005; Hadley *et al.*, 2008). Alongside this picture studies of knowledge among rural Ethiopian adolescents reveals that their understanding of infant feeding runs entirely counter to WHO guidelines, insofar as if they were parents they would not feed their baby entirely by breast-milk beyond 5–6 months, and they would introduce their baby to low protein, vegetable-based meals (Hadley *et al.*, 2008). These reveal cultural norms in the feeding of infants that reserves meat proteins, when they are rarely available for adults, especially men.

Iraq

Iraqi cuisine dates back to the earliest Mesopotamian period in the sixth millennium B.C.E. Although there is a distinct Iraqi cuisine similarities of dishes and customs can be found across the region in the Arab world, including the Lebanon, Syria, Egypt and across the Sahel. There are also similarities with Persian cuisine, and the cuisine of Turkey and the Southern Russian Republics. In that sense, the influence of Mesopotamian culture across a vast region persists to this day.

Wheat, barley, rice, and dates are the staple foods of Iraq. It was the trade in dates that led to the British colonial domination of Iraq in the nineteenth century that later with the discovery of oil there, gave way to strategic interests as the 20th century progressed. These staple crops grow in abundance in the country and the regional variation between the deserts of the South and the mountainous North means that the climate is well suited to different animal husbandry and an abundance of food crops across the year. Mutton from sheep and goats is the most common meat, but lamb, beef, chicken and fish are commonly eaten, and as across Arabia, Somalia and Ethiopia, sometimes camel meat is eaten, the meat of young male camels are preferred, and they of course are less valuable, not being able to reproduce young.

To Iraqi's hospitality is of the highest importance and it is a distinctive cultural asset. They admire and value generosity and meals are set out to be times of enjoyment and conviviality. Again, rather in common with the rest of the Arab world, one is expected to partake of every dish, and food does not stop coming to the table until everyone has stopped eating.

Meals often begin with *mezze*, which are small snack or appetiser dishes. Soup, drunk from the bowl, may follow. Lunch and dinner are similar, with meat and vegetables cooked served with rice and accompanied by salad and flat bread. In some parts of Iraq, food is often served onto communal dishes from which everyone serves themselves and it is eaten with the hands. Because of the high value placed on hospitality, the hosts will very often pay special attention to serve guests, to invite them into conversation and enjoyment of the meal. Children participate in meals with the mother, and older siblings, very often serving food to them.

Iraqis will say, 'there is never a meeting without food'. As a consequence visiting someone for business or calling at the home of an Iraqi friend or associate will mean that coffee and sweets snacks will be brought out, things such as baklava and fruits, often oranges and whatever other fruit is in season.

Religious practice and food in Iraq

Across the Muslim world fasting is understood as a pre-requisite of Ramadan, and across the Muslim world from sunrise to sunset the community fasts. But there are exceptions and these include children, the elderly and the sick. Furthermore, mothers who are breastfeeding are not expected to fast, although some may choose to do so, and Islamic scholars advise mothers to be careful in recognizing their own vulnerability and the needs of their child. For instance, there is an awareness of a nursing mother's need for a higher than usual fluid intake and the child's need for adequate hydration, particularly when Ramadan, which is a festival that moves across the calendar from year to year, falls at the hottest time of the year.

During Ramadan, believers try to follow the moral code of Islam very strictly both in practice and spirit. It is looked upon as a time of forgiveness and a time to reach out with charitable acts. At its heart of Ramadan a time for self analysis and reflection and the fast itself and the heightened ethical demands of the period are a test of believer's sincerity to Allah (Woodcock, 2001). This means that families are enjoined to be generous, to provide food and alms to the poor, and to refrain from lying or slander. At the heart of the festival is the fact that it celebrates the descent of the words of Allah enshrined in the Koran from the highest heaven to the lowest, where they were revealed to Muhammed.

For every family that celebrates Ramadan each day involves very close attention to food and its preparation. So typically women rise early in the morning to prepare food for the first meal of the day before daybreak, which in Iraq may consist of dates, nuts and bananas, which are considered very nutritious and sustaining. Similarly, a great deal of attention is focused on the meal after sunset that breaks the fast, which again may be started with the eating of dates. Meals often have a celebratory quality with family and friends eating communally, which is particularly true of the feast of Eid ul-Fitr that marks the very end of the fast.

Children and food in Iraq

An informant about Iraqi children's feeding said, 'often children from poorer classes are better fed. For richer families, one of the ways to show you are modern is to bottle feed'. Children can begin to be weaned at 3 months, but the general custom is for them to continue on the breast until they grow their first teeth, and occasional breastfeeding can continue until a child is at least three years old. Children will be weaned with a mixture of rice, honey and goat's milk, mixed into soft porridge; using mashed fruit is also common. Children sit on the floor with adults at meals and someone will be deputed to look after the baby, perhaps an older sibling, an unmarried sister or the mother herself. Their task will be to see that the baby eats adequately, and in situations of food scarcity, where there is little food to go around, to see that the baby eats well from the communal food available, which will be served all together on the floor. It is believed that children who are fussy eaters tend to come from families who are doing well. In the general run of other families, children will always be encouraged to eat, with demonstrations from the adults and remonstrations such as, 'if you don't eat you will never grow. You will remain small forever'.

Food is incredibly important and whenever possible meals are never eaten alone; it is important to eat in large groups. In more traditional families, men and boys and women and girls will eat separately, but it seems this happens as a matter of family custom rather than of wider cultural tradition. Before the invasion of Iraq, as Iraqi's tend to refer to the two Gulf Wars, there was little if any pre-packaged food, even tinned tomatoes were a rarity. Now that is slowly changing, but pre-packaged food, other than traditionally dried foods such as fruits and fish, remains rare. Therefore, food is always cooked from scratch, and when an animal is available everything is eaten, the bowels, feet and ears, and children eat everything along with the adults. Meat is valued because it is quite a rarity, and in mountainous areas, people eat fox, wild boar and even wolves. Farmed animals would be chosen before slaughter and kept separately and fed well for a few days. It is quite usual for two or three to slaughter the beast so it could be accomplished quickly and humanely and to say as it is killed, 'My brother or sister, forgive me, this is a fight for survival, thank you for giving us your life'.

Food and culture in the diaspora

People from India, West African, Ethiopia, Iraq and the Middle East are commonly found in diasporas across the world, and when gathered in sufficient numbers it is always possible for their collective food customs to be preserved, and also to change and develop in response to the new influences of migration. Thus, the enormous diversity of food culture in the urban West is utterly commonplace. Food embodies intercultural exchange, and no doubt we are aware that the Indian, Japanese, Chinese or Lebanese food eaten in restaurants of the diaspora has altered to suit the food habits and palates of host countries. Furthermore, that trade and travel in those countries and our own has had an enormous influence on food culture. There is no such thing as a pristine food experience: food culture adapts to circumstances. Similarly, children growing up in families who have migrated will find themselves straddling food cultures, possibly eating one food at school, another at home; eating with knives and forks at school, eating with their hands at home; eating sitting in a chair at school, possibly eating sitting on the floor at home. Mostly children will shift between different food habits with apparent ease, and when they do not, it needs to be considered whether difficulty with food embodies a more general resistance and dissatisfaction with the experience of migration.

Woman from Africa in a 'Hearth and Storytelling' group, which they attended with their children, who were struggling to come to terms with enforced exile. They spoke of the way food in the West tasted 'insipid', how it seemed as if it was cooked without salt, and furthermore how in their culture it was an insult to a woman's cooking to add salt after it had been brought to the table (Campbell-Johnston and Woodcock, 1993). After searching to find a place to eat in London when newly arrived, one woman spoke of how in Uganda and Kenya, 'All restaurants are open, while here they are closed.' In this, she compared the actual physical difference of restaurants and eating habits, which back home spilled out onto the street, where as in London one eats behind closed doors. It was also a comparison in her mind of the openness of food culture in Africa, the welcome and hospitality she felt it embodied, compared with the more ambiguous hospitality she experienced in London. The women noticed with affection and amusement how their children balanced the demands of different cultures. For some though, there was a struggle to maintain the value of their cuisine when compared with Western fast food, which was sometimes desired, and seen as superior, by their children. Very often the bridge between one's original homeland and the food culture of the West for school age children is manifest in the commodified products of fast food outlets and pre-packaged foods sold in supermarkets; this contrasts strongly with the food cooked at home, which is made from scratch. This may also be true of school dinners, which often attempt to mimic fast food offerings, rather than Western food cooked from fresh using raw ingredients.

WOMEN'S REFLECTIONS ON FOOD CULTURE AND CHILDREN'S FEEDING

Women from Africa and Asia who had recently migrated to Britain agreed that it was their custom to introduce mashed fruit at 3 months and to begin to wean off the breast at 6–7 months. Breast milk was considered best, and water was considered definitely unwise before a child was 3 months. The Asian women described how it was the custom to stay with their mothers for 3 months after the birth. She would help them with the new baby and pass on childcare lore to them by example. They later described how their husbands could be helpful, taking part in the feeding but never the preparation of food. One of the Asian women described how her mother, the baby's grandmother, would make the food for her mixing fruit, papaya, banana and avocado with fine cereal porridge, and through this she had learned how to prepare food herself, although she felt she already knew but found her mother's help supportive and invaluable. All women agreed that no sugar or salt would be added to baby food. If the child pushed food away, they just stopped feeding. Often mothers would introduce food by smearing a little mashed food on the breast so the child would get a taste. They also rubbed food onto the baby's gums and placed some on the tongue. Later to deter a child from feeding from the breast it was often the custom to put something bitter on the nipple.

They described how it is easy to provide food for their babies in Britain, 'It's easy here, everything is available'. An African woman described how poorer mothers from her community thought it is important to make their babies fat, 'It is good to have a fat baby, but once they are weaned we don't want our babies to be fat. The uneducated women want to make their babies stomachs full and for their babies to be fat, even after they are weaned'. They did not feed their babies or children ready-made snacks, which they considered to be too expensive. Spicy foods were introduced, and from 12 months, babies were expected to eat the family's food mashed up for them.

A Caribbean mother described how she turned to her mother for advice and was told that she, the grandmother, had fed all her children spicy food from the very beginning of weaning. She reckoned that African-Caribbean mothers generally probably found it easier to wean because there is a general acceptance that children eat the same food that adults eat, and as a result, there is less specialisation of foods, and less processed foods, 'There were never tins or powdered milk in our house when I was growing up', she described, as she recalled being raised as the daughter of a first-generation migrant to the United Kingdom. Furthermore, food was never pre-packed, it was always cooked from scratch and leftovers would go into the next meal. When she wondered to her mother if she put less pepper into her babies' food, she recalled how her mother just laughed. She said, 'My daughter and son were never faddy eaters, it wasn't until my son went to school that he became socialised into what other kids didn't like, for instance, he became reluctant to eat bacon and liver, and he started to ask for processed foods. Now, when we return to the Caribbean, his grandmother looks out for processed food for him'. But in the Caribbean food is really enjoyed. 'Caribbean people do not eat food alone on a tray, food is too important to the whole social make-up. People are proud of what they grow and what they eat; they share it through exchange and cooking. People praise each other for what they eat. If anything is left on the plate it is seen as an insult. There is a culture of nurturing, of seeing people grow, of loving them. I don't feel children enjoy food in this country, there's too much anxiety around. Food is sensory, not like pre-packed food in shops. We like food: we love food, because of our mothers. Food is respected, it is not taken for granted. Mum's garden in Jamaica is full of cassava, coconut, fresh fruit, pineapple, and nearly everything eaten is cooked from scratch'.

Social dislocation, racism and food

Most ethnic minority families in the United Kingdom have experienced social dislocation some time during their current or previous generations. This has meant not only being exposed to unfamiliar ways of doing things but also a loss of extended family, other important social networks and institutions, such as schools, neighbourhood, distant relatives, film and other media. All of these things offer support and comfort in times of need and reinforce their cultural values. Many have experienced this dislocation as extremely traumatic, especially those who have been expelled from their countries as a result of political turbulence. Experiences of racism, both in the form of racial disadvantages and physical and verbal aggression, have also been the norm for many along with the feeling that their cultures and value systems are undermined by the major institutions, even poisoning their children's minds. Goldberg and Hodes (1992) highlight how self-poisoning by many Asian adolescent girls symbolises the acting out of the dominant culture of the ethnic majority group that the minority is 'poisonous' or 'harmful'.

Most toddlers in ethnic minority families develop a taste for and relish the food usually prepared in their families, but as they begin to attend school, they take on their peer group's (and sometimes their school staff's) negative attitudes towards ethnic minority foods. Similarly, children from vegetarian families often begin to insist on becoming non-vegetarian. Many parents give in to their children's wishes but find it difficult to make the same emotional investment in these food dishes or to make these foods overflow with their love. In some families, conflicts around food can create difficulties. These sorts of conflicts (which are, of course, both internal and external) often give rise to the types of feeding problems encountered by healthcare professionals.

THE ROLE OF PROFESSIONALS

In the Western culture, as has already been discussed, there is an emphasis on individuality as the prime value rather than relatedness. Often teachers, social workers, counsellors and various health professionals, because of their cultural conditioning, tend to perceive their role as that of facilitating individuality, self-expression and independence. An adolescent or a child not expressing such independent views, likes and dislikes may arouse concern in such a professional and at times, a passionate wish to 'rescue' the youngster with the assumption that their family might be repressive and over-restrictive. Professional attitudes can have an extensive impact on cultural practices and family relationships in transcultural situations (Dwivedi, 1996d). This can be illustrated by the attitudinal balance model proposed by Heider (1946, 1958). According to Heider's model, a triadic relationship can be in a state of balance if:

(a) all the dyads are positive
(b) all the dyads are negative (although a vacuous balance)
(c) one dyad is positive and two dyads are negative.

Thus, a triadic relationship is in a state of imbalance if one dyad is negative and the other two are positive. In such a situation, in order to balance the system either the negative relation should turn into positive or one of the positive relationships has to turn into negative.

For example, the professional and parent may have different attitudes towards certain feeding practices. In such a triadic situation (i.e. professional, parent and feeding practice), if any of the three relationships (such as the relationship between the professional and the cultural practice) is negative, a state of imbalance will be created (*see* Figure 6.2). Things will have to change in order that a balance can be achieved. There are at least three possibilities:

(a) the professional changes their attitude towards the feeding practice (*see* Figure 6.3)
(b) the parent changes their attitude towards the feeding practice (*see* Figure 6.4)
(c) the relationship between the professional and the parent changes (*see* Figure 6.5).

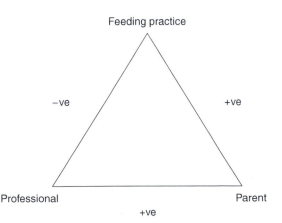

FIGURE 6.2: A state of imbalance.

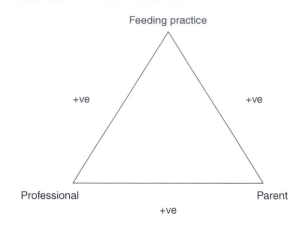
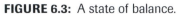

FIGURE 6.3: A state of balance.

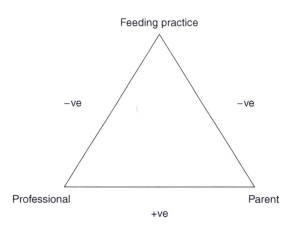
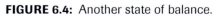

FIGURE 6.4: Another state of balance.

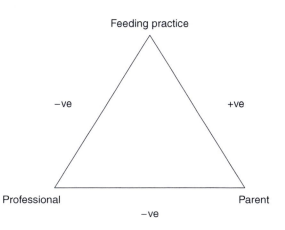

FIGURE 6.5: Yet another state of balance.

Similarly, if the relationship between the parent and the professional is negative, it can negatively affect the relationship between child and parent or the child and professional.

The professionals have an important role to play in enhancing parenting skills including those of ethnic minority parents (Dwivedi, 1997; Stewart-Brown, 1998). Understanding of their cultural context and eliciting of their enthusiasm are, therefore, essential for achieving this (Kemps, 1997).

DIALOGUES ABOUT DIFFERENCE

Engaging with children and families from different cultures at best involves an approach that can be described as enquiring, dialogical and iterative (Ryde, 2009), and which is sensitive to the cultural and power dynamics of the clinical encounter. By this we mean there needs to be an acknowledgement from the professional that it is likely that the power that they embody by virtue of their professional position is likely to lead non-Western people to defer to them, and to agree to observations made by the professional in the clinical setting that do not reflect their true beliefs or practices. This can lead to situations where the client seemingly agrees with a course of action only to discard the advice once they are out of the consultation. How to overcome this? In effect what dialogical enquiry does is to somewhat discard the power and assumed knowledge of the professional in favour of the patient. It means we come to the clinical encounter where there is cultural difference with the ability to hold onto our knowledge but with an ability to use it as the basis for heuristic enquiry that leads to genuine dialogue, and in so doing is open about our own thinking processes, so the patient can be invited into the unfolding process of enquiry. For instance, when seeing a mother and child, referred by a health visitor because the child is a faddy, with an apparently poor appetite, the clinician might be well advised not to use the terms faddy or poor appetite, at least initially, but to begin with the mother's description of the child's behaviour, and to evaluate what she is likely to have said that led the health visitor to refer in those terms. Open questions about how the mother might expect her child to be feeding, and what her beliefs are about feeding her child can be interspersed with remarks like, 'I have some experience of mothers and babies from Kenya, but I am just wondering if you can describe to me how you might be expecting her to be feeding at the moment?' This positions the mother as somewhat of an expert in her own culture and of her own child, who is able to inform the genuine enquiry from the professional of what is going on in that particular instance. It also gives away some of the power of the professional and makes the consultation into a genuine process of discovery. The iterative process also requires repetition, such as 'I wonder, do you mean it's like this, or is it like that?' Making use of small multiples of possible questions to keep the process of enquiry open but well focused. One might also ask, 'If you were in my shoes, what questions would you want to ask a mother like you at this moment and what answers would you want me to give?'

Each clinical encounter has its own complexity. To have one's imagination populated by some knowledge of the cuisine of the patient, and some understanding of the multiple and interacting layers of food, belief and culture and how these might be played out in the relationships of children and their parents or carers where there are feeding problems is enormously helpful.

SUMMARY

Food is not just food. In the Indian culture, emotions are grounded in food (along with other things). Furthermore, in East and West Africa, Iraq, the Middle East and the Caribbean food and cultural life are inseparably connected. In those cultures, food is important because in daily reality or in recent cultural memory food scarcity gives it a high value. Furthermore, in all these cultures, food is something to be shared and celebrated, not merely on special occasions but every day meals are eaten communally. Children are raised within the communal values of cuisine and hospitality in these cultures and the shared experience of food means that fussy or faddy eating is something that is rarely encountered, and when it is, the influences on the child are so varied that fussiness is challenged and ameliorated by the communal experience. Furthermore, the diversity of food means that children have choice over what they might eat. Conversely, food scarcity means food is valued and fussiness has little emotional purchase.

However, many ethnic minority families in the West have also experienced traumatic social dislocation with loss of adequate social, cultural and extended family support, and loss of community inevitably impacts on their feeding patterns. Similarly, racism and professional attitudes towards various aspects of their lives, including food, are also bound to influence their feeding and eating practices. In helping ethnic minority families with their children's feeding problems, it is essential for the professionals not only to be aware of but also to be sensitive to the cultural aspects that provide a complex framework in which feeding may be understood.

REFERENCES

Bennett P. In Nanda Baba's house: the devotional experience in Pushti Marg Temples. In: Lynch OM, editor. *Divine Passions: the social construction of emotion in India*. Berkeley, CA: University of California Press; 1990.

Campbell-Johnston J, Woodcock J. A hearth and story telling group for women in exile. Themes from this paper presented to: *Boundaries and Barriers: European conference of the group analytic society*. 1993 September; Heidelberg.

Carsten J. The substance of kinship and the heat of the hearth: feeding, personhood and relatedness among the Maly of Pulau Langkawi. *Am Ethnol*. 1995; **22**: 223–41.

de Bary WT, Hay S, Weiler R, *et al. Sources of Indian Tradition*. New York, NY: Columbia University Press; 1958.

De Waal A, Tafesse A, Carruth L. Child survival during the 2002–2003 drought in Ethiopia. *Global Pub Hlth*. 2006; **1**(2): 125–32.

Dwivedi KN. Eastern approaches to mental health. In: Ahmed T, Naidu B, Webb-Johnson A, editors. *Concepts of Mental Health in the Asian Community*. London: Confederation of Indian Organisations (UK); 1992; pp. 24–30.

Dwivedi KN. Coping with unhappy children who are from ethnic minorities. In: Varma VP, editor. *Coping With Unhappy Children*. London: Cassell; 1993a; pp. 134–51.

Dwivedi KN. Emotional development. In: Dwivedi KN, editor. *Group Work with Children and Adolescents: a handbook*. London: Jessica Kingsley; 1993b.

Dwivedi KN. The Buddhist perspective in mental health. *Open Mind*. 1994a; **70**: 20–1.

Dwivedi KN. Mental cultivation (meditation) in Buddhism. *Psychiatr Bull*. 1994b; **18**: 503–4.

Dwivedi KN. Social structures that support or undermine families from ethnic minority groups: eastern value systems. *Context*. 1994c; **20**: 11–12.

Dwivedi KN. Culture and personality. In: Dwivedi KN, Varma VP, editors. *Meeting the Needs of Ethnic Minority Children*. London: Jessica Kingsley; 1996a.

Dwivedi KN. Children from ethnic minorities. In: Varma V, editor. *Coping with Children in Stress*. Aldershot: Arena Publishers; 1996b.

Dwivedi KN. Race and the child's perspective. In: Davie R, Upton G, Varma V, editors. *The Voice of the Child: a handbook for professionals*. London: Falmer Press; 1996c.

Dwivedi KN. Introduction. In: Dwivedi KN, Varma VP, editors. *Meeting the Needs of Ethnic Minority Children*. London: Jessica Kingsley; 1996d.

Dwivedi KN, editor. *Enhancing Parenting Skills*. Chichester: Wiley; 1997.

Dwivedi KN. Meeting the needs of ethnic minority children. *Transcult Ment Hlth*. On-line at www.priory.com/journals/chneeds.htm.

Dwivedi KN, Gardner D. Theoretical perspectives and clinical approaches. In: Dwivedi KN, editor. *Therapeutic Use of Stories*. London: Routledge; 1997.

Dwivedi KN, Prasad KMR. The Hindu, Jain and Buddhist communities; beliefs and practices. In: Lau A, editor. *Asian Children and Adolescents in Britain*. London: Whurr; 1999.

Dwivedi R. Community and youth work with Asian women and girls. In: Dwivedi KN, Varma VP, editors. *Meeting the Needs of Ethnic Minority Children*. London: Jessica Kingsley; 1996.

Dwivedi S. Putative use of Indian cardio-vascular friendly plants in preventive cardiology. *Ann Nat Med Acad Med Sci (India)*. 1996; **32**(3–4): 159–75.

Geertz C. *The Interpretation of Cultures*. New York, NY: Basic Books; 1973.

Goldberg D, Hodes M. The poison of racism and the self poisoning of adolescents. *J Family Ther*. 1992; **14**: 51–67.

Hadley C, Lindstrom D, Belachew T, *et al*. Ethiopian adolescents' attitudes and expectations deviate from current infant and young child feeding recommendations. *J Adoles Hlth*. 2008; **43**(3): 253–9.

Hadley C, Lindstrom D, Tessema F, *et al*. Gender bias in the food insecurity experience of Ethiopian adolescents. *Soc Sci Med*. 2008; **66**(2): 427–38.

Haider J, Abate G, Kogi-Makau W, *et al*. Risk factors for child under-nutrition with a human rights edge in rural villages of North Wollo, Ethiopia. *East Af Med J*. 2005; **82**(12): 625–30.

Heider F. Attitudes and cognitive organisation. *J Psychol*. 1946; **21**: 107–12.

Heider F. *The Psychology of Interpersonal Relations*. New York, NY: Wiley; 1958.

Kakar S. *The Inner World: a psychoanalytic study of childhood and society in India.* 2nd ed. Delhi: Oxford University Press; 1981.

Kemps CR. Approaches to working with ethnicity and cultural differences. In: Dwivedi KN, editor. *Enhancing Parenting Skills.* Chichester: Wiley; 1997.

Laungani P. Cultural variations in the understanding and treatment of psychiatric disorders: India and England. *Coun Psychol Quart.* 1992; **5**(3): 231–44.

Lynch OM. The social construction of emotion in India. In: Lynch OM, editor. *Divine Passions: the social construction of emotion in India.* Berkeley, CA: University of California Press; 1990a.

Lynch OM. The Mastram: emotion and person among Mathura's Chaubes. In: Lynch OM, editor. *Divine Passions: the social construction of emotion in India.* Berkeley, CA: University of California Press; 1990b.

Marglin FA. Refining the body: transformative emotion in ritual dance. In: Lynch OM, editor. *Divine Passions: the social construction of emotion in India.* Berkeley, CA: University of California Press; 1990.

Meyer-Rochow V. Food taboos: their origins and purposes. *J Ethnobiol Ethnomed.* 2009; **5**: 18. Doi:10.1186/1746-4269-5-18.

Ogbeide O. Nutritional hazards of food taboos and preferences in Mid-West Nigeria. *Am J Clin Nutr.* 1974; **27**: 213–16.

Onyesom I, Onyesom C, Ofili MI, *et al.* Effect of cultural beliefs and forbidden foods on the ABCD parameters of nutrition among some children in Nigeria. *Middle-East J Sci Res.* 2008; **3**(2): 53–6.

Osseo-Assare F. *Food Culture in Sub-Saharan Africa.* Westport, CT: Greenwood Press; 2009.

Rai PH, Dwivedi KN. The value of 'Parhej' and 'sick role' in Indian culture. *J Inst Hlth Edu.* 1988; **16**(2): 56–61.

Reat NR. *Origins of Indian Psychology.* Fremont, CA: Asian Humanities Press; 1990.

Roland A. Psychoanalytic perspectives on personality development in India. *Int Rev Psychoanal.* 1980; **1**: 73–87.

Ryde J. *Being White in the Helping Professions: developing effective intercultural awareness.* London: Jessica Kingsley; 2009.

Shweder RA, Bourne EJ. Does the concept of the person vary cross-culturally? In: Marsella AJ, White GM, editors. *Cultural Conceptions of Mental Health and Therapy.* Dordrecht: D Reidel Publishing Company; 1982.

Stewart-Brown S. Evidence based child mental health promotion: the role of parenting programmes. In: Dwivedi KN, editor. *Evidence Based Child Mental Health Care.* Northampton: Child and Adolescent Mental Health Service; 1998. pp. 33–42.

Stocking GW, editor. *Malinowski, Rivers, Benedict and Others: essays on culture and personality.* Wisconsin: The University of Wisconsin Press; 1986.

Tamura T, Lau A. Connectedness versus separations: applicability of family therapy to Japanese families. *Fam Proc.* 1992; **31**(4): 319–40.

Trawick M. The ideology of love in a Tamil family. In: Lynch OM, editor. *Divine Passions: the social construction of emotion in India.* Berkeley, CA: University of California Press; 1990.

Vatuk S. To be a burden on others. In: Lynch OM, editor. *Divine Passions: the social construction of emotion in India.* Berkeley, CA: University of California Press; 1990.

Woodcock J. Trauma and spirituality. In: Thom S, editor. *Trauma: a practitioners guide to counselling.* London: Routledge; 2001.

UNICEF. *The State of the World's Children.* New York: United Nations Children's Fund; 2008.

CHAPTER 7

Family and wider system perspectives

Angela Southall

INTRODUCTION: WHY WORK WITH THE FAMILY?

From the day we are born we are engaged with the social environment in which we live. Everything we do is part of an interactive process. As children, we develop through this process of interaction, with new knowledge being continually assimilated. The result is a process of constant transformation within and between individuals and relationships. Human development is primarily social, with infants and caregivers caught up in a complex 'dance', the nature of which is itself organised by a myriad of connecting processes and influences. At the centre of this intricate web is the parent–child relationship, the quality of which shapes every aspect of our functioning and determines how we develop as individuals (Hughes, 2006; Van der Kolk, 2005).

This complex process means that behaviour does not occur in a vacuum: for every action there is a reaction, with constant feedback between the two as we adapt to others' responses to us. We have no choice in the matter: just as we cannot *not* influence (Griffin, 2006) we cannot *not* respond. In other words, this process of being, interacting and relating is dynamic and reciprocal. These considerations make the family context critical to our understanding of children's problems.

The importance of the family as the focus of treatment is not a new idea, nor even a recent idea. We were being advised by Bowlby as early as 1949 that we should be 'concerned not with children but with the total family structure' when looking at children's problems. What Bowlby recognised is that the difficulties experienced by children cannot and should not be taken in isolation. Thankfully, this view has come to be widely shared amongst health, education and social care practitioners to the extent that parenting and family life are now accepted as legitimate areas of focus whenever there are concerns about individual children. Psychosocial emphases have been matched by increasing attention on the family at the social and political levels both in Europe and in North America, where evolving attitudes towards family life over the past 50 years have been reflected in legislation and policy emphases on parental partnership and family support[1]. More recently, increased pressure on international healthcare systems to prioritise interventions that have an evidence base has led to broad endorsement of family interventions (Carr, 2009).

This chapter discusses some of the core characteristics of systemic therapy[2], which have something to offer everyone who works with families. Case examples illustrate how this approach can be effective with parents and children, other professionals and complex groups involving families and multiple professionals. It has the broad aim of being informative and helpful to anyone wishing to take more of a family focus in their own work, as well as challenging to those who don't! Its aim will be to give a 'flavour' of systemic work, providing something of a framework in which to think about feeding and feeding-related issues.

WHAT'S DIFFERENT ABOUT SYSTEMIC WORK?

Despite some similarities and areas of overlap between systemic therapy and other forms of therapy, there are important differences. Basically, no other therapeutic approach has the same sort of emphasis on the family and its extended relationships. Whereas other approaches may focus on individuals, couples or groups, systemic therapy is unique in taking as its 'client' the family system as a whole and uses a range of distinct methodologies to achieve change within that system. This focus on relationships serves as an effective counterpoint to the notion of 'maladjustment' or individual pathology. As Hedges (2005) puts it, 'systemic psychotherapy starts from the premise that humans influence each other'.

Defining Systemic Therapy

Family therapy originated with the idea that an individual's problems begin to make a different kind of sense when examined in the context of the nuclear and extended family. That idea can be extended into an even more complex meaningful system, composed of individuals, families and larger systems, existing in a wider social context that shapes and guides mutual expectations, specific interactions and outcomes (Evan Imber-Black, 1988).

---

[1] In the United Kingdom, these have been made explicit in The Children Act, 1989 and the Every Child Matters programme, launched in 2003.
[2] Systemic therapy, or systemic psychotherapy, is the term that tends to be most used nowadays to describe what used to be referred to as family therapy.

Systemic psychotherapy has as its fundamental concern the person as a whole. Central to this whole-person view is the concept of 'the system', which is defined by the connectedness of those within it and by enduring patterns of relationships, behaviours and beliefs. The term *systemic* therapy refers to this focus on systems and has come to be preferred by many practitioners to that of 'family therapy', as it is less likely to imply work only with families. Systemic therapists are, in fact, well known for their work within and between all sorts of systems, such as schools, hospitals, residential establishments and other professional networks – not just that of the family. This makes systemic therapy especially applicable to working with children with feeding problems, as there are often many different systems involved, including the (extended) family system, the educational system, the social care system and the medical system, to name but a few.

For the systemic therapist, relationship patterns exist within a framework of beliefs, made up of an amalgam of traditions, myths, prejudices and expectations. The family belief system is both an outcome and an initiator of behaviour. For example, a family with a long history of involvement with social services agencies may tend to repeat patterns of crisis in which they will ask their social worker to take one of the children into care. There may be a belief that this is the only solution to the crisis. The more the family believes this, the more they will use it as a solution next time there is a crisis, and so the process continues (Street, 1994).

The discussion thus far implies that feeding one's child not only involves the giving of food but also encompasses a huge interactive area of emotions, beliefs, behaviours, social and cultural processes and pressures. All of these things impact on family relationships and may make feeding difficult. Since the parents have the primary responsibility for feeding their child, the greatest impact is on their relationship with him or her. To focus in a mechanistic way on food or weight only is therefore to deny the importance of the relationship. Unfortunately, this can happen only too readily once the professional system is accessed: too often, there is a focus on food, rather than the feeding, on weight rather than on relationships.

FAMILY CONTEXT AND FEEDING

With the birth of their first baby, the mother and father cease to be a couple and become, with their new child, a family. They have to adjust to their new roles and new definitions about themselves, as they create a new story for themselves about their family. Feeding even a new baby involves other members of the family, whether directly or indirectly. Other family members may take on tasks to enable the new mother to spend time with her baby and in many cultures there is a tradition of grandmothers coming to stay. There is a general acknowledgement that new parents need time to bond with their babies. Fathers often participate in feeding by giving the baby a bottle feed, either with formula or expressed breast milk, allowing the new mother to rest and the new father to enjoy this valuable bonding experience.

As soon as the baby is able to join the family for meals, this involvement becomes even more direct, with meal times serving an important family function. Meal times have long served as regulators of family life; often they are the only times that all family members come together. Traditionally, these are occasions when family roles and tasks become defined and where not only is food made and shared together but so, too, are conversations and experiences. Mealtimes therefore serve important functions in practical, social and meaning-making terms.

In recent years, there have become fewer opportunities for families to sit down and eat together, as the pressures of modern life have encroached on 'family time', leaving, for many, something of a vacuum in family life (Southall, 2007). At the same time, changing attitudes to food and eating can make mealtime issues complex and difficult. Family members may have different routines, mealtime preferences and even different meals. Our thoughts and feelings about food and eating have become more complex as we are subject to the many different and sometimes contradictory influences within modern society. For women, these include the media pressure to be slim, eat healthily and keep busy, whilst also making nutritious meals for happy sit-down family meals, as exemplified by the classic 'TV advertisement families'. The conflicts generated by these pressures actually make us much less likely to sit down and eat together, which is unfortunate, as the importance of family mealtimes has been stressed by a number of studies as being important for family cohesion and adolescent adjustment as well as helping to determine healthy eating (Delaney and Warren, 2009).

WORKING CREATIVELY WITH THE FAMILY

The preference of the systemic therapist is usually to see the family together, at least initially, to get a sense of the relationships. Although every effort is made to do this, it is not the case that all members of the family have to be seen together all of the time. In troubled families, it has been found most helpful initially to see whoever decides to come. Where there are feeding difficulties this often means seeing the parents or carer separately to begin with: this is also helpful in that it enables parents to speak freely about their child, uninhibited by concerns that they are talking 'in front' of them.

In some families, it might be important to see the parents alone. The child may be absent for some reason (e.g. in foster care or in hospital) or perhaps it has been agreed that some work needs to be done without the child being present. Some excellent work may be done with the adults on their parenting and their experiences of being parented, which are wholly connected to the present difficulties. They may agree to undertake tasks that either directly or indirectly involve the feeding of their child. Contrary to popular opinion, systemic therapists do see individuals and a number of authors have written on this subject (Boscolo and Bertrando, 1996; Hedges, 2005).

Many systemic therapists working with feeding problems find themselves meeting initially with the mother. The notion of mothers having the responsibility to feed their families is embedded within many cultures, along with that of personal failure when there is a problem. Not only does the mother often identify it as 'her' problem but others do too, explicitly or not, often by framing it in terms of some kind of a failure in the mother–child relationship.

Feeding problems have an immediate impact on the parents' goal of raising 'competent and intuitive eaters' (Tribole and Resch, 2003). Instead, parents become increasingly anxious about their child's eating, and this leads more and more to mealtimes that are, in effect, battles for power and control. As a result, children fail to develop the self-awareness and autonomy needed to regulate their own eating, develop their own preferences and enjoy the experience of eating.

Mothers, in particular, may find themselves conflicted and confused, with their own attitudes and approaches to food brought sharply into focus. These things can amplify the sense of shame they already experience about failing in what is still regarded by many to be one of their most important jobs – that of feeding their child.

THE FAMILY INTERVIEW

Systemic therapy is predicated on openness towards and an appreciation of the family's perspective. There is an emphasis on therapy as not being about 'doing things to' a family but rather as a process of negotiation between the therapist and family (Dallos and Trelfa, 1993). For many practitioners, this suggests a more respectful way of working with families. Great care is taken to reassure families that an invitation to be seen together is given not because the family is seen as 'the problem'; rather, it is being seen as part of the solution, and a very important part at that. This is always a very important message to get across to families at the first meeting, particularly to parents who may feel – understandably – sensitive about being 'blamed' for the problem.

Family-focused approaches are usually concerned primarily with the here and now, and this is especially true for systemic therapy. At the initial meeting, the focus will be on what is happening now with regard to eating and meal times in the family and on helping the family to tell their story of what is the problem and what has led to the present situation. Questions are framed to raise everyone's awareness of relationships and sequences of events. There is an emphasis on questioning which arises from the recognition that *how* you ask the question is important, not just what you ask.

Although there will undoubtedly be some discussion of past events and some sharing of family stories, for the most part, there will be a 'past-into-present' focus in terms of how past experiences have helped to shape present roles and behaviours. For example, there may be some useful exploration of how childhood experiences of being parented have contributed to beliefs and ideas around parenting as well as parenting practices themselves. The following excerpt is from a conversation with the parents of Lauren, a very selective eater:

> *Mother: In our house, we always had to eat everything on the plate. It was almost a sin to leave food to go to waste. My mother had a saying, 'waste not, want not'. I think that, looking back on it, she saw it as her responsibility to get everyone to eat up all their food. I can see that I've taken on this job for myself! I always swore that I would do things differently but I can see that, actually, I'm doing the same thing.*

This conversation continued as follows, with the therapist wondering aloud what might be some of the reasons for doing the same thing.

> *Mother: I don't know. It's just what a mother does.*
> *Therapist: All mothers do this?*
> *Mother: Well, good mothers (laughs).*

The therapist was then able to reflect that a good mother is one who gets her child to eat.

> *Therapist: (to father) What effect do you think having that belief might have on Sue when it comes to Lauren's eating?*
> *Father: (long pause) I think she probably feels like a complete failure. I think we both do, really, but it's got to affect Sue more than me, because she's the mother…*

Here, careful questioning helped elicit a powerful belief in both parents that a good mother is one who can get her child to eat (and a child has to be 'got' to eat). By definition, therefore, a mother who 'can't' do this has to be bad. The parents felt that this belief was held by the extended family, particularly both grandmothers by whom the mother felt constantly undermined. The more undermined and disempowered she felt, the more effort she put into 'trying to get it right'. This, in turn, affected the way she approached Lauren, leading Lauren to experience meal times as even more aversive. Predictably, she responded by eating less.

BEING SOLUTION FOCUSED

In families such as Lauren's, there is usually a strong sense of hopelessness by the time they come into contact with one of the specialist helping agencies. The tendency to feel hopeless and helpless in the face of an enduring problem has been well documented in the mental health literature. As a result, a number of therapeutic approaches have emphasised the importance of helping people to challenge their thinking as a key to changing behaviour. One of the ways of doing this is to avoid the common trap of focusing too much on what has gone wrong and not enough on what has gone right: this has the effect of exacerbating feelings of helplessness and inadequacy. The alternative is to side-step the problem-focus trap and to have instead the sort of conversation that is more orientated towards solutions. In Lauren's case, this meant that the questioning looked for 'unique outcomes' that contradicted the 'bad mother' story, which was so dominant for them.

Questions that are solution focused rather than problem focused and those that help identify unique outcomes tend to be most effective in helping to challenge dominant stories such as the 'failed mother story' told by Lauren's parents. This mother, for example, had not given herself credit for having managed her younger daughter's feeding very well, so that there was neither conflict nor concern about her eating.

Through a process of considered questioning, both parents agreed that their experiences with Lauren had, indeed, made them 'more expert' at feeding their second daughter. The father agreed that the mother had become even more expert than him.

In addition to 'engaging', validating, information-gathering and exploring, assessment also involves determining which other outside systems are involved and what relationship family members have with them. This is essential in determining who might come to meetings and can form the first stage of an intervention at the professional system level, an illustration of which is given later in this chapter.

APPRECIATING DIFFERENCE

A number of writers and practitioners have highlighted the importance of understanding cultural factors on families and their professional helpers (Fatimilehin and Hassan, 2010; Dwivedi and Woodcock, *see* chapter 6), whilst the wider concept of 'difference' has been much emphasised as a significant factor in the therapeutic relationship. An example is the idea of the 'social GRRAACCES', developed by Burnham (1993). GRRAACCES is an acronym that stands for gender, race, religion, age, abilities, culture, class, ethnicity and sexual orientation. These are all social differences that the therapist should be aware of (including those relating to him or her), and all of them have a reflexive relationship to one another (Campbell and Mason, 2002).

In a similar vein, the issue of awareness (or lack of it) of difference when meeting families is highlighted by Baker (1999), who describes attempting to retain a systemic awareness by viewing client, family and difficulties through three different 'lenses': one's own professional lens, the lens of differing cultures and the lens of the larger social system. The following case vignette is a good example of what happens without that awareness. It emphasises the need to attend to cultural factors, in order both to be able to hear the family's story and to add to our own understanding as helpers.

> ### Sadia
>
> Sadia was an 11-year-old Asian girl who had been first admitted to hospital aged five for food refusal and despite the enduring focus on her eating there had been very little change. She was a highly selective eater with an extremely small appetite, a tiny child who, nevertheless, managed to eat just enough to remain in reasonable health.
>
> Sadia's parents were very involved with their daughter's eating and such was their anxiety to get it right that they had also begun spoon-feeding their 8-year-old son (who was, in fact, very well grown). On spending some time in conversation with them, it emerged that with each successive episode of professional help, Sadia's eating seemed to get worse. This ensured that the parents not only continued to focus on it but they became more and more anxious and had resorted to coercion, force feeding and other aversive methods to try to get their daughter to eat.

As I talked to the parents about what sorts of things had been tried, I became aware of my own overwhelming sense of frustration: they did not seem to want to talk about the present at all, only the future. I was puzzled about this and by a sense that we were speaking different languages. I was to discover that we were, of course. As a white English woman I had not been able to appreciate their fears for Sadia's future, which were firmly focused on marriage and childbearing. Their all-encompassing concern was that Sadia would be too thin to develop fully as a woman and would be unable to have children, and that, ultimately, this would lead to her being rejected as a potential bride. This quite detailed fantasy had its origin in reality: they explained to me that a cousin had been divorced because of her inability to have children. This was the dominant family story that maintained their extremely high levels of anxiety and ensured that they remained over-involved with Sadia's eating, to the extent that she never managed to achieve the autonomy experienced by much younger children in relation to food.

EMPLOYING AN EXTERNALISING LANGUAGE

One of the most important contributions of the systemic school has been to make us conscious of the importance of language in therapy and that how we ask questions and the words we use when we do so can become interventions in themselves. A good example of this is the use of externalization.

Systemic therapists have promoted externalisation as a powerful technique for supporting change. Externalisation personifies or objectifies a problem and places it 'out there', rather than inside one particular individual. Perhaps one of the most famous examples is Michael White's use of 'Sneaky Poo' when helping children with soiling problems (White, 1984). White's externalisation of the soiling enables the whole family to be enlisted in the fight against 'Sneaky Poo', who is terrorising them all. Using this methodology to identifying a difficulty as outside of a person or family creates an immediate cognitive shift in terms of guilt, blame and 'ownership' of the problem. It not only makes it easier to talk about it, it also makes us think differently about it. As Parry and Doan (1994) explain: 'Problem externalisation involves talking about problems as problems rather than people as problems.'

Many systemic practitioners would agree with Parry and Doan that it is possible to employ an 'externalising language' from the very start of therapeutic contact. For example, there is an important difference in asking the question 'Can you tell me when Lauren started to have feeding problems?' and an externalising question, such as 'How long do you think you have all been struggling with this feeding problem?' Externalising conversations often personify the 'problem', as in White's example, above. One example might be talking with a family about the feeding monster who keeps muscling in on family life, no matter what they do to try to keep him out. This way of talking and thinking about difficulties, although on the face of it quite simple and straightforward, contrasts with the traditional way of thinking about people's problems. To summarise from Parry and Doan (1994):

> Although this seems quite a simple notion, it is in direct contrast to the dominant 'mental health story', which pathologises people via placing their problems inside of them.

A SYSTEMIC APPROACH TO SELECTIVE EATING

Adam

Adam was referred to at 3 years for help with very selective eating, where he would eat only a certain brand of chocolate bar, bread and butter and plain crackers and would drink only lemonade. He was in poor health, with frequent 'minor' ailments, coughs, colds and tummy upsets. He was also anaemic and receiving an iron supplement in syrup form, which he was 'force fed'. Although a small, slight child, Adam's weight remained fairly stable and was not a cause for concern.

In common with many families, it was the mother who attended the first appointment, even though the invitation had been explicit in including both parents or carers and whoever lived at home. The father's involvement was elicited by persevering in inviting him through carefully worded letters[3]. When we met, it was

---

[3] 'Therapeutic letters', carefully worded letters which serve as interventions in themselves, are another powerful tool used by systemic therapists.

evident that there was parental conflict not only about Adam's feeding but also in terms of the general approach to bringing him up. The father, who was in the forces, took a more traditional 'hard line', whereas the mother took the opposite approach. One of her core beliefs about parenting was that parents should strive not to 'upset' their children. The parents' relationship was complementary in that the more the father toughened up, the more gentle the mother became. It was not known whether this complementarity preceded the feeding difficulties or resulted from them. Certainly, by the time we met they had become very stuck in a cycle in which Adam's poor feeding led them to take an ever stronger position on this 'see–saw'. The pattern was that the mother would seek 'expert' help from a range of healthcare professionals, while the father's view was that these professionals were there as a source of support for the mother, confirming to him that she could not cope. However, he also saw them as not helping. The result was that he distanced himself from them and took up an even 'tougher' position with regard to his son's feeding.

It is easy to see how the outside systems contributed to this cycle. The mother was, in fact, quite depressed and isolated, the enforced mobility of the father's work limiting opportunities for maintaining her social and support networks. Helping everyone to shift from their 'stuck' positions therefore involved both the coordination and partnership with professionals in other systems with regard to the feeding difficulties and the separation of the issue of support for the mother (via a community nurse counsellor). Involving the father was an essential first step in trying to effect the movement in the parents from complementarity to a more symmetrical relationship.

Adam's eating progressed slowly, with evening meals being focused upon as a time for the family to come together and eat together. Adam was offered a little of what his parents were eating (something that necessitated a great deal of compromise, as both parents were fairly insistent that their meals were 'unsuitable' for Adam). Previously, meal times had simply not happened. Adam had been fed whenever he had expressed any hunger. He was given food wherever he happened to be, in a very functional way. Neither his father nor mother ate with him, although they did eat together 'sometimes' when Adam was in bed. Having a meal time when the family ate together introduced a structure and routine that they all began to enjoy and that enabled both parents to participate in meal-time preparation. It also changed the context of the eating, from being purely functional to being a more relaxed, social time.

It was very hard for the parents when there was not an immediate improvement in Adam's eating and when he chose not to sit with them for very long. They were encouraged to persist, however, and acknowledged that the alternative strategy (which they had given a good try) did not work. Adam's parents were also encouraged to give themselves 'time off' from being parents by getting a babysitter so that they could go out together. This, too, had not been happening. No doubt this was another factor that led to them being able to be more united in their management of Adam generally.

Adam's eating improved, and he became more adventurous in trying new foods. He continues to be clear about his likes and dislikes, however, and remains what many parents would call a 'fussy' eater. Adam's parents admit that they would still like him to eat more but their lives are not dominated by his eating in the way that they once were. They have other things to do and think about. They are now expecting another baby.

CHILDREN ON THE AUTISM SPECTRUM

The kinds of approaches and techniques offered by systemic therapy can be very helpful for families who have a child on the autism spectrum and offer a way to change the family's position in relation to the feeding problem.

Children with an autism spectrum condition often experience hypo- or hypersensitivity that can make the taste, smell and/ or texture of food abhorrent to them. This can lead to very rigid preferences, extreme selectivity and food refusal (see Dovey and Martin, this text). The need for these children to feel safe (i.e. from fear and anxiety) tends to express itself in the need for sameness, routine and ritual. These issues can make them reluctant to extend their repertoire of foods in the way that non-spectrum children typically do and to become fixed on certain aspects of the food and the routines associated with mealtimes. The following list includes examples which will be familiar to any practitioner working with feeding problems: it is by no means exhaustive.

- Children who will eat only round food.
- Children who will eat only green food (readers may have come across children with other colour preferences).
- Children who will eat only one type of food (e.g. soup).
- Children who are phobic of certain foods.
- Children whose mealtimes have become extremely ritualised, for example, they will only eat from certain plates and with certain utensils in a specific place and with specific people.

The above features often occur in combination with each other; for example, the child who would only eat round food also had a strong preference for the colour green. His favourite food was peas.

It can be particularly helpful to 'uncouple' the autism from the child, using techniques such as externalisation: for example, '…so what you're really telling me is, this is not Stefan making mealtimes difficult: this is Autism making the mealtimes difficult for all of you'. When the parents can give themselves permission to accept this position, there is not quite the same pressure to change behaviour and the impact can be immediate.

Autism is a lifelong condition, and there is not quite the same drive to change the child; rather, the challenge is to manage the condition. Many families talk about finding ways around 'the brick wall' rather than trying to crash through it – and this can actually be fun. For example, in the case of the child who would only eat round food – the parents decided to make it all round. They started from where their child was, joining him in his position *vis a vis* his autism. They moved on to make other shapes (cookie-cutters are wonderful for this). He is still pedantic, but what is lovely about this family is that are happy to join him in his pedantry and that their acceptance of his difficulties have enabled him to make social and communication progress through inclusion and involvement. For example, from the very beginning of our involvement, he joined his family at the dinner table with a single round biscuit on his plate and moved on from there: the mealtime experience was always pleasant and always social. Critically, he wanted to be there. And they wanted him. This is also an illustration of how behavioural and systemic approaches work so well together. Whilst the evidence shows that behavioural approaches work well with children with feeding problems, it also suggests that family based behavioural programmes are particularly effective (Carr, 2009).

THE FAMILY-PROFESSIONAL SYSTEM

Some of the most important work done by systemic therapists has been by way of helping us understand that it is not possible to stand outside the family system as an independent observer. Professionals working with families become part of what is known as the family-professional system. They bring with them their own stories about feeding, based on their own life experiences. These will invariably have an impact on the situation with which they are helping, just as the situation itself will help reshape their stories. Furthermore, the processes taking place in the family-professional system echo those in the family, with similar types of coalitions being established. A common observation is that the professional system may often come to 'mirror' the family one. For example, a family might have different helpers who form a coalition with either parent, taking a complementary position to each other and becoming ever more anxious and hostile towards each other. The very emotive nature of feeding problems inevitably adds considerably to the tension and complexity of the situation.

FAMILIES WITH FEEDING DIFFICULTIES AND MULTIPLE HELPERS

Many families with feeding difficulties have a great many helpers. Children with medical problems, who are premature or who have feeding problems from birth can be said to be born into a system of multiple helpers. It is not unusual for there to be several healthcare professionals, such as a paediatrician, community paediatric nurse, health visitor and dietician, as well as a social worker (sometimes more than one), speech and language therapist and clinical psychologist. At other times play therapists, child psychotherapists or child psychiatrists may also be involved. Often, the anxiety of the parents is mirrored in the professional system in such a way as to lead them to invite more and more professionals to join them. Professional culture expectations support this. As Imber-Coppersmith (1985) notes:

> Our present culture supports the entry of multiple helpers, first by promoting specialisa-
> tion which identifies a specific kind of helper for every aspect of a problem…and second
> by deeming that helpers do their job well when they uncover a multiplicity of problems
> to address.

Multiple helpers may be engaged routinely by families over time, sometimes over generations, as 'their way' of responding to crises. The helpers may fulfil a variety of roles for the family. Reder *et al.* (2005) suggest that these helpers will often refer to other sources of help when they feel defeated by the problem. Having done so, however, they do not withdraw as they have become 'entangled' by the problem – hence, the professional system becomes ever-larger. Relationships may then develop between different groups, as well as competition, to see who can offer the 'best' help and who can solve the problem.

The situation often gets worse as more helpers become involved: the greater the number of professional helpers, the more helpless the family feels. Among the professionals, there are not only competing and conflicting beliefs, allegiances and affiliations but conflicting advice to the family. Amongst other things, such systems can lead to a diffusion of responsibility and, perhaps not surprisingly, have been implicated in child protection 'failures' (Reder *et al.*, 2005).

One of the strengths of the systemic approach is in helping to acknowledge and explore some of these conflicts in a way that is professionally non-threatening. This is achieved by focusing on processes rather than problems, an openness to adopt a number of positions and alternative viewpoints, and by using techniques such as externalisation, already described, which separates the problem from the individual helper and places it 'outside', where it becomes something for everyone to work on. This type of contribution of family therapy to working more effectively with larger systems is described by Imber-Coppersmith (1985):

> Applying the systemic model to families and multiple helpers has widened the conceptual
> base for understanding human problems. Just as family therapy initially provided a move
> away from individual blame concepts, so the family-multiple helpers view provides a move
> away from family blame concepts. The attempt here is not to blame professionals but rather
> to grasp the complexities that evolve when families and multiple helpers interact…

Such an approach encourages a mutual curiosity about one another's place in the macro-system, enabling movement from hostile or negative views of other helpers. It also emphasises the therapist as part of the system, rather than outside it. Many find that the work in the professional system is not only an important prerequisite to working with the family but essential in helping what may be a 'stuck' situation. Only then can things begin to move forward.

A PROFESSIONAL SYSTEM INTERVENTION WITH A TUBE-FED CHILD

Matthew

Matthew was referred at 3 years. He was in long-term foster care and had been tube-fed since his reception into local authority care 2 years previously on 'failure to thrive' grounds. He was the subject of a child protection order and was on the child protection register on the grounds of physical abuse and neglect. There had been several previous attempts by other agencies to help with Matthew's feeding with no success. Typically, those who had become involved had stayed involved, resulting in a huge professional system. Different agendas, emphases and working practices made the ground ripe for conflict. The professional groupings were characterised by poor communication and conflict, with open hostility between some professional groups, each blaming the other for the failure to make any progress.

Each successive failure meant that the foster parents became increasingly regarded with suspicion. There had even been suggestions from medical professionals that Matthew's case was an example of Munchausen's syndrome by proxy. This created conflict between the social care and medical systems. The foster parents, for their part, found themselves in a complementary relationship with the outside systems: the more help they were offered, the more helpless and defeated they became. Their increasing anxiety and confusion made them less inclined to cooperate, thus creating further suspicion and frustration in the medical system.

The author became involved following a referral from the hospital paediatrician. Although there was an army of helpers already attached to Matthew and his carers, there was not, at that point, any involvement of a child psychologist: the referral was probably an attempt to redress this 'oversight' and lack of inclusiveness by involving yet another professional, regardless of the kind of contribution they might make. It is also a good illustration of how others may be invited to join the professional system when it has become 'stuck'.

THE PROGRAMME
To change the parents' position *vis-a -vis* the 'expert' systems
The first part of the intervention consisted of a meeting with the foster parents on their own. This was, in itself, difficult to arrange and necessitated careful and

sensitive negotiation with other professionals, some of whom insisted that they needed to come, too. At the initial meeting, great care was taken to listen to the parents and value what they said. It was explained that this meeting was to agree on a strategy to help Matthew. It was then suggested that as there were so many people involved it was necessary to have a 'core' group representing the 'feeding experts': this would be the parents, therapist and dietician.

Although we would all be meeting together to discuss Matthew's progress, no one else would call at the house and no one else would give advice. The parents' response to this was a mixture of surprise, relief and apprehension. Although they clearly felt swamped by all of the help they were receiving and expressed a keenness to see fewer people and have fewer appointments, they had also got used to having a lot of helpers.

The meeting of the family-professional system

This was followed by a meeting of the family and professional system, during which the rationale for having the core group was explained and the flow of information and coordination of different services were negotiated. This meeting proved to be the most fundamental component of the plan to help Matthew and his family. An important function of this meeting was to help the professionals to hold their own feelings of anxiety and impatience for change.

Physically, having a large group of professionals in the room together can be a powerful way of making a statement. The response from the professionals is invariably 'I never realised there were this many of us'. As a facilitator, it is often useful to make the point to the family: 'I can't believe there are this many people involved with Matthew's feeding. How ever do you manage to talk to us all?'

The externalising language, mentioned earlier, which is so helpful to families and individuals is also extremely useful when working with larger systems. A conversation employing this way of thinking and talking about the problem enabled those present to move from defensiveness about what was perceived as their own therapeutic failures. This was a focus from the onset, with helpers asked to introduce themselves in terms of their relationships with Matthew and his family and then to say something about the way they had been helping with the feeding problem. The effectiveness of this technique has already been highlighted. It is important to note that this is also the case for groups, where it can have similarly powerful effects, as summarised below (White, 1988/1989):

> **The power of externalising**
> - it decreases conflict between people over who is responsible for the problem
> - it reduces the sense of failure people have in not having solved the problem
> - it unites people against the problem, rather than against each other
> - it frees people to think about the problem in different ways.

The 'core group' meeting to plan/clarify the feeding regime

By carefully limiting professional involvement, there was automatically less advice giving. At the same time, there was acknowledgement of the foster parents' coping and the skills they had developed during the period they had been caring for Matthew. Through a process of consulting with them as experts on Matthew's feeding, the meetings became a process of empowering them, as well as offering support and encouragement on a practical level. A key moment in therapy came when the foster mother informed us with great pride of a change she had made: previously, she would not have felt confident enough to initiate this change without consulting the health professionals 'in charge'; she now felt expert enough in her own right. The core group continued to follow the agreed plan together, using a combined approach based loosely on behavioural management techniques and 'shaping up' Matthew's feeding while maintaining an overarching systemic focus. This enabled Matthew to gradually resume oral feeding. The process was long, taking about 10 months in all.

As can be seen from the above description, the plan for helping Matthew (as well as Adam and Lauren) involved attending to both meaning and behavioural change. Dallos and Trelfa (1993) remind us that people engage in thinking and behaving simultaneously and caution against giving one primacy over the other. Furthermore, there is, of course, a reciprocal relationship between the two, with beliefs influencing our behaviour and behaviour, in turn, affecting our thoughts, attitudes and beliefs. For this reason, they suggest that therapy must inevitably involve both:

> A helpful re-frame should lead to behavioural change which can lead to further conceptual change. Likewise, a behavioural task, such as the parents changing roles for a week, should also lead to new ways of seeing events, new behaviours, new constructions and so on.

PROFESSIONAL COLLABORATION

It is important to distinguish collaboration from the kind of haphazard involvement of different professionals that results in the (unintentionally) large professional system described earlier. Collaboration is a purposeful activity. It should therefore also be contrasted with the notion that the presence of different professionals together in a 'team' will somehow make them effective co-workers. This does not happen unless attention is paid to key processes.

Effective collaboration needs dedicated work. Core issues, according to Salmon and Faris (2006) are a 'common purpose' and a 'shared view', both of which help group members to manage their differences. The experience of this author suggest that clarity of roles is also important in order to achieve collaboration from the perspective of systems theory, which is, in a nutshell, 'the idea that the whole is more than the sum of the parts' (Salmon and Faris, 2006).

SAFEGUARDING: A CAUTIONARY NOTE

An underlying theme of this chapter is that of empowering rather than blaming parents. However, it is important to acknowledge that feeding problems may be one of the first signs that all is not well in the parent–child relationship and to ignore this is to ignore a significant and potentially serious issue. There are some children whose poor feeding arises out of a disastrous collision of relational, environmental and psychosocial factors and who are at risk of abuse and neglect.

The systemic approach can offer new perspectives on how the various systems interact and, critically, what are the past and present influences on the parent. These considerations deepen our understanding of the nature of risk and help us to intervene in ways that are different in order to break the cycle of neglect and abuse, which is often inter-generational.

STORY REVISION: HOW WOULD YOU LIKE THINGS TO BE?

Systemic practice has been very much influenced by a school of therapy arising out of the constructivist domain, known as narrative therapy. One of the important and challenging emphases of the narrative therapists is on what they term 'story revision'. This idea is also apparent in solution-focused therapy, where the process of therapy begins with the therapist using his or her skills to facilitate a description of the client's 'preferred future' and then proceeding to work towards that.

Both approaches emphasise the importance of 're-storying' as an essential part of the helping process. Parry and Doan (1994) suggest that those of us in the so-called 'helping professions' need to be aware of the limits and pitfalls of our training. They suggest that we are very good at analysing things and taking them apart, but less good at putting them back together:

> We have been increasingly concerned that, to a large extent, our training has inadvertently predisposed us…to be much better at story deconstruction than at story revision. This is especially true of training that attempts to emulate the medical science model.

Parry and Doan make a strong case for the importance of story revision, warning against leaving those 'deconstructed' clients in a state of 'psychological freefall' (i.e. the problem has been well and truly taken apart but scant attention has been paid to life without it). For those of us involved with helping families resolve their feeding problems, this means that the end point should not be the resolution of the feeding problem but the reconstruction of the entire episode that leaves parents and child with a more positive view of themselves and their capabilities.

In practical terms, this entails enabling the family to construct a new story about themselves and about the problem, perhaps as an ongoing process throughout. For example, Lauren's parents were able to move from a position of seeing themselves as parental failures with a 'sick' child to that of having become expert at feeding their children and having a very independent daughter with strong views of what she liked and disliked. Matthew's foster parents moved from a similar story of being inadequate to one of being expert enough to 'sort out' the experts. Interestingly, when they retell their story, they now recall that they were 'chosen' to parent Matthew because of their skill in managing tube-fed children (which was the case, but somewhere along the line this became forgotten).

The emphasis in family therapy methodology on *how* questions are asked remains. There are questions that help re-story the past and have the effect of immediately facilitating a different way of thinking about past events and one's part in them. For example, 'Despite having a really difficult few years, you have managed to find ways of helping Lauren to become much more confident about making choices. What do you think other people would say about you that made it possible for you to get to this point?' It is important to remember that, as Epston (1993) emphasised, 'each time we ask a question, we are generating a possible version of life'.

SUMMARY

This chapter has highlighted the importance of working with the family and has outlined some of the useful ways that systemic therapies can be applied to helping families with feeding problems. It highlights the importance of being able to take account of and be responsive to other professional systems and demonstrates that interventions at this level can often be very powerful and effective. It introduces the important dimension of 'us' as professionals and means that we have to consider our part in the drama. It also raises the issue of helping people to reconstruct their stories, often the very point at which many helpers exit the stage. Overall, the chapter has, hopefully, reflected some of the richness and diversity of systemic working as well as the complexity of issues related to feeding. The whole picture is not only rarely seen but is rarely even sought. This may be an unfortunate by-product of our 'expertness', against which we must remain eternally vigilant (Parry and Doan, 1994):

> There is a strong, historically dominant story in our culture that true understanding involves being able to reduce something to its essential elements. This can be a very useful model for many areas of interest, but in dealing with the problems that humans encounter in the process of living, a wide angle lens is often more useful.

REFERENCES

Baker KA. The importance of cultural sensitivity and therapist self-awareness when working with mandatory clients. *Fam Proc.* 1999; **38**(1): 55–67.
Boscolo L, Bertrando P. *Systemic Therapy with Individuals.* London: Karnac Books; 1996.
Bowlby J. The study and reduction of group tensions in the family. *Hum Relations.* 1949; II(2): 123–9.
Burnham J. Systematic supervision: the evolution of reflexivity in the context of the supervisory relationship. *Hum Syst.* 1993; 4(3,4): 349–81 (special issue).

Campbell D, Mason B. *Perspectives on Supervision.* London: Karnac Books; 2002.

Carr A. The effectiveness of family therapy and systemic interventions for child-focused problems. *J Fam Ther.* 2009 Feb; **31**(1): 3–45.

Dallos R, Trelfa J. To be or not to be: family beliefs, madness and the construction of choice. *J Fam Ther.* 1993; 4(3): 63–82.

Delaney K, Warren L. *Creating Health Family Eating.* 2009. www.peopleintransition. com/?cat=19 last accessed 26.07.09.

Dwivedi KN, Woodcock J. Cultural aspects of feeding: some illustrations from Indian and other cultures: In: Southall A, Martin C, editors. *Feeding Problems in Children: a practical guide.* Oxford: Radcliffe Publishing; 2010.

Epston D. Internalising discourses versus externalising discourses. In: Gilligan S, Price R, editors. *Therapeutic Conversations.* New York, NY: Norton, 1993.

Fatimilehin I, Hassan A. Working with children of African heritage: the implications of extended systems. *Clin Psychol Forum.* 2010 Jan; **205**: 46–50.

Griffin EA. *A First Look at Communication Theory.* 6th ed. New York: McGraw Hill; 2006.

Hedges F. An introduction to systemic therapy with individuals: a social constructionist approach. *Basic Texts in Counselling and Psychotherapy.* Hampshire UK: Palgrave MacMillan; 2005.

Hughes DA. *Building the Bonds of Attachment: awakening love in deeply troubled children.* 2nd ed. New York, NY: Jason Aronson; 2006.

Imber-Black E. *Families and Larger Systems: a family therapist's guide through the labyrinth.* New York, NY: Guilford Press; 1988.

Imber-Coppersmith E. Families and multiple helpers: a systemic perspective. In: Campbell D, Draper R, editors. *Applications of Systemic Therapy.* London: Grune and Stratton; 1985.

Parry A, Doan RE. *Story Revisions: narrative therapy in the post-modern world.* New York: Guilford Press; 1994.

Reder P, Duncan S, Gray M. *Beyond Blame: child abuse tragedies revisited.* New York: Routledge; 2005.

Salmon G, Faris J. Multi-agency collaboration, multiple levels of meaning: social constructionism and the CMM model as tools to further out understanding. *J Fam Ther.* 2006 Aug; **28**(3): 212–92.

Southall A. *The Other Side of ADHD: attention defecit hyperactivity disorder exposed and explained.* Oxford: Radcliffe Publishing; 2007.

Street E. A family systems approach to child-parent separation: 'developmental closure'. *J Fam Ther.* 1994; **16**: 347–65.

Tribole E, Resch E. *Intuitive Eating: a revolutionary program that works.* New York, NY: St Martin's Griffin; 2003.

Van Der Kolk BA. Developmental trauma disorder. *Psychiatr Annal.* 2005 May; **35**(5): 401–9.

White M. Pseudo-encopresis: from avalanche to victory, from vicious to virtuous cycles. *Fam Sys Med.* 1984; **2**(2): 150–60.

White M. The externalisation of the problem and the re-authoring of lives and relationships. *Dulwich Centre Newslett.* 1988/1989; **Summer**: 3–200.

PART II

Applications

CHAPTER 8

Biological nurturing: a new approach to breastfeeding initiation

Suzanne Colson

INTRODUCTION

Breastfeeding is recognised as the biological norm, the most natural way to feed a baby, conferring both short- and long-term health benefits (Lawrence, 1997). In several English-speaking countries, breastfeeding is referred to as *nursing*, integrating ideas of feeding and mothering. Many new mothers say that nursing the baby lays the foundations for attachment and trust, helping them to establish the give and take of their relationship (La Leche League, 2004). Practically speaking, mother's milk is economical, saving both money and time spent on shopping. Mother's milk is species-specific, personalised for the baby, ecological, plentiful, always ready to serve and always at just the right temperature. These are only some of the reasons why mothers, the world over, are encouraged to breastfeed exclusively for 6 months (WHO, 2001).

Today, across the industrialised world, there is great disparity in breastfeeding rates with almost 100% initiation in the Scandinavian countries and less than 65% in France and Ireland. Nevertheless, widespread global programmes, like the baby-friendly initiative (BFI), have been promoting breastfeeding for more than two decades. These concentrated efforts are starting to achieve good effect! For example, in the United Kingdom, static and low rates of breastfeeding initiation increased significantly from 69% in 2000 to 77% in 2005 (Bolling *et al.*, 2007). However, we must not be complacent. Compared with current initiation rates in other English-speaking countries, like Australia (90%), New Zealand (88%) and Canada (84%), UK rates are some of the lowest in the world, only slightly higher than those in the United States (75%) (OECD, 2009). Furthermore, British mothers remain some of the most reluctant to sustain any breastfeeding, let alone exclusive breastfeeding for 6 months with 17% of mothers stopping during the first postnatal week (6% during the first two days). By 6 weeks, every third British mothers (37%) have given up. Consecutive national feeding surveys demonstrate that few (1%) British mothers plan to stop.

These statistics suggest that it makes sense to focus upon the first postnatal week, where, for over 20 years, there has been a small but steady increase in early unintended breastfeeding cessation. Surprisingly, this occurs at a time when, in the United Kingdom, breastfeeding support from health professionals is at its greatest. For over 20 years, continuance rates, the world over, have never met public health targets suggesting an urgent need to re-examine early support practices.

What causes this early unintended breastfeeding cessation? Although society at large promotes breastfeeding as the easiest and most natural way to feed a baby, in practice many mothers disagree saying that breastfeeding does not feel natural at all. Statistics in successive UK feeding surveys show that the most frequent problems causing premature breast weaning during the first week include: breast rejection (35%), milk insufficiency (25%), sore nipples or breasts (24%) and maternal exhaustion (10%) (Bolling *et al.*, 2007). If breastfeeding is natural and the biological norm, why then would so many mothers encounter these problems? When mothers are asked if they want to breastfeed most say they do … *if they can.* What causes this scepticism?

This chapter is divided into two sections. First, we will address these questions by reviewing the traditional cultural and social-economic influences within a nurturing perspective that are associated with early breast weaning in the recent mainstream literature. Then, the history of some time-honoured beliefs concerning the ontogeny of breastfeeding will be summarised, shedding light on how lactation management became best practice; attention will be drawn to concurrent trends found in infant feeding surveys for the immediate problems prompting mothers to switch to bottle feeding during the first week. Finally, it will be suggested that in view of static and low rates of breastfeeding duration, there is a need to explore other more spontaneous approaches and support strategies.

In the second part of the chapter, biological nurturing (BN) will be defined as a newly developed approach to breastfeeding initiation optimising positional interactions to release innate breastfeeding behaviours. BN is not really 'new' but the laid-back maternal postures central to the concept are rarely portrayed in the mainstream literature except to illustrate 'incorrect' maternal posture or 'important things to avoid' (Inch *et al.*, 2003, p. 17; Renfrew *et al.*, 2004, p. 60). The development of BN, through 15 years of clinical experience and research, will be related and the BN feeding positions compared with traditional ones standardised in the1980s within the management approach. The reflex theory that underpins BN will be introduced and the mechanisms summarised introducing some implications for practice.

SECTION I: CULTURAL AND SOCIAL PRESSURES: BREASTFEEDING IN A BOTTLE-FEEDING CULTURE

A range of subtle factors in a wide social context have been identified as exerting an often unconscious pressure on women to switch from breast to bottle feeding (Bolling *et al.*, 2007; McConnville, 1994; Palmer, 2009). These include changing family structures, attitudes and values that reflect the fast-food needs of an industralised, bottle-feeding culture. Other factors range from the over-sexualisation of women's breasts, educational level and socio-demographic and maternal factors to age, social class and peer influences. The ubiquitous promotion of artificial milk feeds as baby milk has also had a subliminal impact upon baby feeding expectations, conveying images of convenience and health outcomes equivalent to breast-feeding. Taken together, these have had an insidious effect contributing to reduced breastfeeding duration (Howard *et al.*, 2000). Bottle-fed babies are fatter and the values of a consumer society equating 'biggest with best', associated with the purchasing power that often characterises industrialised societies, also biases maternal choice towards bottle feeding. It can be argued that the word 'choice' in itself introduces consumer parity between breast and bottle requiring decisive action. As early as 1995, Hytten, a British obstetrician used factory metaphors to highlight the power of choice:

> The defining characteristic of mammals is their ability to manufacture and deliver a complete food to their newborn young in the form of milk (…) Breastfeeding obviously requires lactation, but lactation does not in itself lead to breastfeeding, and although all women are able to manufacture at least some milk in the immediate puerperium, the human species is unique in exercising the option of whether or not to use it for infant feeding.

These largely subconscious factors have been compounded by a broad cultural loss in confidence in mothers' natural ability to breastfeed. A nature or biological perspective suggests that a mother's body is innately designed for both normal birth and breastfeeding. It makes sense that both mothers and babies be genetically pre-programmed to ensure the survival of the species, yet in the recent literature it is only the baby who is acknowledged to have hardwired breastfeeding behaviours. Mothers, it is believed, require environmental education: they need to observe 'normal' breastfeeding as children or be taught the skills of breastfeeding as adults (Gunther, 1955; Klaus and Klaus, 1985; Matthiesen *et al.*, 2001; Renfrew *et al.*, 2004; Widstrom et al., 1990; Woolridge, 1986a).

This environmental or nurture rationale abounds, dominating explanations of maternal breastfeeding failure. As early as 1954, Gunther, a British obstetrician and breastfeeding expert, stated categorically in the Lancet, an internationally recognised scientific medical journal, that 'modern' mothers lack innate breastfeeding behaviours, although human babies, like other mammals, are born with three innate reflexes, rooting, sucking and swallowing enabling them to find the breast, latch on and feed. Gunther did not base her observations on research. Rather clinical experience informed her belief together with what was known at the time about innate behaviours from the work of Tinbergen (1951) and Lorenz (1952) who studied fish, insects and birds for the most part, not mammals. Gunther (1955) sought to clarify the causes of what she considered 'maternal deficiency', theorising that in primates including man, mimicry takes the place of instinct. She supported her argument by citing, what was at the time, recent findings from chimpanzees born and reared in captivity where the mother could not breastfeed. It seems the chimp babies would have died of starvation if the kindly zoo keepers had not fed them! The chimps were deprived of the early visual breastfeeding experience, and this resulted in mothering failure. In bottle-feeding environments, the mimicry thesis had instant success, and it was widely accepted across the world, firmly anchoring the ontogeny of breast-feeding or how mothers acquire breastfeeding behaviours within the nurture camp of that age-old debate between nature and nurture.

Initially, reactions to Gunther's (1955) work from experts like Pryor (1963), an American marine biologist, continued to promote a combination of both nature and nurture to be at the root of breastfeeding ontogeny, suggesting that a cocktail of the right hormones underpins breastfeeding initiation and make mothers feel motherly.

However, during the 1960s, increasing experimental evidence suggested that the word 'instinct' was inappropriate in the human adult context. Although some psychologists suggested that human adults had 'biological predispositions', they argued that it was inappropriate to call these behaviours instincts (Morris, 1977). Therefore, the maternal instinctual component of the ontogeny of breastfeeding was never fully investigated. Today, building upon Gunther's (1955) early clinical speculations but without any supporting research evidence, it has become an established 'fact' that mothers lack breastfeeding instincts (Wells, 2006).

This was the professional context within which Woolridge (1995), following his landmark research examining the anatomy of infant suckling, suggested that for mothers breastfeeding is learned, rather than innate. Assuming that mothers should sit upright to breastfeed, Woolridge illustrated and explained the mechanisms of milk extraction using a fixed system of correct neonatal positioning and breast attachment. Although Woolridge only studied what was happening in the baby's mouth during latch and milk transfer, leading authorities illustrated the application of his work with pictures of mothers sitting upright to breastfeed. Lactation management was developed to apply the Woolridge findings to achieve successful breastfeeding (RCM, 1986).

Management, a business term, is essentially a problem-solving approach involving plans, organisation, leadership and control and the concept was introduced into the UK modern maternity services in the 1960s. O'Driscoll, an Irish consultant obstetrician, coined the term 'active management of labour', an explicit plan to promote and achieve effective uterine contractions, resulting in a quick 'normal' birth. Subsequently, advocates of this medical approach standardised routine interventions within a fixed positional system using strict medical criteria for the diagnosis of labour, followed by early artificial rupture of the foetal membranes and regular vaginal examinations to ensure mandatory cervical dilatation of one centimetre per hour, failing which labour was immediately augmented with intravenous oxytocin (syntocinon). Later, continuous foetal heart monitoring was introduced to assess the effect of the contractions upon the foetus. Using this approach mothers were usually confined to a 'bed labour' but guaranteed the attendance of a support person and a speedy (10 h) delivery. Although O'Driscoll claimed good outcomes, since the introduction of many of the components of the active management of labour into hospital policy, we have seen soaring rates of caesarean section and birth-related morbidity. Today, it is recognised that any first intervention leads to a cascade of interventions resulting in poor birth outcomes and increased morbidity (Tew, 1995).

A PROBLEM-BASED PERSPECTIVE

Lactation management was developed in the 1980s by breastfeeding experts like Woolridge (1988) practicing in feeding clinics where 'women with seemingly intractable breastfeeding problems' were taught step-by-step skills. Like the active management of labour, lactation management quickly became the breastfeeding watchword, the cornerstone of good practice. Using a fixed system of verbal instruction, midwives first enabled mothers to position themselves (back upright at right angles to lap, feet flat on the floor) or lying on their sides. Then mothers were taught how to place the baby on a pillow on their laps and to attach the baby to the breast correctly, bring the baby to the breast, nipple to nose and leading in with the chin following mouth gape. In that way a close 'asymmetrical' latch was achieved where more of the lower part of the maternal areola is in the baby's mouth. Mothers were taught demand feeding where the baby takes the lead. Mothers were therefore told to put the baby to breast following specific cueing or fussing behaviours indicating hunger. It was believed down through the years that because this breastfeeding management consisted of repeatable teaching interventions, it would reduce conflicting advice and increase breastfeeding duration (Renfrew *et al.*, 2005). However, five recent trials suggest little benefit associated with these lactation management routines (De Oliveira *et al.*, 2006; Forster *et al.*, 2004; Henderson *et al.*, 2001; Labarere *et al.*, 2003). Although breastfeeding experts, writing in the mainstream literature today, no longer explicitly say that laid-back maternal positions are incorrect, photos or line drawings still illustrate mothers either upright or side-lying (Inch, 2009; BFI UK, 2009b). The BFI UK appears to welcome input from a BN perspective; nevertheless, the teaching and assessment of positioning and attachment within the management approach remains at the forefront of their support policies (BFI, 2009a). Teaching positioning and attachment skills continues to be promoted as the single most effective intervention to target and reduce those problems causing early unintended breast weaning.

Interestingly, scrutiny of concurrent longitudinal data from consecutive feeding surveys reveals surprising trends. Although from 1985 to present day, fewer mothers wean their babies because of sore nipples and perceptions of milk insufficiency, this difference does not appear to be significant. However, a sharp increase in mothers having difficulty getting their babies to the breast, from just under a quarter (24%) in 1985 to 35% in 2005, can be seen. Termed 'latch refusal' or 'breast fighting', this problem often makes mothers think that the baby does not like breastfeeding or does not like her milk. This sharp 11% increase commenced at the time when lactation management was introduced as the way to achieve successful breastfeeding.

Breastfeeding duration is the index often used to measure success. Continuance statistics have not increased since the introduction of lactation management; however, it can therefore be suggested that the routine teaching and assessment of the positioning and attachment skills central to the management approach might not comprise all the indicators appropriate for evaluating or predicting breastfeeding success. Taken together, these facts suggest there is a need for new ways of looking at breastfeeding initiation.

SECTION II: BIOLOGICAL NURTURING, A NEWLY DEVELOPED BREAST-FEEDING APPROACH

WHAT IS BIOLOGICAL NURTURING?

Biological nurturing (BN) is a mother-centred approach consisting of mother and baby positions in which maternal comfort is the priority. BN aims to increase maternal enjoyment addressing specifically the early unintended breastfeeding cessation occurring during the first postnatal week. However, BN can also be used as a rescue strategy for the older baby (up to 8–12 postnatal weeks).

Nurturing is a verb meaning to nourish, develop, to bring up (or raise) and to educate (Brown, 1993). It is often associated with the nature/nurture origins of behaviour debate. Those supporting the nature perspective argue that a person's potential is pre-determined at birth by genetic predisposition, whereas the advocates of nurture consider environmental and cultural variables like ethnicity, age, geographic situation, education, income, social class and other socio-economic factors as central to the origin of behaviour and determination of human achievement (Slater *et al.*, 2003). Today, in many disciplines, researchers agree that both nature and nurture act and interact to influence behaviours and developmental outcomes (Elman *et al.*, 1998; Slater *et al.*, 2003).

The definition of BN draws upon both of these meanings, but the BN concept attempts to counteract the dominance of the nurture perspective underpinning breast-feeding practices during the past 50 years. BN brings 'nature to the fore' (Colson, 2008). The concept has evolved through 15 years of constant appraisal and feedback from the practice area as well as from research. Today, BN is used as a collective term for a range of mother–baby breastfeeding positions whose interactions appear to release both maternal and infant innate behaviours, aiding breastfeeding initiation.

What is different in BN is that mothers neither sit bolt upright nor do they lie on their sides or backs. Instead, they simply lean back in semi-reclined postures usually placing the baby on top of their bodies so that the entire frontal aspect of the baby's body is facing, touching and closely applied to a maternal body contour or to a part of the environment (Colson, 2000).

NEW WAYS OF THINKING

Although BN is easy to describe and quick to do, the concept is multifaceted, intro-ducing new ways of thinking about breastfeeding. Its conceptual framework draws upon both the nature and nurture determinants referred to above taken together with biological theories of early behaviours and research evidence, where available. The BN concept also interprets and applies the anatomy and physiology of lactation in new ways. These numerous perspectives offer a strong, scientific theoretical frame-work underpinning BN, which has been published elsewhere (Colson, 2007).

Inspiration from a landmark research video

In the 1990s, as a baby feeding adviser responsible for two busy postnatal wards, a 6-minutes videotape (Righard and Frantz, 1992) stimulated me to think about new ways to support breastfeeding. The video displayed clips from an observational study and showed mothers and babies in the postnatal hour following birth. The aim of the research was to examine the effects of two routine labour ward inter-ventions (pharmaceutical pain relief during labour and early mother/baby separa-tion at birth) upon breastfeeding and sucking technique. Seventy-two mothers self-selected to one of the two groups: a contact group, where they had at least an hour of uninterrupted skin-to-skin contact with their babies following birth or until the first breastfeed, or a *separation group*, where the infant had skin-to-skin contact with the mother for about 20 minutes after the birth but was then removed for measuring, bathing and dressing before being returned to the mother.

The infants in the contact group displayed crawling movements, the rooting reflex and mouthing movements after about 20 minutes. At 50 minutes, most had self-attached and were sucking. Ten infants in the contact group, whose mothers received intramuscular injections of pethidine, a narcotic analgesic for

pain relief during labour, did not self-attach spontaneously during the first postnatal hour. Most infants in the separation group, when returned to their mothers,
had no sense of direction and displayed a poor sucking technique. The authors
concluded that babies should be left undisturbed in skin-to-skin contact with
their mothers during the first hour following birth and that narcotic analgesia
should be restricted (Righard and Alade, 1990).

These recommendations were challenged at the time as the relatively small groups
were drawn from a convenience sample and not randomised; variables such as type
of pain relief were poorly controlled, because they were not held constant across the
groups. Furthermore, breastfeeding definitions were not made explicit, and observ-
ers of sucking technique were not blinded to the group allocation (WHO, 1998).
However, the video clips were incredibly appealing and stimulated discussion during weekly antenatal education sessions for parents. Frequent viewings prompted
practice-related thinking and further reflection led to concepts central to the development of BN as an early postnatal intervention. For example:

1 The maternal body appeared to provide some continuity from foetus to neonate
   suggesting that it would, perhaps, be an ideal nurturing environment not only for
   the first hour following birth but also during the establishment of breastfeeding.
2 In the videotape, a clip showed the behaviour of a baby who had been separated
   from his mother; although he did not appear to have a sense of direction and
   did not latch, he did make some gross head movements from side to side.

BEYOND THE FIRST POSTNATAL HOUR

Mothers and babies are often separated immediately following birth for a variety
of baby-centred reasons including foetal distress, birth asphyxia, caesarean section,
ventouse or forceps deliveries, prematurity and any intercurrent situation demanding facial oxygen or full resuscitation. Some mothers also require care necessitating
separation or where baby-holding is difficult; other mothers request a meal, a bath
or shower, or they feel 'spent' and too exhausted to hold the baby.

Viewing and reviewing this video led to two theoretical questions:

1 Could prolonged baby-holding in close body contact during the first postnatal
   days help to compensate for such delays in breastfeeding initiation?
2 Would it be possible for reluctant, slow feeders or those babies recovering from
   birth in mothers' arms to self-attach as the babies did in the video and feed well
   at a later stage?

The early patterns of crawling and mouthing movements looked like involuntary
reflex activity and appeared to be triggered by neonatal positions on the maternal
body even when the baby seemed to be in sleep states. Another question surfaced:
could all babies latch on in sleep states, as the one on the video appeared to do?

The Righard video resulted in subtle changes in the clinical practice of the author: mothers were encouraged to hold their babies more often and for longer periods of time, especially when the baby was asleep.

ARTICULATING BIOLOGICAL NURTURING

Metabolic research projects

In 1998, while working as a research midwife, I had the opportunity to articulate the BN intervention in London. Under the guidance of Jane Hawdon, a pioneering consultant neonatologist, I recruited and drew blood samples in studies examining the effect of breastfeeding upon metabolic adaptation. Specifically, for an MSc in midwifery studies, I examined the clinical management and the effects of using a mother/baby suckling diary for a subset of the 12 pre-term babies studied who avoided transfer to special care.[1] At the time, I was unaware of the central role played by the mother's posture. Nevertheless, during episodes of BN, I observed and described ten primitive, neonatal reflex-like movements, appearing to stimulate feeding behaviours in the babies. The presence or absence of the reflexes helped determine clinical management as well as breastfeeding support. Even if a reflex was only weakly present, it appeared it could release a cascade of innate baby behaviours. Seven of the 12 at-risk babies studied required no supplementation with artificial milk from birth. The mean age at hospital discharge was six days, and all 12 infants were exclusively breastfed at that time. At four postnatal months, 11 of the 12 infants were still breastfed, 10 of these exclusively (Colson, 2000). These results were unusual at the time for healthy but moderately pre-term babies.

Although study numbers were too small to enable comparisons, the outcomes looked encouraging when viewed alongside the UK national breastfeeding rates and suggested that further research on BN was warranted (Colson *et al.*, 2003).

WHAT ABOUT SKIN-TO-SKIN CONTACT?

During BN, maternal activity is similar to *Kangaroo Mother Care* (Anderson *et al.*, 2003), a method originally designed for pre-term infants where mothers incubate their nappy clad babies in skin-to-skin contact, lying prone on their chests offering unrestricted access to the breast.

---

[1] The MSc dissertation was awarded a distinction in June, 2000 and a bound copy is available for consultation in London, South Bank University Library. In addition, methodology and results are published in a research paper (Colson *et al.*, 2003).

Research observations (Colson, 2002; Colson *et al.*, 2003, 2008) suggest that, for any healthy baby, whether in skin-to-skin contact or lightly dressed, close juxtaposition with maternal body contours, in full ventral and front body contact, be it upright between mother's breasts or not, stimulate a range of what appear to be innate, involuntary behavioural activities such as:

- mouthing, licking, smelling, nuzzling and nesting at the breast
- crawling movements
- rooting movements
- latching onto the breast
- sucking and swallowing
- sleeping and active searching and sucking behaviours.

In close body contact during episodes of BN, mothers often appeared to elicit these behaviours spontaneously. Maternal cues appeared to trigger infant responses which in turn stimulated further cueing/responding behaviours (Colson, 2000).

PRIMITIVE NEONATAL REFLEXES

The three primitive neonatal reflexes (PNRs), rooting, sucking and swallowing, have been studied extensively in the feeding context. However, little is known about the role that a range of perhaps 50–100 other innate movements might play in the feeding context.

PNRs

PNRs is a collective term for a group of innate reactions, responses as well as simple reflexes that paediatricians currently use as part of a screening test to evaluate nervous function and assess gestational age. Four schools of thought inform the neurological assessment of the term and pre-term infant, and each gives detailed description of the reflexes and the releasers. In particular Prechtl (1977), a Dutch physician, studying over 1500 babies, standardised the evaluation procedures, neonatal behavioural states and positions that would enable inter-assessor reliability. These procedures were understandably inflexible as the PNRs formed an integral part of the evaluation of neurological well-being. Most of the PNRs are examined when the baby is in a quiet alert behavioural state, and three neonatal positions are used by paediatricians to release the reflexes: supine, prone and ventral suspension whereby the examiner holds the baby around the thorax with feet dangling. For example, finger grasping, sucking, rooting and the Babkinski reflex are examined when babies are supine. When babies lie prone such responses as spontaneous head righting, lifting and crawling are released. In ventral suspension, automatic walking movements and placing are triggered. Placing is described as a lifting and placing movement in response to brushing the top of the baby's foot top against a hard surface, usually the examination table.

When people look at pictures of these reflexes in the neurological books, they are often puzzled, wondering what such movements as placing or the Babinski toe fan could possibly have to do with infant feeding. For the answers to this question, we need to look closer at BN.

EVIDENCE FROM INFANT OBSERVATION

In a study of 54 mother–baby pairs conducted by the author,[2] 20 PNRs were identified, described, compared and validated in the feeding context with high (0.8) inter-rater agreement. PNRs were categorised into four types: endogenous, rhythmic, motor and anti-gravity. Three feeding functions were suggested: cueing, finding and sustaining milk transfer. Initially, the reflexes were believed always to be stimulants, but the role of PNRs was infinitely more complex. Surprisingly, analysis revealed that PNRs could either help or hinder, that is, they were observed to either aid latch or sustain milk transfer, or they appeared to be barriers thwarting a successful feed.

This negative function has been documented in the literature (Gunther, 1955) as 'breast refusal' or 'fighting the breast', although objective descriptions of what is visible or audible are sparse. Nevertheless, many health professionals are familiar with a to and fro horizontal head shaking behaviour observed thwarting latch. The UK BFI (1997) suggest that mothers often interpret these movements as the baby 'saying no' to breastfeeding, and they are quick to reassure the reader that it is 'normal behaviour'. Another form of latch refusal is termed breast boxing, first documented as a new breastfeeding behaviour observed during engorgement. Here, Gohil (2006, p. 268), an Indian paediatrician offers an objective description of a behaviour that is familiar to mothers and health professionals:

It was observed that the infant does not suckle and pushes himself away with his fisted hands at the breasts or abdomen of the mother, and kicks away at the mother's abdomen and avoids feeding.

---

[2] This PhD thesis won the inaugural Akinsanya award in 2006 and a bound copy is available for consultation in the Royal College of Nursing Library Steinberg Collection. In addition, methodology and results are published in a research paper (SD Colson *et al.*, 2008).

TRADITIONAL MATERNAL POSTURES

Over half the babies in the study displayed these behaviours, preventing them from latching onto the breast. Close scrutiny of the mother's posture and how she held her baby revealed some common points: first, mothers having difficulty sat upright, bolt upright or leaning slightly forward as they were taught to do, often placing the baby on a pillow; the baby usually was lying across the mother's body, and although baby was often 'tummy to mummy', the entire front aspect of the babies' bodies were not completely applied to the mother's. Thighs, calves and feet were often in contact with thin air; importantly, back pressure was always a requirement keeping the baby in place at breast level. This positional phenomenon is termed 'dorsal feeding' in the literature by Peiper, a German physician who suggested that the human infant is an obligate dorsal feeder always requiring this back pressure no matter if the mother is upright or if she lies on her side.

As soon as mothers lay back, and only three mothers did this spontaneously, another reflex was observed, a pendular or head bobbing movement in the babies, which appeared to be released from a fixed point in the baby's spine. This movement was also documented previously by Schielct and Prectl (Peiper, 1963) who suggested that pendular movements were observed to have a feeding function in non-human, ventral feeding mammals, those animals such as puppies, kittens, rats and hamsters whose ventrum usually lies on the ground during feeding. Interestingly, one of the mothers in the study characterised this movement by saying that her baby latched onto the breast like a little woodpecker.

OBSERVED COMMONALITIES

Like the mothers whose babies rejected the breast, those whose babies attached quickly and easily had some common points. First, they were laid-back but not all to the same degree of body slope. Their babies were often lying longitudinally or obliquely on top of the mother's body. Babies then naturally seemed to lead in with the chin or sometimes the approach involved the entire trigeminal area. Babies also appeared to achieve their own positional stability and often self-attached suggesting that breastfeeding in BN positions is a proprioceptive activity for the baby. Importantly, gravity appeared to have a positive effect holding the baby on top of the mother's body so that back pressure was not required. Indeed, understanding the positive and negative effects of gravity was key to elaborating the mechanisms of BN.

Of course, some babies do latch on when mothers are sitting upright or slide-lying, and it would not be helpful to prescribe laid-back postures as the only way to initiate breastfeeding. Nevertheless, more PNRs were observed as breastfeeding stimulants, aiding latch and sustaining milk transfer when mothers lay back then when mothers sat upright or lay on their sides, and this difference was statistically significant (Colson *et al.*, 2008). Similar to the discovery of the benefits associated with being vertical during labour and birth (Balaskas, 1983; Kitzinger, 1970), BN or 'laid-back' postures appear to be optimal to initiate breastfeeding, and the mechanisms have to do with the positive effect of gravity together with maternal body slope and neonatal body weight, tilt and angle of approach or the direction of the baby's position.

THE MECHANISMS OF BIOLOGICAL NURTURING

When mothers sit upright, their bodies are closed at right angles (90°). As soon as they lean back, the dimensions of the body space (in the midriff) available to the neonate is increased, full frontal ventral positions enable body brushing, which releases the motor reflexes enabling neonatal locomotion. Babies manoeuvre themselves on the maternal body, often finding a position similar to how they lay in utero. The laid-back posture also increases the number of positions available to the neonate, because the breast is round and the baby's can lie around the breast like the hands of a clock. The approach is determined by the lie or the direction of the baby's position, and this is important particularly for mothers who have had caesarean sections. When the baby approaches the breast in an over the shoulder lie, mothers appear to worry less about pain from the recent wound. The numerous possibilities of neonatal lie also appear to work well for the obese mother or one who has dysmorphic characteristics, short arm length, for example.

The positive use of gravity appears central to a pain-free effective latch and also seems to increase maternal enjoyment as the angle of the body slope that releases latching behaviours looks like it is at just the right distance to enable eye-to-eye contact and maternal baby gazing without placing strain on the mother's neck.

Last but certainly not least, results of this study demonstrate that the positional interactions release the PNRs as stimulants, even when the baby was observed to be in sleep states. Putting the baby to the breast in BN positions while asleep (without waking him or her) was the single most important factor aiding those mothers who were struggling with breastfeeding. As soon as those mothers who experienced problems (latch refusal, sore nipples, postural pain (sore shoulders, aching necks and backs), breast fighting, etc.) held their sleeping babies in laid-back postures, the immediate pressure to feed was reduced, and many mothers appeared to focus on the baby, not the problem.

THE MECHANICAL EFFECTS OF SLEEP

BN is first and foremost underpinned by reflex theory. The mechanisms enabling latch and milk transfer when babies are in sleep states are the same with any other simple reflex activity, e.g. the knee jerk. Nurses know this as we are taught how to assess reflex activity in the unconscious patient. So, it is for babies in light sleep and drowsy states, the body brushing releases the motor and searching PNRs blunting them somewhat which in turn helps the mother make adjustments to alleviate the problem. Laid-back breastfeeding is hands-free and mother's hands spontaneously stroked neonatal feet releasing the Babinski reflex as well as the toe grasp or curl. Both of these PNRs were observed to activate neonatal latching behaviours.

CLINICAL APPLICATIONS

Taken together, these findings suggest widespread clinical applications for those 35% of mothers experiencing the latch refusal or breast fighting that so frequently prompts early unintended breastfeeding cessation during the first postnatal week.

Hospital doctors and midwives are reluctant to release new mothers without the baby having had at least one 'good' feed. Suggesting BN, therefore, often has immediate effect on another 'at risk' group or those 52% of mothers who are mixed feeding during the hospital stay as it is likely that these mothers are 'failed' breastfeeders; many introduce a bottle to hasten hospital discharge. My clinical experience suggests that releasing the foot to mouth connection, mentioned earlier, by applying simple pressure along the outer aspect of the sole of the baby's foot (releasing the Babinski reflex) or on the ball of the baby's foot (releasing the toe grasp) triggers a latch. I do this having asked the mother's permission while the baby is asleep on her in full BN positions. As soon as a baby experiences the trigeminal facial/breast experience, he appears to be hardwired to seek it again. Mothers often remark 'What did you do?' However, few mothers need explanations: when in BN postures, their behaviours appear to be as spontaneous as their babies'.

Results from qualitative work carried out in Scotland suggest that first-time mothers believe that hospital midwives favour breastfeeding spending more time helping nursing mothers to the detriment of bottle-feeding mothers. To make matters worse, even after hours invested in skills learning, breastfeeding mothers often continue to experience the same problems prompting them to switch to bottle feeding, which in turn often leads to maternal feelings of incompetence, failure and sometimes to postnatal depression.

On the other hand, BN is quick and easy to do. Health professionals simply suggest laid-back maternal postures and assess positional interactions at a glance. Many midwives using BN say that the approach is rewarding. Mothers appear more relaxed and often proudly share their babies' achievements. BN also helps midwives prioritise their work identifying those mother/baby pairs who require help. For example, those babies in whom no reflexes can be observed over a two to four-hour period of BN will probably require a paediatric referral. BN is a natural screening test because the presence or absence of the PNRs, of course, still serves as an early indicator of a neurological problem.

Last but not least, because no teaching is involved, there may be untold costs-saving benefits to the NHS concerning midwifery time.

CONCLUSION

In recent decades, within our English-speaking bottle-feeding cultures, breastfeeding has been considered problematic requiring lactation management, which offers a consistent, repeatable and one-way approach. Before 2000, some small studies suggested that the routine teaching of positioning and attachment skills central to lactation management was promising as an intervention to promote breastfeeding continuance. However, there were no randomised controlled trials (RCTs) examining the cause and effect relationship. Since then five trials have shown equivocal results and few if any benefits to routine skills teaching (De Oliveira *et al.*, 2006; Forster *et al.*, 2004; Henderson *et al.*, 2001; Labarere *et al.*, 2003). Indeed Henderson *et al.* (2001) found that mothers who were in the 'managed' experimental group had shorter duration and enjoyed breastfeeding less than those mothers in the control group who had not been managed.

Spontaneous breastfeeding can be compared to giving birth spontaneously; there will always be a small percentage of mothers who will encounter problems that require management. However, like eating, drinking and sleeping, breastfeeding is not and should not be considered as a problem for the majority. Rather, it is a public health perspective together with a medical need to regulate and manage that underpins the kind of prescriptive routine breastfeeding advice that so often creates self-doubt and other problems that decrease maternal breastfeeding competence and enjoyment. As Greiner (1993, p. 7), well-known breastfeeding activist suggests:

> The term [breastfeeding management] was chosen in order to attract the attention of the largely male body of physicians whose lack of understanding and interest in breastfeeding has in the past only been surpassed by their power over it. Unfortunately the term implies that this power is somehow correct and necessary.

Today, mothers often think they will fail even before they start! In response, instead of sharing our confidence in the unique biological design of a mother's body to nourish her baby, health professionals suggest 'helpful' metaphors saying that breastfeeding is like typing, riding a bike, dancing or driving a car. These activities are learned skills and/or enhancements to increase enjoyment of life or to get ahead professionally. They are neither necessary to sustain life nor integral to a lifelong relationship.

Breastfeeding, on the other hand, is comparable to those activities of daily living as defined in the Roper *et al.* (2000) model of nursing. Breastfeeding in itself maintains a safe environment and is an activity that is associated with breathing, communication, personal hygiene, mobility, eating and drinking and expressing sexuality among others. The suggestion that breastfeeding is similar to learned activities often creates a 'helpless' mother dependent upon advice from experts at the very time when new-mothers feel most vulnerable. Biologically and in countries untouched by lactation management, breastfeeding remains an activity of daily living for an average of 4 years for both mother and baby. During the time of lactation, there is a pre-programmed mutual biological dependency, occurring when it is supposed to happen at just the right time in the life span.

Breastfeeding is certainly not something that the baby does by himself as Righard (2008) has suggested. The word relationship implies, by definition, interaction, communication and the give and take of two people. Mothers are active breastfeeders! They guide and protect their babies, aiding latch as necessary through, what we have observed as, 'emerging patterns of maternal instinctual behaviours' (Colson *et al.*, 2008, p. 446). Furthermore, mothers' participation is essential as mothers constantly assess their babies' well-being, protecting their babies and detecting as soon as possible any deviation from the normal or potential problems. Indeed, there is a strong argument suggesting that, rationally, mothers should take the lead.

The breastfeeding relationship, like any relationship, comprises both innate and acquired behaviours. However, for about a century, the 'breastfeeding as an acquired skill' or the nurturing approach has dominated our understanding and informed practice about how mothers should best initiate breastfeeding. Innate behaviours depend upon the right hormonal environment. The BN approach emphasises first and foremost the importance of maintaining an environment conducive to the release of the primary breastfeeding hormones, oxytocin and prolactin, and then observing maternal behaviours, learning from mothers and trusting maternal instincts to release baby behaviours. BN aims to restore the balance bringing the nature or innate component back into breastfeeding.

REFERENCES

Anderson GC, Moore E, Hepworth J, *et al.* Early skin-to-skin contact for mothers and their healthy newborn infants. *Cochrane Db Syst Rev.* 2003; (2).

Baby Friendly Initiative UK. Statement 18. *The BFI Position on Biological Nurturing.* 2009a. Available on line at: www.babyfriendly.org.uk/items/item_detail.asp?item=558 (accessed 21 December 2009).

Baby Friendly Initiative UK. *Information Sheet Word Free Picture Pack.* 2009b. Available on line at: www.babyfriendly.org.uk/pdfs/infosheets/word_free_teaching_pack_infosheet.pdf (accessed 21 December 2009).

Balaskas J. *Active Birth.* London: Unwin Paperbacks; 1983.

Bolling K, Grant C, Hamlyn B, *et al. Infant Feeding Survey 2005.* London: The Information Centre; 2007.

Bragg M. Review No. 901031 in MIDIRS Midwifery Digest Standard Search L46PN101. Available at: www.MIDIRS.org (accessed 20 March 2006).

Brown L. *The New Shorter Oxford Dictionary.* 5th ed. Oxford: Oxford University Press; 1993.

Colson S. *Biological Suckling Facilitates Exclusive Breastfeeding from Birth a Pilot Study of Twelve Vulnerable Infants.* Dissertation submitted as Course requirement of MSc in Midwifery Studies. London: South Bank University; 2000.

Colson S. Womb to world: a metabolic perspective. *Midwifery Today.* 2002; **46**(1): 12–17.

Colson S. Biological nurturing: the physiology of lactation revisited (2). *Pract Midwife.* 2007; **10**(10): 14–19.

Colson S. Bringing nature to the fore. *Pract Midwife.* 2008; **11**(10): 14–16, 18–19.

Colson S, DeRooy L, Hawdon J. Biological nurturing increases breastfeeding duration. *MIDIRS Midwifery Dig.* 2003; **13**(1): 92–7.

Colson SD, Meek J, Hawdon JM. Optimal positions triggering primitive neonatal reflexes stimulating breastfeeding. *Early Hum Dev.* 2008; **84**(7): 441–9. Available at: http://linkinghub.elsevier.com/retrieve/pii/S0378378207002423 (accessed 10 March 10).

De Oliveira LD, Giugliani ERJ, Santo LCDE, *et al.* Effect of intervention to improve breastfeeding technique on the frequency of exclusive breastfeeding and lactation-related problems. *J Hum Lact.* 2006; **22**(3): 315–21.

Elman JL, Bates EA, Johnson MH, *et al. Rethinking Innateness: a connectionist perspective on development.* Michigan: MIT Press Paperback; 1998.

Forster D, McLachlan H, Lumley J, *et al.* Two mid-pregnancy interventions to increase the initiation and duration of breastfeeding: a randomized controlled trial. *Birth.* 2004; **31**(3): 176–82.

Gohil JR. Boxing neonate on an engorged breast, a new behavior identified. *J Hum Lact.* 2006; **23**(3): 268–9.

Greiner T. Infant and young child nutrition: a historic review from a communication perspective. In: Koniz-Booher P, editor. *Communication Strategies to Support Infant and Young Child Nutrition.* Cornell International Nutrition Monographs; 1993. pp. 24–5 (combined); 7–15. Available at: www.geocities.com/HotSprings/Sp 3156/Ted.html (accessed 10 March 10).

Gunther M. Instinct and the nursing couple. *Lancet.* 1955; **265**(6864): 575–8.

Henderson A, Stamp G, Pincombe J. Postpartum positioning and attachment education for increasing breastfeeding: a randomized trial. *Birth.* 2001; **28**(4): 236–42.

Howard C, Howard F, Lawrence R, *et al.* Office prenatal formula advertising and its effect on breast-feeding patterns. *Obs Gynecol.* 2000; **95**(2): 296–303.

Hytten F. *The Clinical Physiology of the Puerperium.* London: Perrand Press; 1995.

Inch S. *How to Breastfeed, a Visual Guide.* 2009a. Available at: www.babycentre.co.uk/baby/breastfeeding/visualguide/ (accessed on 18 December 09).

Inch S. *Good Positions for Breastfeeding.* 2009b. Available at: www.babycentre.co.uk/baby/breastfeeding/positions/ (accessed on 18 December 09).

Inch S, Law S, Wallace L. Hands off! The breastfeeding best start project (1). *Pract Midwife.* 2003; **6**(10): 17–19.

Klaus MH, Klaus PH. *The Amazing Newborn.* Reading, MA: Addison-Wesley Publishing Company Inc; 1985.

Kitzinger S. *The Experience of Childbirth.* 1st ed. London: Penguin; 1970.

La Leche League International. *The Womanly Art of Breastfeeding.* 7th ed. Chicago: Schaumburg; 2004.

Labarere J, Bellin V, Fourny M, *et al.* Assessment of a structured in-hospital educational intervention addressing breastfeeding: a prospective randomized open trial. *Br J Obstet Gynecol.* 2003; **110**: 847–52.

Lawrence RA. A review of the medical benefits and contraindications to breastfeeding in the United States. *Maternal and Child Health Technical Information Bulletin.* New York: HRSA; 1997.

Lorenz K. *King Solomon's Ring.* London: Methuen and Co; 1952.

Matthiesen AS, Ransjo-Arvidson AB, Nissen E, *et al.* Postpartum maternal oxytocin release by newborns: effects of infant hand massage and sucking. *Birth.* 2001; **28**(1): 13–19.

McConville B. *Mixed Messages Our Breasts in Our Lives.* London: Penguin Books; 1994.

Morris D. *Manwatching: a field guide to human behaviour.* London: Triad/Panther; 1977.

O'Driscoll K, Jackson RJA, Gallagher JT. The active management of labour. *BMJ.* 1969; **2**: 477.

Organization for Economic Co-operation and Development. *Breastfeeding Rates* on line at OECD Family Data Base. 2009. Available online at: www.oecd.org/dataoecd/30/56/43136964.pdf (last accessed 18 December 2009).

Palmer G. *The Politics of Breastfeeding: when breasts are bad for business.* 3rd ed. London: Pinter & Martin; 2009.

Peiper A. *Cerebral Function in Infancy and Childhood.* 3rd ed. New York, NY: Consultants Bureau; 1963.

Prechtl H. *The Neurological Examination of the Full Term New Born Infant. Clinics in Developmental Medicine No 63.* 2nd ed. Spastic International Medical Publications. London: William Heinemann Books; 1977.

Pryor K. *Nursing Your Baby.* 1st ed. New York: Harper & Row; 1963.

Renfrew M, Dyson L, Wallace L, *et al. The Effectiveness of Public Health Interventions to Promote the Duration of Breastfeeding Systematic review.* 1st ed. London: National Institute for Health and Clinical Excellence; 2005.

Renfrew M, Fisher C, Arms S. *Bestfeeding: Getting Breastfeeding Right for You.* 3rd ed. Berkeley, CA: Celestial Arts; 2004.

Righard L. The baby is breastfeeding – not the mother. *Birth.* 2008; **35**: 1.

Righard L, Alade MO. Effects of delivery room routines on success of first feed. *Lancet.* 1990; **336**: 1105–7.

Righard L, Frantz K. *Delivery Self Attachment* [Videocassette]. Sunland, CA: Geddes Productions; 1992.

Roper, Logan WW, Tierney AJ. *The Roper Logan and Tierney model of nursing based on activities of living.* 4th ed. London: Churchill Livingstone; 2000.

Royal College of Midwives. *Successful Breastfeeding.* 1st ed. London: RCM; 1986.

Slater A, Hocking I, Loose J. Theories and issues in child development. In: Slater A, Bremner G, editors. *An Introduction to Developmental Psychology.* Oxford: Blackwell Publishing; 2003. pp. 34–64.

Tew M. *Safer Childbirth: a critical history of maternity care.* 2nd ed. London: Chapman & Hall; 1995.

Tinbergen N. *The Study of Instinct.* Oxford: Clarendon Press; 1951.

Wells J. The role of cultural factors in human breastfeeding: adaptive behaviour or biopower? In: Raj K, editor. *Hum Ecol.* 2006; SI No. **14**: 39–47.

Widstrom AM, Wahlberg V, Matthiesen AS, *et al.* Short-term effects of early suckling and touch of the nipple on maternal behaviour. *Early Hum Dev.* 1990; **21**(3): 151–63.

Woolridge MW. The 'anatomy' of infant sucking. *Midwifery.* 1986a; **2**: 164–71.

Woolridge MW. Aetiology of sore nipples. *Midwifery.* 1986b; **2**: 172–6.

Woolridge MW. Baby controlled breastfeeding. In: Stuart-Macadam P, Dettwyler KA, editors. *Breastfeeding Biocultural Perspectives.* New York: Aldine de Gruyter; 1995. pp. 217–42.

World Health Organization. *Evidence for the ten steps to successful breastfeeding* (Revised). Family and Reproductive Health Division of Child Health and Development. Geneva: World Health Organization; 1998.

CHAPTER 9

The management of selective eating in young children

Jo Douglas

INTRODUCTION

Selective eating, faddiness or 'picky' eating is a common behavioural problem in young children. It is often transient and short-lived, with food preferences altering every few weeks or lasting for a few months at most. In some children, it becomes a severe and chronic problem that can affect their health, socialisation and ability to mix with peers. It also causes considerable stress and inconvenience to parents. These children refuse to go to parties, are unable to eat out in public or will not eat all day at school. They are extremely rigid and controlling about what they will eat, i.e. texture, colour, brand, smell and will gradually reduce the range of foods that they will accept over time. They can often create a situation where the parent has to cook a separate meal or only provide the very limited range of food that the child will eat in order to ensure that the child actually eats something. They are not prepared to try new foods, and this food 'neophobia' impairs their ability to extend their range (Russell and Worsley, 2008).

This eating problem is common throughout the life span and is not specific to early childhood. Once the behaviour pattern becomes entrenched, it can be very difficult to treat in adult life. Selective eating is not considered to be an eating disorder but more of a behavioural problem (Jacobi *et al.*, 2009).

Children who are severely selective eaters fall into two major categories.

1   Children in the first category may drink excessive quantities of milk or squash, which reduces their appetite and consequently reduces the range of food they are prepared to eat (Wright *et al.*, 2007). They have developed a habit pattern and mistake the signal of hunger for that of thirst. These children frequently are highly dependent on bottles and gain a lot of comfort and satisfaction from sucking.

2   The second group of severely selective children are those who tend to eat a highly restricted range of food, which are usually the carbohydrate range, i.e. crisps, biscuits, bread, cereal and chips, but they will also frequently drink milk or eat fromage frais, which maintains a balance in their diet and also maintains their weight. The most frequently refused foods are fruit, vegetables, pulses, meat and fish (Russell and Worsley, 2008). Some eat an excessive amount of sweet foods and chocolate.

PREVALENCE OF SELECTIVE EATING IN PRE-SCHOOL CHILDREN

In a large British retrospective population study, 4% of 5-year-olds were described as being 'faddy' by their parents. There was an equal prevalence in boys and girls. Around 30% of the faddy eaters had feeding problems as a baby (Butler and Golding, 1986). Richman *et al.* (1982) found that 12% of 3-year-olds were faddy eaters, as identified on the behaviour screening questionnaire. When the rate of faddy eating was examined in a group of children defined as having behaviour problems, this percentage increased to 31%. Results from the Gateshead Millennium Baby Study showed that 8% of children at 30 months were described as definitely 'faddy', while 17% said their children ate a limited variety and 13% preferred drinks to food (Wright *et al.*, 2007). Being faddy was only weakly associated with poor growth and simply eating a limited variety of foods was found to be unrelated to growth.

Severe selective eating in young children is not well described in the clinical literature as it does not fit into existing diagnostic categories (Nicholls and Bryant-Waugh, 2009, Timimi *et al.*, 1997). It is often included in general samples of children treated as food refusers (Douglas, 1995a, b). Douglas and Bryon (1996) found that a one-third of their clinic-referred sample of young children with severe eating problems showed selective eating. However, the sample did not permit definitive classification as some of the same children also had co-morbid features of severe problems with quantity or texture of food for their age. The concept of 'picky eating' is associated with a consistent pattern of inhibited and selective eating beginning in infancy, but this does not indicate the level of severity and longevity of the symptoms shown by some children.

Chatoor (1997) has attempted to provide a classification of feeding disorders and describes extreme food selectivity as food refusal. She sees this as a disorder of separation with onset between 6 months and 3 years of age during the transition to self-feeding. There is variable food refusal, which is often situational. The child frequently bargains about food and has conflicts about eating with the parents, who are extremely anxious about the food refusal. She sees this problem developing from conflicts in autonomy and control and by lack of appropriate limit setting by the parents.

AETIOLOGY OF SELECTIVE EATING

Children who are highly selective over long periods in early childhood can maintain reasonable weights, as they often eat large quantities of foods that they prefer.

Alternatively, they supplement their diet by drinking large quantities of milk. These children often present as being phobic of their non-preferred food. If it is presented to them they may physically shake and cry or become aggressive and confrontational in an effort to avoid it. They appear to feel extremely anxious about food. This heightened state of arousal also affects other eating-related behaviours.

These children are often reported to be meticulous about the presentation of food (Timimi et al., 1997). They may become upset if one food touches another on the same plate, demand different foods to be placed on separate plates, are specific about brands of food or particular flavours they will eat or demand that it is cut in a particular way. They may be concerned about food or 'mess' on their fingers. They may eat certain foods only in certain places or demand that the parent takes their 'home' food or own utensils whenever they go out. Some children who are anxious about the wetness of food and cannot tolerate sauces or 'messy' food, may have seen this modelled by fastidious mothers who wipe up the slightest mess immediately and do not allow their child to play or get their hands into food.

This 'obsessional' behaviour can affect other areas of behavioural development, and the child can show compulsive traits, e.g. rituals about falling asleep, excessive tidiness, concern about clothes matching or shoelaces being tied exactly the same. They may have difficulties with separation and with socialisation at nursery or school.

It is possible that there is a continuum of severity of selective eating, ranging from the food faddiness of pre-school children through the severely selective children to children with severe difficulties with social communication, i.e. autism spectrum disorders (ASD). Selective eating has now being well described in children with ASD (Kodak and Piazza, 2008; Ledford and Gast, 2006; Lockner et al., 2008), and it may be part of their symptomatology of inability to cope with change or newness.

Laurie

Laurie, aged 4 years, had been diagnosed with ASD, but he had started to speak in the previous 6 months and could communicate reasonably at assessment. He had a significant number of behaviour problems, including obsessional and repetitive play with specific toys, sleeping difficulties and severe tantrums twice a day. The parents, with behavioural management advice, had been able to set clear limits for his behaviour and had resolved his night waking. His diet had become progressively restricted by the age of 18 months of age. At assessment, he would eat only 'smiley face' potato shapes, bananas and milk. His weight was between the 75th and 90th percentiles. He was extremely avoidant of any other food and vehemently refused to try new foods.

It is not clear why children become severely selective eaters, although certain hypotheses can be considered and revealed through the assessment process. Parents frequently report early onset under the age of 2 years in pre-school children. Most of this age group show onset of symptomatology at the introduction of lumpy stage 2 baby foods, although it can appear earlier with infants 3 months of age rejecting different tastes of stage 1 purees. Breast- or bottle-feeding usually presents no problems. Parents can often identify events that triggered the start of the problem, such as choking on a specific food or after an illness of diarrhoea and vomiting.

Children who have had a delayed introduction to lumpy food in their first year of life do show a more restricted diet later in childhood. The Avon Longitudinal Study of Parents and Children has shown that 18% of the children were introduced to lumpy solids after the age of 9 months. They ate less of many food groups at age 7 years in including all fruit and vegetables and also had more eating problems at age 7 years than children introduced to lumpy food earlier (Coulthard *et al.*, 2009). The difficulty with this type of survey is that it is not clear whether the reason for the late introduction of lumpy food is due to the child's avoidance and refusal or due to the mother's reluctance and fear of the child choking.

In a another treatment sample of 34 children diagnosed as selective eaters, 100% of the children had started to be selective by the age of 2 years, 85% by the age of 1 year and 47% by 6 months of age. The transition to the lumpier stage 2 baby food had created a problem for most of the children (Douglas and Bryon, 1996).

Other children show onset after they have accepted solid and finger foods and they become progressively more selective over time. They start to refuse foods offered and lose these from their diet. They will gag, choke and retch on non-preferred food and will refuse to swallow it.

A more recent diagnostic category of tactile defensive children show picky eating as part of their symptomatology (Smith *et al.*, 2005). They tend to avoid unfamiliar foods, do not eat in other people's houses and refuse certain food because of the smell and temperature. They often gag and show a pronounced aversion to certain textures and consistencies. Work on their tactile or oral defensiveness can be effective and aid their eating pattern.

TASTE PREFERENCES AND AVERSIONS

Studies that have attempted to understand how children develop taste preferences all cite the finding that there is a heightened preference for sweet-tasting and greater rejection of bitter-tasting food in infants (Birch, 1998, 1999). Genetic findings show that different taste receptor genes are associated with sensitivity to bitter and sweet tastes (Mennella *et al.*, 2005). Parental influences have also been considered to be important in the development of taste preferences (Scaglioni *et al.*, 2008). Harris (2008) combines both approaches and suggests that there is a strong-to-moderate heritability of willingness in children to accept new food and specific foods, which is moderated by cultural differences and gives rise to different patterns of food acceptance. She considers that modelling and flavour conditioning may also contribute to food acceptance.

Aversion to trying new foods (neophobia) is a significant clinical symptom of children who show selective eating (Dovey *et al.*, 2008). Twin studies indicate that neophobia is a strongly heritable characteristic while food preferences show some genetic influence and are also influenced by family environment (Wardle and Cooke, 2008). Galloway *et al.* (2003) have attempted to identify separate predictors for food neophobia and picky eating in girls and found that girls with neophobias were more anxious and had mothers with food neophobia while picky eaters had mothers with less variety in their vegetable intake and less time to eat healthy foods. The inter-relationship between these two symptoms is important in therapy and techniques that take both into account are likely to be most successful.

ASSESSMENT OF THE PROBLEM

A detailed account of the date of onset of the problem, the medical history and the eating history of the child is an essential feature of assessment. There is usually no concern about their physical health, although some children who drink excessively large amounts of sugary fruit squash or eat large quantities of chocolate may have dental caries. For example, Jack, aged 5 years, had 15 teeth removed because of severe dental caries as his diet consisted of chocolate and milk. Some children may have a history of repeated ENT problems and enlarged tonsils while others may show some sensitivity to dairy products.

Observation of a meal time with the parents will provide information about the behaviour patterns and how they are being maintained. Observation of how the child reacts to non-preferred foods being on their plate will often provide clear guidance as to how the existing pattern of behaviour has become entrenched. Children are frequently uncooperative, will not come to the table or sit down; they may push the plate away, whine and moan, or cry and become upset. The parents often give in very quickly if they are unable to cope with the child's distress; they may be unable to get the child even to come and sit at the table and they may rapidly offer a preferred alternative food to reduce both the child's and their own anxiety.

Jamie

Jamie aged 4 years refused to sit down and eat the crisps that were on his plate with other food. The parents requested that the packet of crisps be brought in to show him that they were his preferred brand and he agreed to eat some tipped out of the packet in front of him. He then demanded that the parents shut their eyes while he ate the first one and sat on the floor under the table to do so. Once he had tasted the first crisp, he accepted that they were his type of crisp and proceeded to eat the rest perfectly well and even took the original ones from the main plate of food.

The child's distress and protestations will suddenly disappear when the preferred food is offered. The child may eat it rapidly in large mouthfuls as they feel confident and relieved. They frequently ask for more. But some children will nibble around the edges of even their preferred food and eat relatively slowly. Observing these differences in eating style is important for the development of a hypothesis about how to treat the child. Children who nibble could be considered to have a mild oral-motor dysfunction and find that they prefer the bite-dissolve foods that this easy range of carbohydrates provides.

Parents may also have very different styles of coping with the child, one often being more lenient and compliant than the other. Parents may disregard each other's attempts to encourage the child to eat, undermine the actions of the other parent or be more impatient and less tolerant than the other. They may be very positive with the child encouraging them to try food, but they often ask questions rather than make statements or give clear instructions about what is expected and leave themselves open to a clear refusal. The tentative nature of the request to try a food only reinforces the child's power in the situation. Some parents will not comment if their child does try a new food for fear of making too big an issue out of it, of making the child embarrassed or of putting him or her off repeating the attempt. In general, the parents are extremely anxious about the child's food refusal and may try excessively to encourage the child to eat, or alternatively give the child anything that he or she wants to eat at any time.

TREATMENT STUDIES

Werle *et al.* (1993) describe the treatment of three chronic food-refusing children, two of whom are selective eaters while the third has difficulties with eating age-appropriate textures of food, where a home-based behavioural programme was successfully implemented. Single case studies of children with food aversion, which had elements of selective eating, are described by Archer and Szatmari (1990) and Blisset and Harris (2002). Singer *et al.* (1992) describe three boys with food phobias one of who is a selective eater. A single session psychoeducational approach in a community setting is described by Fraser *et al.* (2004). The other end of the spectrum of severity of eating problem is the more intense day centre treatment programme described by Douglas and Harris (2001). Behavioural treatment for children with ASD is described by Ahearn (2003) and Najdowski *et al.* (2003).

TREATMENT APPROACHES

When families attend for treatment, there are several major characteristics that the clinician should take into account.

- The parents have a long experience of their child not eating a wide range of foods and have already accommodated to this.
- The parents will have tried a wide range of methods to try and encourage their child to eat a wider range and feel helpless and impotent.
- The parents are usually upset about other people's comments about their child (e.g. that he or she is naughty or should be starved or that anyone can get a child to eat) but feel helpless.
- The parents' anxiety about maintaining the child's weight is managed by giving the child a lot of the limited range of food he or she will eat.
- Most parents are concerned that they might have caused the problem in some way.
- The child is used to getting his or her own way about what he or she eats and how he or she eats.
- The child is very strong willed.
- The child is very fearful of new foods and does not want to try them.
- The child does not know why he or she cannot eat a wide range of foods and probably does not want to change.
- The child has a repertoire of food-avoidant behaviours that are effective in the family.
- The child and the family do not know how to change the existing state of affairs.

Recognition, acceptance and reassurance about the problem are important. Parents' concerns need to be taken seriously. Most of these children are not unwell and are not failing to thrive: the problem is really a social and psychological one. Parents often say that they owe it to their child to try and solve the problem and are usually very motivated for treatment. They worry about the long-term outcome and do not want to be blamed later by their child because he or she is still on a restricted diet.

A BEHAVIOURAL MANAGEMENT APPROACH

Taking a behavioural perspective, it is possible to identify both classical and operant conditioning experiences that may have influenced the development of the child's selective eating (*see* Chapter 3). Classical conditioning would have occurred when the child's experience of eating has been paired repeatedly with an unpleasant experience, perhaps force, pain, nausea or fear. Operant conditioning would have occurred when the child's difficult behaviour has resulted in parents giving in to his or her demands or providing only preferred foods. Treatment strategies therefore need to take into account stimulus control issues, i.e. events or stimuli that precede the intake of food and elicit fear reactions, as well as contingent events aimed at reinforcing the acceptance of new foods.

Parents, similarly, have a learning history with their child and have evolved a method of keeping their anxiety as low as possible. The mother rapidly learns not to offer food the child does not like. She reduces the behavioural disturbance, the emotional upset and her concern about adequate nutritional intake by offering the child his or her preferred foods. The child equally learns that if he or she causes enough disruption and upset then he or she will get his or her own way.

The focus of treatment is at several levels:

- to build up the child's confidence and self-esteem about trying new foods
- to desensitise the child's fear of new food and change
- to enable the parents to set clear limits for their child and to expect compliance
- to introduce a graded system of new foods including texture, range and quantity
- to increase the range of foods eaten in a systematic manner
- to reinforce the child's success at trying new foods
- to maintain the child's weight and growth.

If the child is old enough or has sufficient language, it is often helpful to gauge his or her level of motivation for change by enquiring directly. Some will indicate that they would like to be able to eat some other foods some day, others will give a complete denial or even refuse to talk about the issue. The child will usually be happy to talk about the range of foods that he or she can eat and this can be confirmed by the parents. A list of preferred foods is important in planning the changes that need to take place.

TREATMENT PLAN

Planning treatment requires full co-operation and motivation from the parents as they need to apply the plan on a regular basis at home two or three times a day at meal times. They need to acknowledge that it is going to be a long, slow process of change that will require consistency and firmness of resolve. The child will be reluctant to change and requires help to face up to the challenge in small, manageable steps.

Stimulus control methods to reduce fear of new food by desensitisation prior to the child learning to put a new food into his or her mouth may be necessary if the child is extremely anxious or the parents are unable to cope with the child's level of resistance. A systematic plan of initially just touching the new food, putting it to lips, kissing it, licking it, sucking it and then putting it in his or her mouth over several days or weeks can be successful. This 'shaping' procedure helps the child learn all of the necessary skills before eating. Once the child has become less fearful then the next stages of change are as follows:

1 Choose a new, non-preferred food to taste that is close to the range that the child already eats easily, e.g. a new type of bread, biscuit, or a new flavour of crisp. (This reduces the likelihood of coming up against a genetic taste preference or a textural difficulty.)

2 Expect the child to eat a tiny piece or crumb of the new food (approximately half a centimetre in size) at each meal and snack time before they are allowed to eat

the preferred food or drink. (This reduces the child's level of anxiety in relation to parental expectations that they should eat a large amount of a new food.)

3 Offer the same new food for 4 days before changing to a new one. (Repeated presentation reduces anxiety by increasing familiarity.)

4 Increase the size of the piece of the new food on successive presentations once the child starts to eat it without distress. (Anxiety is kept low and positive reinforcement of coping helps the child feel successful.)

5 Develop a reward program associated with success, e.g. an *Eat Up* book where the child sticks in a picture or labels of food that he or she can eat and has tasted, or sticker charts for trying a new food. (This increases the child's motivation to co-operate and creates a win/win situation.)

6 Introduce new foods outside the carbohydrate range once the child has accepted the new pattern. (Reduced anxiety and improved self-confidence in child and parent permits a more challenging food to be tried.)

The aim is for the parents to be successful in instructing the child in what to do. Having a clear expectation and goal that is within the ability of the child to achieve is vital. Both the parent and the child need to feel success: the parents by realising that they can set limits for their child and achieve compliance; the child for having managed a new skill. Some children are very fearful of change and require resolute and firm control from their parents. Others will need to learn skills to cope orally with the new food, putting larger amounts in their mouths, learning to chew and move food around their mouths.

The success of the changes achieved depends on the parents' ability to set limits and establish boundaries about food. It is often a long and slow struggle to achieve change with the child readily reverting to preferred foods if given a chance. It is rare for a child to be able to eat all types of food at the end of treatment but they are usually able to eat a wider range of children's-type foods, including some vegetables and other forms of protein such as fish fingers, chicken fingers, sandwiches with different fillings, and cheese. They are not so confined by brands and eat a wider range of foods than they had previously eaten, e.g. all different types of biscuits, crisps and breakfast cereals. The increase in range of foods eaten makes it easier for them to eat socially at friends' houses or to go out for a meal with their family.

Case study 1: David

David was eating wheat cereal with hot milk for three meals a day at age 5 years. In addition he would eat two specific brands of crisp, frozen chips, a couple of teaspoons of spaghetti hoops, sandwiches without filling, smooth yoghurt, milk chocolate, jelly or gum sweets and a specific brand of chocolate sweet. His problems had started when lumpy foods had been introduced. He would gag, choke and vomit on the lumpy textures. In addition his range of food dramatically reduced at the age of 2.5 years when his sister was born. The aim of treatment was for meal times to become calmer and less aversive, and for the parents to be able to set expectations about what David should eat and the quantity he should eat. The family chose the reinforcer to be 15 minutes on the computer with father after having tried a new food, but if he made a scene for the reward to be withdrawn without anger or reproach. He was expected to eat a tiny amount of the new food before his preferred food. At times he would take over an hour to try the speck of new food, but his parents persevered and kept to their plan despite the strain. David gradually began to try more foods, and a star chart was introduced where he could earn one star for eating a particular size of a new food and one for eating it in a set time limit. Gradually, two new foods were introduced every other day and the resistance to meal times reduced.

About halfway through the program, there was a slight setback as David started to store food in his mouth. His parents' expectations had accelerated slightly faster than David's ability to change. His father started to shout at him for slow chewing and he was starting to receive more attention for bad behaviour than appropriate behaviour at the table. The chart system was modified to give him a silver star for eating half of the amount in a certain time and a gold star for finishing his plate in the agreed time. His mother also started a game of counting to swallow a food. By the end of treatment (12 attendances), David was starting to ask for new foods and was willing to try. The range of foods he was eating had increased to include sausages, fish fingers, spaghetti bolognese, rice, pasta and biscuits.

Case study 2: Sam

Sam, aged 7 years, was referred as he was eating only liquidised foods prepared by his mother in her food blender, plus particular brands of biscuits, yoghurt and crisps. His problem had started at the age of 7 months when he had choked on a rusk. He had demonstrated significant oral-motor delay and gagged when solid food was placed in his mouth from that time. Sam also had a moderate developmental delay but his language was in keeping with his other developmental skills. He disliked mess on his hands and was reluctant to touch food. His weight was in the average range.

The aims of the treatment plan were:

- to encourage him to touch foods by handling food at home, putting fruit and vegetables into bags in the supermarket, giving his hamster pieces of lettuce and cucumber
- to thicken the texture of the blended food by adding more potato and reducing the liquid content
- to introduce new brands of preferred foods, i.e. biscuits and crisps, and avoid buying his preferred brands
- to introduce tiny portions of new foods
- to stop him gagging and choking by clear instruction
- to use an *Eat Up* book as a reward
- to increase his tolerance to new textures of food.

Sam's progress

Sam was extremely avoidant of new foods, would argue and refuse to eat. Initially, to encourage him to eat some thickened puree, it was necessary to offer a crisp as a reinforcer for each mouthful. His mother decided early on that if he gagged and tried to vomit she would make him eat an extra spoonful. This had the effect of rapidly stopping the gagging. Gradually over the course of 10 sessions, Sam managed to learn to eat small quantities of a variety of foods. His mother stopped liquidising his food after six sessions, by which time he had started to eat small quantities of soft food, e.g. soft cheese, spaghetti hoops, toast and cooked carrots. His pattern of eating the more solid foods was one of nibbling small pieces and chewing them thoroughly before swallowing, which made the meal times very prolonged.

His mother was extremely committed and persevered with each new stage of change. She acknowledged the immense amount of effort it took to encourage change in Sam. By the end of the program, Sam could eat a small amount of a wide range of foods, including fish fingers, sausages, chips, baked beans and pasta. He still needed approximately half of his calorie intake from his preferred range of food after having eaten the new range.

At follow-up 5 years later, at the age of 12 years, he was still eating a variety of food and the good progress had been maintained and extended. His mother still had to be firm about varying his range so that he does not become fixed on to any one type of food. He had made little further progress with vegetables and would still gag if given them.

PROGNOSIS AND OUTCOME

A simple telephone follow-up of seven children, referred for severe and chronic selective eating, 3 years after completing a day centre treatment program revealed that three children had totally normal diets, three children were the same as they were at the end of treatment and had not extended their range of foods further, while one child was eating a more limited range than he had at the end of treatment. These children had been able to extend the range of foods eaten with behavioural management techniques, but it required great effort and commitment from the parents to carry out the treatment program and then to continue with it after leaving the treatment program.

The natural outcome of severe selective eating in early childhood has not been documented. From clinical experience, it is clear that many of these children continue their selective eating throughout childhood and some into adult life but the epidemiology of this problem is not known. Anecdotal evidence and retrospective information from adults who were selective eaters as children point to the possibility of the child or adolescent deciding to extend their range of foods at a significant life change, for example starting secondary school, going out on the first date, leaving home or getting married. Severe selective eating exists in the adult population but it is not clear whether this originated in early childhood or infancy. A long-term follow-up study would be valuable to document the progress of these children.

It is possible that there may be a co-morbid association with obsessional and ritualistic behaviour and that there may be continuity with the selective eating seen in many children with autistic spectrum disorders. Children on the autism spectrum are much more difficult to treat, so it may be possible to see a continuum of severity and prognosis dependent on the presence of co-morbid features.

REFERENCES

Ahearn WH. Using simultaneous presentation to increase vegetable consumption in a mildly selective child with autism. *J Appl Behav Anal*. 2003; **36**: 361–5.

Archer LA, Szatmari P. Assessment and treatment of food aversion in a four year old boy: a multidimensional approach. *Can J Psychiatr*. 1990; **35**: 501–5.

Birch LL. Development of food acceptance patterns in the first years of life. *Pro Nutr Soc*. 1998; **57**: 617–24.

Birch LL. Development of food preferences. *Annu Rev Nutr*. 1999; **19**: 41–62.

Blisset J, Harris G. A behavioural intervention in a child with feeding problems. *J Hum Nutr Diet*. 2002; **15**: 255–60.

Butler NR, Golding J, editors. *From Birth to Five. A Study of the Health and Behaviour of Britain's Five Year Olds*. London: Pergamon Press; 1986.

Chatoor I. Feeding disorders of infants and toddlers. In: Noshpitz JD, Greenspan S, Wieder S, Osofsky J, editors. *Handbook of Child and Adolescent Psychiatry*. Vol. 1. *Infants and Pre-schoolers: development and syndromes*. New York, NY: Wiley; 1997.

Coulthard H, Harris G, Emmett P. Delayed introduction of lumpy foods to children during the complementary feeding period affects child's food acceptance and feeding at 7 years of age. *Matern Child Nutr*. 2009; **5**: 75–85.

Douglas JE. Behavioural eating disorders in young children. *Curr Paediatr*. 1995a; **5**: 39–42.

Douglas JE. Behavioural eating problems in young children In: Davies P, editor. *Nutrition in Child Health*. London: Royal College of Physicians, BPA; 1995b.

Douglas JE, Bryon M. Interview data on severe behavioural eating difficulties in young children. *Arch Dis Child*. 1996; **75**: 304–8.

Douglas JE, Harris B. Description and evaluation of a day centre based feeding programme for young children and their parents. *Clin Child Psychol Psychiatr*. 2001; **6**: 241–56.

Dovey TM, Staples PA, Gibson EL, *et al*. Food neophobia and 'picky/fussy' eating in children: a review. *Appetite*. 2008; **50**: 181–93.

Fraser K, Wallis M, St John W. Improving children's problem eating and mealtime behaviours: an evaluative study of a single session parent education programme. *Health Educ J*. 2004; **63**: 229–41.

Galloway AT, Lee Y, Birch LL. Predictors and consequences of food neophobia and pickiness in young girls. *J Am Diet Assoc*. 2003; **103**: 692–8.

Harris G. Development of taste and food preferences in children. *Curr Opin Clin Nutr*. 2008; **11**: 315–19.

Jacobi C, Schmitz G, Agras WS. Is picky eating an eating disorder? *Int J Eating Disord*. 2009; **b**: 626–34.

Ledford JR, Gast DL. Feeding problems in children with autistic spectrum disorders. *Focus Autism Other DevDisabil*. 2006; **21**: 153–5.

Lockner DW, Crowe TK, Skipper BJ. Dietary intake and parents' perceptions of mealtime behaviours in preschool age children with autism spectrum disorder and in typically developing children. *J Am Diet Assoc*. 2008; **108**: 1360–3.

Kodak T, Piazza CC. Assessment and behavioural treatment of feeding and sleeping disorders in children with autism spectrum disorders. *Child Adoles Psychiatr Clin N Am*. 2008; **17**: 887–905.

Mennella JA, Pepino MY, Reed DR. Genetic and environmental determinants of bitter and sweet preferences. *Pediatrics*. 2005; **115**: 216–22.

Najdowski AC, Wallace MD, Doney JK, *et al*. Parental assessment and treatment of food selectivity in natural settings. *J Appl Behav Anal*. 2003; **36**: 383–6.

Nicholls D, Brynat-Waugh R. Eating disorders of infancy and childhood: definition, symptomatology and comorbidity. *Child Adolesc Psychiatr Clin N Am*. 2009; **18**: 17–30.

Richman N, Stephenson J, Graham PJ. *Pre-school to School. A Behavioural Study*. London: Academic Press; 1982.

Russell CG, Worsley A. A population based study of preschoolers' food neophobia and its associations with food preferences. *J Nutr Edu Behav*. 2008; **40**: 11–19.

Scaglioni S, Salvioni M, Galimberti C. Influence of parental attitudes in the development of children's eating behaviour. *Br J Nutr*. 2008; 99(Suppl. 1): 22–5.

Singer LT, Ambuel B, Wade S, *et al*. Cognitive-behavioural treatment of health impairing food phobias in children. *J Am Acad Child Adoles Psychiatr*. 1992; **31**: 847–52.

Smith AM, Roux S, Naidoo NT, *et al*. Food choice of tactile defensive children. *Nutrition*. 2005; **21**: 12–19.

Timimi S, Douglas J, Tsiftsopoulou K. Selective eaters: a retrospective case note study. *Child: Care Health Dev.* 1997; **23**: 265–78.

Wardle J, Cooke L. Genetic and environmental determinants of children's food preferences. *Br J Nutr.* 2008; **99**(Suppl 1): 15–21.

Werle MA, Murphy TB, Budd KS. Treating chronic food refusal in young children: home based parent training. *J Appl Behav Anal.* 1993; **26**: 421–33.

Wright CM, Parkinson KN, Shipton D, *et al.* How do toddler eating problems relate to their eating behaviour, food preferences and growth? *Pediatrics.* 2007; **120**: 1069–75.

CHAPTER 10

The management of feeding in children with neurological problems

Sheena Reilly, Angela Morgan and Alison Wisbeach

INTRODUCTION

This chapter will focus on the management of feeding difficulty in children with neurological problems where there is a readily identifiable organic component. In particular, the chapter focuses on the population of children with cerebral palsy. The first section outlines briefly the prevalence and clinical features of feeding difficulties, or dysphagia, in children with cerebral palsy. The second section provides an overview of the principles of assessment for this group, and the third section focuses on management of these problems. We take an integrationist perspective to managing dysphagia in complex disability, recognising that management by a skilled multidisciplinary team is essential.

PREVALENCE AND CLINICAL FEATURES
OF DYSPHAGIA IN CEREBRAL PALSY

Dysphagia is a condition common to many children with neurological impairment. The term 'dysphagia' is used to describe any disorder of swallowing that occurs in the oral, pharyngeal and/or oesophageal stages of deglutition. Subsumed in this definition are problems positioning food in the mouth and in oral movements, including suckling, sucking and chewing. Dysphagia in children with neurological problems rarely arises from one single cause. The aetiology is likely to be multi-factorial (*see* Figure 10.1) and may involve the whole digestive tract. Aetiological factors include gross motor difficulties, problems of the oral, pharyngeal and oesophageal stages

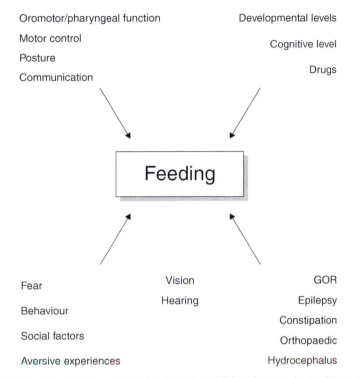

Oromotor/pharyngeal function

Motor control

Posture

Communication

Developmental levels

Cognitive level

Drugs

Feeding

Fear

Behaviour

Social factors

Aversive experiences

Vision

Hearing

GOR

Epilepsy

Constipation

Orthopaedic

Hydrocephalus

FIGURE 10.1: Factors that may affect feeding the child with neurological impairment.

and the process of elimination. Equally important contributory factors include the emotional and psychological aspects of eating and drinking, communication and the preparatory stages of feeding.

Prevalence of dysphagia

Dysphagia may occur as part of a congenital or an acquired condition. It is a particular feature of a number of genetic disorders/ syndromes and of certain types of cerebral palsy. Dysphagia may also arise from insults such as trauma, stroke, brain tumour, infection, metabolic disease and neuro-degenerative conditions. The nature of the resulting problems may be structural, neuromuscular, functional or a combination of all three.

The exact prevalence of dysphagia in many cases remains unknown, as there have been few studies of these conditions. Traumatic brain injury (TBI) is arguably the most common acquired disability of childhood, and dysphagia occurs in up to 68%–72% of children during the acute phase post-trauma (Morgan *et al.*, 2003; Morgan *et al.*, 2010). In many cases, the prognosis for dysphagia following TBI is positive, and typically resolves within a few months following injury (Morgan *et al.*, 2004). However, for children with cerebral palsy, the dysphagia may be present from birth, and the condition may be life-long.

Children with cerebral palsy form the largest group presenting to a tertiary dysphagia clinic (Field *et al.*, 2003). A number of studies have described the nature and extent of dysphagia in cerebral palsy, and the prevalence in children with neurodisability has been reported to range from 58% to 86% (Dahl *et al.*, 1996; Fung *et al.*, 2002; Stallings *et al.*, 1993). However, many studies have been beset by poor methodology, and, in particular, the use of clinical convenience samples rather than whole population studies. A structured mealtime observation was introduced by Reilly *et al.* (1996) and revealed a dysphagia prevalence of 90% in a community cohort of children with cerebral palsy. Most recently, a study by Calis *et al.* (2008) reported a prevalence figure of 99%. Clearly, dysphagia is a common problem and one with potentially deleterious consequences for these children.

Consequences of dysphagia

The consequences of dysphagia are widespread and range in severity. At their most extreme, they may be life threatening. Consequences most commonly associated with cerebral palsy are summarised below.

Failure to thrive

Direct links have been made between reduced calorie intake and poor growth in children with cerebral palsy (Thommessan *et al.*, 1991). Reduced body weight, body protein, linear growth, triceps and subscapular thickness have been found in the majority of children with spastic quadriplegia (Arrowsmith *et al.*, 2006). There are a number of reasons why children with cerebral palsy have difficulty achieving an adequate nutritional intake; whilst adequate calories may be taken, there may be excessive loss due to vomiting and regurgitation (usually as a result of gastro-oesophageal reflux). Caloric intake may be inadequate; oral and pharyngeal function may be so poor that some children may take up to 18 times longer to eat a single mouthful of food. In such cases, even excessively long mealtimes will not compensate for the severity of the dysphagia (Gisel and Patrick, 1988). Whatever the cause, the resulting malnutrition has wide ranging effects that often go beyond physical growth. There may be neuro-developmental consequences for psychomotor development, and brain growth may be directly affected. Furthermore, there are recognised effects on the immune, skeletal and cardiovascular system (Rosenbloom and Sullivan, 1996).

Specific nutrient deficiency

Micro-nutrient deficiencies have been reported in children with cerebral palsy (Patrick and Gisel, 1990). Disabled children are at risk of iron deficiency, especially if their diets are limited to ready prepared baby foods and prolonged use of cows' milk (Rosenbloom and Sullivan, 1996).

Respiratory compromise

Recurrent aspiration in non-ambulant children with neurological disease may result in repeated respiratory tract infections and can eventually lead to chronic pulmonary disease.

Pain and discomfort

Feeding is just one potential cause of pain and discomfort for children with a neurological problem. Many have co-morbid severe communication difficulties, making it vital to consider all the potential sources of pain and discomfort. The presence of gastro-oesophageal reflux can cause pain and irritability as well as damage to the lining of the oesophagus (oesophagitis) resulting in ulceration and bleeding.

Constipation

Constipation is a common problem in cerebral palsy and developmental neuro-disability as a whole (Sullivan, 2008). This may be because of a number of factors including poor fibre and fluid intake, immobility, dysmotility associated with neurological lesions, medication, skeletal anomalies and low tone (Claydon, 1996; Park *et al.*, 2004; Staiano and Del Giudic, 1994). Constipation may be painful and also leads to a decrease in appetite, deterioration in behaviour and concentration, and in some children compromise urinary continence (Claydon, 1996). For further information, the reader is referred to Sullivan (2008).

Dental problems

Both hygiene and structure may be compromised. Dental care may be limited and dental caries therefore develop in children who do not tolerate tooth brushing, cannot completely empty their mouths of food residue and cannot use their tongue to clean particles of food from the teeth or gums. Children who drool excessively are deprived of the cleansing properties of saliva. Some anti-convulsants have an adverse effect on oral hygiene resulting in gingival hyperplasia. Finally, there is an increased incidence of malocculsions (Sandler *et al.*, 1974) and contractures of the temporo-mandibular joint have also been noted in children with spastic quadriplegia (Pelegrano *et al.*, 1994).

Social impact

Mealtimes normally serve an important social function and this may be lost in the child with dysphagia, where the routines, timing and processes associated with feeding may be disturbed. There is no doubt that mealtimes are often stressful occasions for the child, the feeder and the family. Limited empirical data exists reporting on social interaction during mealtimes. In a recent study, the characteristics of mealtime communication between 20 mothers and their children with cerebral palsy (Veness and Reilly, 2008) were documented. Physical, cognitive and feeding abilities varied across this group. The communicative functions used, and method of communication was recorded. Mothers were found to dominate the interactions and used more directive communicative functions than their children. This study highlights that health professionals must consider mealtime interactions as an integral part of the feeding investigation, and in particular to support families in ensuring the child's nutritional demands can be met efficiently so that the parents and the children may enjoy the social aspects of eating.

Clinical characteristics of dysphagia

A recent study of children with severe cerebral palsy by Calis *et al.* (2008) reported that of the 99% of children with dysphagia, 8% had mild dysphagia, 76% moderate to severe dysphagia and 15% profound dysphagia (nil by mouth). At a physiological level, dysphagia may occur due to disruption at one or more of the key stages of feeding, i.e. the oral phase, pharyngeal phase or oesophageal phase. The oral phase involves preparing the food within the oral cavity and transporting it to the back of the mouth in readiness for triggering the swallow. During the pharyngeal phase, food and liquid is moved safely through the pharynx by the swallowing process and transported into the oesophagus (oesophageal stage). Each stage must be considered individually and as an integrated function. An overview of key clinical features of dysphagia for children with cerebral palsy are outlined in Table 10.1 and discussed below.

Oral stage

Oral motor problems are common for children with cerebral palsy, and children with bilateral involvement tend to have more severe oral-motor function (Sullivan, 2008). In a study of pre-school children with cerebral palsy (aged between 12 and 79 months), Reilly *et al.* (1996) found that nine of the ten children had clinically significant oral motor dysfunction. Of this group, more than one third (36.2%) had severe oral motor impairment and these tended to be children with four-limb motor involvement as highlighted in previous studies (Stallings *et al.*, 1993).

Pharyngeal stage

There are few studies that examine the prevalence of pharyngeal stage problems. Gisel (1995) found that 60% of the children assessed with a modified barium swallow were at risk of aspiration.[1]

Oesophageal stage

Oesophageal stage problems are also common; Sondheimer and Morris (1979) evaluated a series of severely affected children and found that up to 75% had

---

[1]Aspiration indicates the passage of food and/or liquid into the airway below the level of the vocal folds. This may occur before during or after swallowing. Penetration is the passage of food/or liquid into the airway but not below the level of the vocal folds.

TABLE 10.1: Clinical features of oral pharyngeal and oesophageal dysphagia in children with cerebral palsy

Physiological stage	Clinical feature
Oral stage	Poor/absent bolus formation
	Poor/absent transportation of bolus
	Poor/absent manipulation of bolus
	Poor/absent tongue lateralisation/elevation etc.
	Poor/absent ability to retain food/liquid bolus within oral cavity
	Poor/absent lip/jaw closure
	Premature overspill into pharynx
Pharyngeal stage	Delayed/absent swallow reflex
	Aspiration/penetration before, during, after swallow
	Incomplete clearance of food/liquid residue
	Pooling of food/liquid in valleculae or pyriform sinus
	Nasal regurgitation
	Poorly co-ordinated ventilatory cycle and swallowing
	Slow pharyngeal transit
	Reduced peristalsis
Oesophageal stage	Gastro-oesophageal reflux
	Oesophageal dysmotility
	Delayed gastric emptying
	Oesophagitis
	Aspiration of GOR

reported gastro-oesophageal reflux.[2] Somerville *et al.* (2009) reported that 270/294 (91%) of children with developmental disability experienced gastro-oesophageal reflux (182 children within this group had cerebral palsy).

ASSESSMENT PRINCIPLES

A comprehensive assessment is crucial to establish a baseline of abilities and difficulties against which change can be measured and as a basis on which to develop treatment regimes. Both the clinical examination and the diagnostic work-up should include assessment of all potential causes of dysphagia in the child with cerebral palsy. As previously highlighted, gastro-oesophageal reflux (GOR) commonly occurs in cerebral palsy and should therefore always be excluded in the child with four-limb involvement. Readers are directed to Sullivan (2008) for further information.

---

[2] Gastro-oesophageal reflux refers to the spontaneous return of the gastric contents into the oesophagus. Gastric contents may be refluxed into the pharynx and cause regurgitation and/or vomiting.

THE MULTI-DISCIPLINARY APPROACH

The multi-factorial nature of dysphagia necessitates the skills and resources of a multi-disciplinary team, and therefore, a large number of professionals may become involved. In order to avoid any confusion or conflicting advice, key workers are recommended to coordinate complex cases.

Assessment procedures

There are a number of areas that should be included in the interview or background to the dysphagia assessment. These are summarised below.

History

As has been emphasised in preceding chapters, a thorough assessment should always start with and include a detailed history. The value of an accurate feeding history cannot be overstated. Nor can it be assumed that the history as described in previous reports is accurate and complete. In some cases, a detailed feeding history may never have been previously established despite the fact that it is critical in understanding the child's current difficulties. The history will naturally focus on feeding, but it is vital that information regarding other aspects of the child's development are also included as they may have particular relevance to the presenting problem (Table 10.2).

As well as information about the history of the problem a clear picture of the current situation is also required and is outlined in Table 10.3.

Clinical examination

The clinical examination should involve both general and specific observations, including observation of the child, a medical and neurological examination as well as evaluation of the child's posture, fine and gross motor abilities and oral and pharyngeal function.

An illustration of the importance of a comprehensive feeding observation is given in the example of Chris.

Chris

In a recent interview, both parents of Chris, a severely disabled boy, reported that he did not vomit and over the years had repeated this to many consultants who had queried if the boy might have had gastro-oesophageal reflux. However, it became clear during the observation that Chris frequently regurgitated and vomited small amounts both throughout and after the meal. This was despite the parent's best efforts to keep him still and upright. When we asked if this was typical, both parents agreed 'he's always like this'; however, they did not recognise that the observed vomiting and regurgitation was abnormal or significant in their son since it had been happening for more than 10 years.

TABLE 10.2: Summary of salient points to be documented in the medical and feeding history

Medical diagnosis	How/when the diagnosis was made Confirmatory tests Known associated impairments What are the child's major difficulties at present
Neonatal history	General concerns Early feeding (methods used) Type and duration of non-oral feeding Establishing oral feeding (difficulties reported) Progression to weaning (difficulties reported) Duration of feeds Vomiting/regurgitation Intervention strategies to date
General medical history	*Developmental history* • Drooling • Motor development • Hearing/vision • Speech/cognitive function *Medical history* • Hospitalisation for significant illness • Surgical procedures (orthopaedic, neurosurgical, etc.) *Review of systems to include* • Respiratory (cough/wheeze/chest infection) • Gastro-intestinal (vomiting/regurgitation) • Mediastinal or abdominal pain/constipation • Neurological – abnormal movements – feed related • General affect – behaviour/sleep, etc. • Seizures • Vision and hearing
Medication	Current (anti-convulsants, laxatives, etc.) Previous trials of treatment (anti- reflux medication, etc.)
Professionals involved	Social Medical Educational
Psychosocial factors	Family structure Support mechanisms

The feeding observation may also alert the clinician to how accurately and sensitively the parent or carer may be interpreting the child's signals during a meal and provides an indicator of how difficult the child is to feed. It may be a useful way of identifying symptoms that the parent has become accustomed to over the years. Parental reports and perceptions may not always match the clinical observation. For example, a study examining the feeding characteristics of a group of pre-school children with cerebral palsy, Reilly *et al.* (1996) found that the children's mealtimes were in reality far shorter than mothers/carers perceived them to be. The more severe the

TABLE 10.3: Specific details to be obtained regarding current feeding

Feeding history	
Current feeding practices	Feeding diary • Typical days intake • Routines • Methods (e.g. who feeds) • Duration/frequency feeds • Tastes/textures
	Oral/non-oral feeding • Ratio oral to non-oral • Bolus vs continuous feeds • Type of tube feed
	Appetite Behaviours and responses at mealtimes
Feeding related issues	Positioning • Special seating • Special routines/equipment/techniques • Who feeds Utensils
Child health and well-being	Sleeping behaviour Bowel habits Growth Respiratory symptoms
Communication	How does the child communicate Does he/she indicate hunger/thirst or pain/discomfort?

child's dysphagia the bigger the discrepancy; children with the more severe problems tended to have the shortest mealtimes. Clearly how questions are asked is very important if clinicians are to elicit accurate information, but there is no substitute for the observation of a mealtime in a child with dysphagia.

Further investigations

Following the clinical examination, some children with dysphagia may require further investigation. Specific groups of children with neurological disease, namely those with four-limb involvement, are at greater risk of dysphagia and are likely to require further investigation of the oral, pharyngeal and oesophageal stages of swallowing. The clinical team may identify clusters of signs and symptoms, which, when combined with the type of cerebral palsy, identify children likely to warrant further investigation.

Where a swallowing abnormality is suspected and aspiration may be a consequence, the existence of any single symptom may warrant further investigation although in the majority of cases there is more than likely to be a cluster of symptoms. Similarly, signs and symptoms suggestive of gastro-oesophageal reflux may be identified during the history taking or the clinical examination and lead to the recommendation of further investigation.

Respiratory signs and symptoms may be indicative of aspiration either as a result of a swallowing problem or as a result of gastro-oesophageal reflux. It can be impossible to differentially diagnose between the two clinically without further investigation. Children presenting with any of the symptoms discussed should be considered for further investigations of their dysphagia.

Co-ordination of results

Throughout this chapter, we highlight the importance of the multi-disciplinary team. It is vital that this approach extends throughout the assessment period and in discussion of the results with the family. A problem-solving approach is necessary; the results may not be clear cut and meaningful management strategies developed in isolation. For example, a decision made solely on the basis of aspiration observed during a modified barium swallow could be very misleading; the barium swallow may not have been representative of the child's normal feeding pattern, and there may be no other evidence or clinical signs and symptoms suggestive of aspiration in the child's history.

The previous section provides an overview of the main difficulties that prevent children with cerebral palsy from achieving an adequate intake of calories and the factors that sometimes make eating and drinking hazardous. It has highlighted the complexity of the problem, the need for a multi-disciplinary team and early diagnosis. Each stage of the feeding process in children with complex dysphagia must be carefully evaluated and then considered as part of the 'whole' picture.

Management of dysphagia

The management of dysphagia in children with neurological problems should begin early in infancy, as soon as problems become evident, and continue throughout childhood and adolescence. Unfortunately, in many instances, children with dysphagia come to the attention of the multi-disciplinary team late in childhood, when crisis management may be necessary. Early intervention is essential, not only for the child's health and well being, but also to help support the child's carers and family members through this process as early as possible. Two critical principles of management that apply to all children include:

- management of dysphagia within the context of the child's other problems
- discussion and agreement of management regimes with parents/carers, other professionals and the child.

In the following section, we focus on the range of problems that might need to be addressed. These include specific management considerations and strategies, including seating and postural considerations, specific feeding strategies for addressing oral motor or pharyngeal phase problems, supplemental feeding decisions, and gastro-esophageal reflux management. The management of feeding in the child with severe and complex neurological problems can also sometimes raise challenging issues for both health professionals and carers, who may not agree on the best treatment course, particularly in reference to the use of tube-feeding.

Sometimes it is necessary to set priorities for management as an intervention is rarely independent in the child with complex and multiple needs. Appropriate seating is almost always a priority to ensure that the child is optimally positioned so that they can feed safely and adequately. A small study by Lanert and Ekberg in 1995 demonstrated that aspiration decreased in children who were positioned with a 30° recline with their necks flexed. As oral-motor control and postural control are very closely related, oral-motor therapy may not be fully instigated until the child's seating needs and equipment have been provided. Its success is almost completely dependent on the child's stable and safe positioning.

Discussion and agreement of regimes with parents/carer givers and the child

Care plans should be discussed openly and fully with parents, care givers and the team. Parents need to be in full agreement with the proposed management regime, understand the rationale behind it and be able to integrate it into home life. The provision of equipment, such as specialised seating, can be costly. If parents are not fully included in the decision-making process about equipment, they may feel it has been imposed on them and they are less likely to use it. This was clearly illustrated in a pilot study of feeding patterns in children with cerebral palsy (Reilly and Skuse, 1992). Only half of the children observed at meal times were actually fed in the seating provided or prescribed by occupational therapists and physiotherapists. As a result, many of the children were very poorly positioned during meal times. Some mothers described the equipment as a nuisance and cumbersome to use; others found it impractical or uncomfortable to use. In just over a quarter of families, the equipment was not used but was stored in a cupboard or another part of the house. Thus, parents need to be partners in treatment decisions.

Decision making

One of the first and often most crucial decisions about feeding children with dysphagia is whether the child can be fed orally. Both the safety and adequacy of oral feeding must be taken into account as well as current dietary management and nutritional requirements. For children unable to achieve an adequate intake via oral means, non-oral methods of feeding might be considered to supplement nutrition taken orally. This may include nasogastric tube-feeds (used for short-term feeding supplementation) or gastrostomy tube-feeding (used for longer-term feeding problems). Decisions regarding the continuation of oral feeding or alternative methods to be used can only be made after a thorough assessment. Failure to do so can result in poor outcome for the child and family.

Positioning and seating

For the child to have the best opportunity to participate in the feeding process, positioning to achieve core stability and optimal head position is essential. This is usually achieved by the provision of a chair. To identify the most suitable seating for the child, it is necessary to assess their physical status and functional abilities. Assessment of physical status will include joint range, particularly of the hips, knees and ankles, shoulder girdle and spine, skin condition, the child's saving and balance reactions, sitting ability, head control and hand use. In addition, it is necessary to assess the child's response to the chair and the child's comfort and safety in the chair. For children with deformities, it is important to identify whether or not these are fixed or mobile, and the plans for their management within the context of the child's overall postural management.

To gain sufficient information to decide on the most appropriate seat, it may be necessary for the child to be seen by a team of professionals who focus on spinal and postural management, since the options for treatment are complex and may include:

- spinal surgery/hip surgery
- spinal bracing
- dynamic Lycra splinting
- special seating
- pressure relief cushioning
- 24-hour postural management.

It is also essential to take into account the physical measurements of the child since this will help in identifying the correct seat size.

The range of potential seating solutions is ever-changing, with new systems being introduced to the market all the time. The principles on which these seats are designed fall broadly into three categories:

- standard seating
- adaptive seating
- moulded seat.

Standard seating

These are conventional seats with support offered only from the seat, backrest and armrests. A child would need to have independent sitting abilities to function in this type of seat. It would generally be unlikely that children with complex dysphagia would have sufficient motor skills to use these types of seats

Adaptive seating

These systems are flexible, offering a variety of support options that can be tailored to the needs of the individual. They comprise individual postural supports within a seat system enabling the individual seat to be customised by selecting size, shape and placement of support.

Moulded seating

These are intimately contoured seats for maximum support and are suitable for children with the most involved movement disorders and/or complex deformities that cannot be accommodated in other forms of seating.

Following evaluation of the child's physical abilities and dimensions as well as their functional needs, the most appropriate type of seating system can be identified. To help select the seat system from within the category, other considerations must be taken into account. These will include the following social and environmental considerations:

- acceptability by the child and carer givers
- reliability
- ease of use
- space within the home/school/social environment
- manoeuvrability
- access to all necessary environments; this will include: steps/stairs, door widths
- transportability in the family, at and school transport and vehicle access
- storage facilities
- heights of tables/chairs for interaction.

Although some children are provided with a chair purely for feeding, it is more usual for the chair to be used for school and leisure activities as well. Once the seating system has been provided and is agreed to be suitable, the child will need to be gradually introduced to the system to give both the child and carers time to accommodate. During this time, observations should be made of the effect stimulation/activity/emotion has on the child's sitting. It may be necessary to make adjustments during this period. Once the child appears comfortable and relaxed in his or her chair, then oral feeding may be introduced. It is important to review the seat regularly to ensure that it continues to meet the child's needs.

MANAGEMENT OF ORAL-SENSORIMOTOR PROBLEMS

Oral-sensorimotor treatment aims to improve the child's oral-motor control of food and liquid. The therapist will identify where there are oral motor deficits and focus on improving control. For example, this might include tongue lateralisation, lip and jaw control and vigour of chewing. Techniques vary widely but have included: physical/manual manipulation of the tongue, lips and jaw in an attempt to encourage chewing and or munching, specific exercises designed to encourage and practise lip-rounding; particular activities to encourage a wider range of tongue movements, such as placing tastes at the outer lip margins; and encouraging the child to lick the substance or placing the food directly on to the teeth in an attempt to encourage chewing. The evidence base for oral-sensorimotor treatment is not extensive, and there are no conclusive studies proving its efficacy. It is difficult to interpret the specific impact of an oral sensorimotor component to feeding intervention in children with cerebral palsy, because published studies usually employ a number of management strategies in parallel (Williams *et al.*, 2007) or are limited by the absence of a control group for comparison (Clawson *et al.*, 2007).

One of the most widely quoted and well-known studies (Ottenbacher *et al.*, 1983) showed no change in oral-motor function or weight gain after a nine-week intensive sensori-motor training period. Erika Gisel (1996) suggested possible explanations for the failure to demonstrate change. First, many studies included children with a range or oral-motor impairments (from mild to severe) and do not focus on a particular group. Second, the specific oral-sensori-motor techniques used in many of the studies varied considerably. Third, different outcomes measures were used to judge success.

Gisel (1996) conducted a methodologically robust study that addressed many of the limitations of other investigations outlined above. She chose a group of children with cerebral palsy defined as having moderate eating impairment to test the efficiency of specific and clearly defined oral-sensori-motor treatment. Gisel compared children who had received oral-sensori-motor treatment with those who did not and the findings are summarised below

- There was no significant decrease in the mean meal-time duration of the treatment groups.
- Some children were able to advance from soft, mashed textures to more solid textures during the treatment period.
- There was no catch-up growth during the treatment period, although the children maintained their weight.

Gisel (1996) argued that longer treatment periods might result in significant change given the trends demonstrated in the study. Although the study demonstrated some benefits to oral-sensori-motor therapy, it is important to weigh up the benefits against the costs. For example, is there a cost in encouraging a more highly textured diet that results in longer meal times for the child with cerebral palsy who is underweight? Common sense tells us that it takes longer to eat foods that require vigorous chewing and that this could fatigue some children. The increased effort and extra time taken (for both the child and carer) to eat more solid foods must be balanced against the child's nutritional requirements, which remain paramount.

Many different oral-sensori-motor techniques have been developed over the years and some of those used for children with neurological impairment are illustrated in Table 10.4. Applying the appropriate management strategy is wholly dependent on understanding the problem, which is only possible after a comprehensive

TABLE 10.4: The management of common oral motor problems in children with dysphagia

Stage	Problem	Management strategy
Oral	Poor absent bolus formation	Modify texture – deliver a cohesive bolus that does not spread throughout the oral cavity
	Poor/absent transportation of bolus	Place bolus carefully within the oral cavity to facilitate swallow initiation*
	Poor/absent manipulation of bolus	Dependent on texture therefore modify texture as necessary and consider bolus placement
	Poor/absent tongue lateralisation/ elevation, etc.	Place food directly on to molars of gum margins
		Avoid food which required munching and/or chewing if child is not able to manage safely
	Poor/absent ability to retain food/liquid bolus within oral cavity	Consider total body position, in particular head and neck position. Modify seating if necessary, to avoid loss due to gravity
		Modify texture – thicker textures may result in reduced loss as compared to liquids Consider bolus placement
	Poor/absent lip closure	Modify position – ensure child has postural stability
		Assist with manual lip closure
	Poor/absent jaw closure	Modify position – ensure child has postural stability
		Provide jaw support
	Lumps swallowed whole	Place food directly on to molars
		Avoid
	Lumps manipulated but not masticated	Avoid
	Lumps remain stationary on the tongue	Avoid
		Try placing food on to molars
	Premature overspill into pharynx	Modify texture – thicken to slow down passage of bolus
		Alter method of delivery to slow down pace

*This can only be achieved if there is sufficient mouth opening and the child is tolerant of posterior bolus placement.

assessment. Oral motor treatment strategies must be applied in conjunction with managing posture and position for eating and drinking. For example, traditional methods for managing poor lip closure include the provision of jaw support while firmly helping to keep the lips closed using the therapist's fingers. The technique was often not successful because the therapist was treating only the most visible component of the problem. Providing manual lip closure will not be successful in the child with a malocclusion (because of the structural abnormality). Similarly, in a child with postural instability, correction may permit the child to develop jaw stability without the need for manual lip and jaw assistance.

Children with cerebral palsy may have difficulty retaining food and/or liquid in the mouth. The child's posture may be such that gravity contributes to liquid/food loss. Structural abnormalities, such as malocclusions or fixed contractures for the jaw, may make closure impossible or very difficult. They may not be able to collect up the liquid/food placed in the mouth. Limited tongue movements (e.g. extension and retraction movements only) might result in some of the liquid/food being accidentally expelled. The problem may be texture specific; that is, there may be greater loss with liquids than with solids. The inability to transport the bolus through the oral cavity may result in the food/liquid remaining on the front of the tongue until it is expelled or falls out.

These examples illustrate that there can be many reasons underlying the presenting oral-motor problem. It is therefore necessary to manage such problems not only from a multi-disciplinary perspective but also to be aware that there may be multiple factors contributing to the presenting problem.

MANAGEMENT OF PHARYNGEAL DYSPHAGIA

In 95% of the referred sample of children with cerebral palsy studied by Mirrett *et al.* (1994), the oral- and pharyngeal-stage problems occurred independently of each other. When a child has difficulty controlling a bolus in the oral stage, this can result in premature overspill into the pharynx and aspiration may occur prior to the swallow being triggered. However, if the oral stage can be controlled (e.g. by slowing down the bolus, changing posture and improving bolus formation), aspiration may be prevented, and the pharyngeal stage may progress well with no obvious dysphagia. It is important therefore to carefully evaluate each stage to ascertain if both stages are affected and, if so, to what extent. Equally, it is important to understand how a deficit in the oral stage may result in significant pharyngeal problems.

Given that the consequences of pharyngeal-stage dysphagia can affect morbidity and mortality, by definition, the strategies employed are more aggressive and it is often necessary to consider non-oral methods of feeding sooner rather than later. Table 10.5 outlines the most common pharyngeal-stage problems and management strategies are suggested.

MANAGEMENT OF OESOPHAGEAL-STAGE PROBLEMS
Medical management

The presence of GOR and/or constipation requires consultation with a paediatrician and/or gastroenterologist. A phased therapeutic approach to the management of GOR is recommended by Vanenplas *et al.* (1993) and Lloyd and Pierro (1996).

TABLE 10.5: The management of pharyngeal dysphagia in children with cerebral palsy

Stage	Problem	Management strategy
Pharyngeal	Aspiration/penetration before swallow	Improve bolus formation in the oral stage, by modifying texture, pacing delivery and altering bolus size
		Alter head position to change calibre of airway. Chin tuck may be useful
	Aspiration/penetration during swallow	Alter head position to change calibre of airway. Chin tuck may be useful
		Change utensil – an angled bottle is sometimes useful
		Supraglottic swallow might be useful for children who are cognitively able
	Aspiration/penetration after swallow	Dry swallow to clear pharyngeal residue
		Liquids may be given to clear residue if safe
		Modify consistency – feed foods that cause least amount of residue and pooling
		Encourage non-nutritive sucking after swallow Palatal training devices reported to be useful
	Absent swallow reflex	Do not feed orally
	Delayed swallow reflex	Improve bolus formation in the oral stage, by modifying texture, pacing delivery and altering bolus size
		Thermal stimulation is useful in some situations
	Pooling of food/liquid in valleculae or pyriform sinus	Alter head position to decrease size of valleculae thus reducing likelihood of pooling – use with caution
	Reduced pharyngeal peristalsis	Modify texture
	Nasal regurgitation	Alter head position
		Modify texture – avoid those which cause significant regurgitation
		Palatal training device
	Delayed/absent cricopharyngeal relaxation	Surgical – cricopharyngeus
		Botulinum toxin injections
	Poorly coordinated ventilator cycle and swallowing	Discourage post-swallow inspiration
		Supraglottic swallow

Three phases are outlined: in phase 1, attention is given to position, dietary advice and thickening agents. Traditionally, thickening feeds and the maintenance of an upright position after feeds were encouraged; however, these are no longer thought to be effective in children with neurological disorder. In addition, antacids may be used to neutralise the gastric acid.

In phase 2, treatments aimed at increasing the tone of the lower oesophageal sphincter and enhancing gastric emptying may be added. A further aim is to reduce acid production. Some children with neuro-disability fail to respond to medical management of GOR as may be illustrated by the persistence or worsening of symptoms. Surgical management is sometimes required. It is a major undertaking and not without potential complications in the child with multiple and complex disabilities. There are a number of different surgical procedures and descriptions may be found in a variety of sources (Lloyd and Pierro, 1996; Sullivan, 2008).

Nutritional intervention

Nutritional therapy should be part of the child's comprehensive care and rehabilitation. It aims not only to improve weight and linear growth but to improve physiological and functional capacity. Caloric requirements are usually estimated from recommended daily allowances (RDAs). However, RDAs assume normal levels of activity and are therefore not always appropriate for children with complex and multiple disabilities. There are a variety of methods used to calculate energy requirements in the child with complex and multiple disabilities. Some clinicians recommend that energy requirements be based on the RDA for their height, age or their weight at the 25th percentile weight for height. Others recommend determining basal metabolic rates that are corrected for activity levels, such as the World Health Organization formulae that allow for more individualised prediction based on gender, age and body weight as well as accounting for activity levels.

It is crucial that a paediatric dietician experienced in the management of children with multiple and complex needs be part of the team to evaluate and establish nutritional plans for each child. Monitoring these plans is of vital importance to ensure that children reach the expected growth targets. However, in the case of some children, particularly those who are gastrostomy fed, it may be necessary to ensure that they do not exceed weight targets (Sullivan *et al.*, 2006).

Utensils

Part of managing dysphagia, particularly the oral phase, involves modifying the manner in which food and/or liquid is delivered and placed in the mouth. This often means experimenting with different types of cup and spoon. As a general rule non-metallic utensils are advised for the child's comfort and safety. Spoons and cups should be non-breakable, as some children may bite on the spoon or glass, which can be dangerous. In addition, cold metallic spoons can be uncomfortable and cause pain if not placed carefully, coming in contact with sensitive teeth or sore mouths. The sudden, uncontrolled movements of some children mean that teeth and gums can contact painfully with metallic utensils despite the caregivers best efforts.

For the young child who is capable of sucking from a bottle, there are a range of teats available, including vented teats that help prevent air-swallowing. Soft, squeeze bottles, such as the Mead Johnson (used for babies with cleft lip and palate), may also help when the suck is weak. Care needs to be taken not to flood the baby's mouth and pharynx. However, for many babies with cerebral palsy, the suck is so weak that this becomes an inefficient method of feeding when the energy and time spent on feeding are measured against the effort. For this reason, early cup feeding is often appropriate. Small, plastic, medicine cups or soft, flexible cups are often very useful. Alternatively, soft trainer spouts are now available, and providing the baby can manage the flow of liquid they can be very successful. The liquid may also be thickened if necessary to slow the flow.

A wide range of spoons is also available, in various shapes, bowl depths, sizes and material. The type chosen depends largely on the individual child. Small tea-spoons coated with a soft plastic are often suitable for the young child taking his or her first solids. Weaning spoons, some with flat bowls and others with deep bowls, with either long- or short-handles are also helpful. Spoons made of bone are also available and suit the requirements of certain children, although they are costly and can be hard to find. Bowl size should be determined by the size of the child's mouth. For children aversive to spoons or those taking very small tastes of food, small plastic spatulas can be used.

Self-feeding

For some children with cerebral palsy independence in self-feeding is not possible. Both Reilly *et al.* (1996) and Thomas *et al.* (1989) found that a high proportion of individuals with cerebral palsy (60% and 56% respectively) had major difficulties in self-feeding. Decisions to introduce self-feeding must be carefully assessed in conjunction with assessment of joint mobility, balance and type of seating. While encouraging independence at meal times is desirable, it must be carefully balanced against an individual's nutritional needs and the time taken to feed. For some children the effort to maintain postural stability and initiate hand-to-mouth actions can cause a decrease in oral-motor control and result in loss of food and/or liquid.

Some children are determined to self-feed. To achieve maximum independence, careful consideration should be given to their posture and position. The relationship of the table and/or tray to the child is vital. It must be of the correct height and position; this is especially important if the child is to stabilise or fix one arm on the tray while feeding with the other. Reach, grasp and hand-to-mouth ability require careful evaluation, and modification of equipment and position may be necessary to accommodate any difficulties. The pace of feeding and delivery of food often change when a child begins to self-feed and it may be necessary to provide verbal prompts to encourage the child to take one to two mouthfuls before pausing. Similarly, head position may alter during self-feeding by the child extending their head further back as the spoon approaches, resulting in increased oromotor difficulties and potential aspiration. All these aspects of self-feeding require monitoring if the child is going to be able to feed safely and take in an adequate amount. It may of course be necessary to continue a combination of dependent and independent feeding and it is sometimes helpful to target less potentially stressful times, such as snack periods, to encourage self-feeding.

Communication/behaviour/interaction

There are many reasons why difficulty communicating complicates the feeding problems in children with neurodevelopmental problems. Owing to severely delayed and/or disordered speech development, many children are unable to request food or drink, make their preferences known, tell if food is offered too fast or too slow, or explain how the process feels. Imagine yourself unable to let your feeder know that you loathe spinach, yet you find it is on the menu every lunch-time! Some children can communicate either verbally or non-verbally (e.g. eye-pointing and gestures), but their attempts may not be easily interpreted. Awareness and sensitivity to the child's method of communication is therefore important. This should include being aware of any non-verbal messages such as change in the child's facial expression, body posture and mood. Understanding and attending to communicative behaviours is time-consuming and demanding for the feeder, who must remember to give the child choices and create opportunities for communication. When not given some means of communication it is not surprising that children develop 'difficult' behaviour at meal times.

Through careful assessment the team should aim to eliminate the possibility of any underlying organic deficit for food refusals and other aversive behaviours evident at meals times. Feeding children with dysphagia can be stressful for their parents and carers and is often not a pleasant experience (*see* Sullivan *et al.*, 2004; Veness and Reilly, 2008 for further reading). Children may cough and choke excessively, lose a large proportion of each mouthful, and regurgitate and vomit feeds. In many cases mothers remain solely responsible for feeding their child, adding to the already considerable burden of care.

Non-oral feeding

The safety of oral feeding is essential. It is often the most pressing issue yet also the most difficult to evaluate and mange in children with dysphagia. The result of the clinical examination, dietetics evaluation, videofluoroscopy and chest X-ray contribute to the decision-making process. In children with neurodevelopmental disorders it is sometimes necessary to consider non-oral methods of feeding. Factors which may contribute to the decision-making process are listed below.

- The child is unable to consume adequate calories orally to meet energy requirements
- There is evidence of ongoing aspiration leading to respiratory complications during oral feeding
- Oral feeding is stressful for either the carer or the child or both
- Meal times are protracted leaving limited time for other daily activities
- Oral supplementation of the diet has failed
- Chronic food refusal or aversive behaviour has developed
- Oral intake is erratic
- Child needs safe route for regular medication (e.g. anti-convulsants)

NASOGASTRIC AND GASTROSTOMY FEEDING

Nasogastric tubes enter the gastrointestinal tract via the nose. Recent developments have resulted in the availability of a much larger range of tubes, which are easier to insert and can be left in situ for longer periods. Nasogastric feeding is often the first choice if enteral feeding is required because it is less invasive and viewed as a temporary measure. Either continuous or bolus feeds may be given and the tube can be used to top up or supplement oral intake (*see* Chapter 11).

Ideally nasogastric tubes should be used for short-term feeding and if prolonged tube-feeding is required then gastrostomy feeding should be considered. Gastrostomy tubes can be placed via a variety of techniques (Sullivan, 2008). The indications for gastrostomy insertion are the same as those already highlighted for tube-feeding. For further reading regarding outcomes for children with CP following longitudinal gastrostomy feeding (Craig *et al.*, 2003, 2006; Sullivan, 2008; Sullivan *et al.*, 2005, 2006).

Protocols for managing unsafe oral feeding

The management of aspiration challenges all clinicians working with dysphagic children and their families. It is important to remember that aspiration is a symptom of dysphagia and not a condition in itself. There is much that we do not understand about managing children who aspirate. However, there is no doubt that it should never be managed in isolation. The whole child must be considered in decision-making and management strategies implemented with the knowledge and agreement of the whole team. Wolf and Glass (1992) established four treatment strategies for infants and children who aspirate. These have been adapted and modified for use clinically (*see* Table 10.6) with children who have complex and multiple disabilities. They help to form the basis for decision making regarding oral feeding and provide a rationale for the approach adopted for the child's parents, carers and other professionals.

TABLE 10.6: Protocols for managing 'unsafe' feeding

Protocol 1	Unrestricted oral feeding • No aspiration/penetration • Trace aspiration/penetration (material cleared from airway) • No history of chest infections • Chest X-ray clear • Good pulmonary status
Aim	Monitor oral and pharyngeal skills and respiratory function May be for trial period
Protocol 2	Restricted oral feeding allowed • Aspiration/penetration observed but texture specific (e.g. liquids only) • Material may/may not be cleared from airway • Respiratory status not compromised • Good parental compliance
Aim	Eliminate texture aspirated or modify so safe. Improve and maintain oral and pharyngeal skills giving as wide a range of tastes and textures as possible. Depending on severity, nutritional intake may be supplemented non-orally.
Protocol 3	Therapeutic swallowing trials and/or tastes • Significant aspiration for more than one texture (material not cleared) • Frequent chest infections • Chest X-ray findings consistent with recurrent aspiration • Improvement expected with improved positioning/treatment of GOR, etc.
Aim	Maintain oral skills, improve swallowing control and minimise tactile aversions. Non-oral feeding required possibly long term
Protocol 4	Eliminate oral feeding • Significant aspiration for all food textures • No attempt to clear material from airway/depressed cough • Frequent chest X-rays/pneumonia • Chest X-ray evidence consistent with recurrent pneumonia • Evidence of micro-aspiration
Aim	Maintain oral skills and minimise tactile aversions. Non-oral feeding probably required long term

CONCLUSION

In 1989 Martin Bax, a distinguished paediatrician, wrote an editorial entitled 'Feeding is important'. He asked why 'feeding', in particular how to get food into young children, had received such scant attention in the paediatric medical literature. He suggested that this apparent neglect might be attributed to the fact that the topic was adequately covered in general childcare books and was therefore not seen as a 'respectable' one worthy of attention in paediatric textbooks. Many years later professional attitudes to feeding the disabled child have changed significantly. Clinicians are now aware of the importance of ensuring that children with cerebral palsy are adequately nourished.

This has resulted in the adoption of a variety of different management strategies, including the increasing use of surgical placement of feeding tubes.

However, these changes have raised clinical dilemmas for clinicians regarding nutritional intervention in children with severe cerebral palsy. Stronger evidence for decision making is urgently required (*see* series of case studies presented by Cass *et al.*, 2005). The use of gastrostomy feeding in this population of children seems to have become a particularly contentious issue for both professionals and parents. In discussing the ethics and implications of treatment programmes for disabled children with feeding problems, Rosenbloom and Sullivan (1996) suggested that:

> 'The provision of appropriate nutrition has to be set within the context of their overall needs, their prognosis and the perceptions and wishes of their parents and other carers'.

Clearly there is a range of complex issues for parents, carers and the professionals involved with the child's care. It is beyond the scope of this chapter to discuss these in detail and the reader is referred to Sullivan *et al.* (2004), Sleigh *et al.* (2005) and Stoner *et al.* (2006) for further information. It is vital that clinicians working with children who have cerebral palsy are familiar with the complex management issues that may arise.

ACKNOWLEDGEMENTS

This chapter condenses two chapters prepared for the first edition of this book. We sincerely thank Dr Lucinda Carr, Consultant Paediatric Neurologist at Great Ormond Street Hospital, for her contribution to the earlier chapters and acknowledge her contribution.

REFERENCES

Arrowsmith FE, Allen JR, Gaskin KJ, *et al.* Reduced body protein in children with spastic quadriplegic cerebral palsy. *Am J Clin Nutr.* 2006; **83**: 613–18.

Calis EAC, Veugelers R, Sheppard JJ, *et al.* Dysphagia in children with severe generalized cerebral palsy and intellectual disability. *Dev Med Child Neurol.* 2008; **50**: 625–30.

Cass H, Wallis C, Ryan M, *et al.* Assessing pulmonary consequences of dysphagia in children with neurological disabilities: when to intervene? *Dev Med Child Neurol.* 2005; **47**(5): 347–52.

Clawson EP, Kuchinski KS, Bach R. Use of behavioral interventions and parent education to address feeding difficulties in young children with spastic diplegic cerebral palsy. *Neuro Rehabil.* 2007; **22**: 397–406.

Claydon G. Constipation in disabled children. In: Rosenbloom L, Sullivan P, editors. *Feeding the Disabled Child. Clin Dev Med.* 1996; **140**: 106–16.

Craig GM, Carr LJ, Cass H, *et al.* Medical, surgical, and health outcomes of gastrostomy feeding. *Dev Med Child Neurol.* 2006; 48: 353–60.

Craig GM, Scambler G, Spitz L. Why parents of children with neurodevelopmental disabilities requiring gastrostomy feeding need more support. *Dev Med Child Neurol.* 2003; 45: 183–8.

Dahl M, Thomessen M, Rasmussen M, *et al.* Feeding and nutritional characteristics in children with moderate or severe cerebral palsy. *Acta Paediatr.* 1996; b: 697–701.

Field D, Garland M, Williams K. Correlates of specific childhood feeding problems. *J Paediatr Child Hlth.* 2003; 39(4): 299–304.

Fung EB, Samson-Fang L, Stallings VA, *et al.* Feeding dysfunction is associated with poor growth and health status in children with cerebral palsy. *J Am Diet Assoc.* 2002; **102**: 361–8, 373.

Gisel EG. Effect of sensorimotor treatment on measures of growth and efficiency of eating in the moderately eating-impaired child with cerebral palsy. *Dysphagia.* 1996; 11: 59–71.

Gisel EG, Applegate-Ferrante T, Benson JE, *et al.* Effect of oral sensorimotor treatment on measures of growth, eating efficiency and aspiration in the dysphagic child with cerebral palsy. *Dev Med Child Neurol.* 1995; 37(6): 528–43.

Gisel EG, Patrick J. Identification of children with cerebral palsy unable to maintain a normal nutritional state. *Lancet.* 1988; 1: 283–6.

Lloyd DA, Pierro A. The therapeutic approach to the child with feeding difficulty: III Enteral feeding. In: Rosenbloom L, Sullivan P, editors. *Feeding the Disabled Child. Clin Dev Med. No. 140.* London: MacKeith Press; 1996. pp. 132–50.

Mirrett PL, Riski JE, Glascott MA, *et al.* Videofluoroscopic assessment of dysphagia in children with severe spastic cerebral palsy. *Dysphagia.* 1994; 9: 174–9.

Morgan AT, Mageandran SD, Mei C. Incidence and clinical presentation of dysarthria and dysphagia in the acute setting following paediatric traumatic brain injury. *Child Care Health Dev.* 2010; 36(1): 44–53.

Morgan AT, Skeat J. Evaluating service delivery for speech and swallowing problems following paediatric brain injury: an international survey. *J Eval Clin Pract.* In press.

Morgan AT, Ward E, Murdoch B, *et al.* Incidence, characteristics and predictive factors for dysphagia following paediatric traumatic brain injury. *J Head Trauma Rehabil.* 2003; 18(3): 239–51.

Morgan AT, Ward EC, Murdoch BE. Clinical progression and outcome of pediatric dysphagia following traumatic brain injury. *Brain Injury.* 2004; 18(4): 359–76.

Ottenbacher K, Bundy A, Short MA. The development and treatment of oral motor dysfunction: a review of clinical research. *Phys Occup Ther Pediatr.* 1983; 3: 147–60.

Park ES, Park CI, Cho SR, *et al.* Colonic transit time and constipation in children with spastic cerebral palsy. *Arch Phys Med Rehabil.* 2004; 85: 453–6.

Patrick J, Gisel EJ. Nutrition for the feeding impaired child. *J Neurol Rehabil.* 1990; 4: 115–19.

Pelegrano JP, Nowysz S, Goesfered S. Temporomnandibular joint contractures in spastic quadriplegia: effect on oral motor skills. *Dev Med Child Neurol.* 1994; 36: 487–94.

Reilly S, Skuse D. Characteristics and management of feeding problems in young children with cerebral palsy. *Dev Med Child Neurol.* 1992; 34: 379–88.

Reilly S, Skuse D, Poblete X. Prevalence of feeding problems and oral motor dysfunction in children with cerebral palsy: a community survey. *J Pediatr.* 1996 Dec; **129**(6): 877–82.

Reilly S, Skuse DH, Poblete X. The prevalence of feeding problems in pre-school children with Cerebral Palsy. *J Pediatr.* 1996; 877–82.

Rosenbloom L, Sullivan P, editors. Feeding the disabled child. *Clin Dev Med. No. 140.* London: MacKeith Press; 1996. pp. 1–10.

Sandler ES, Roberts MW, Wojcicki AM, *et al.* Oral manifestations in a group of mentally retarded patients. *J Dent Child.* 1974; **41:** 207–11.

Sleigh G. Mothers' voice: a qualitative study on feeding children with cerebral palsy. *Child Care Hlth Dev.* 2005; **31**(4): 373–83.

Somerville H, Tzannes G, Wood J, *et al.* Gastrointestinal and nutritional problems in severe developmental disability. *Dev Med Child Neurol.* 2009; **50:** 712–16.

Sondheimer JM, Morris BA. Gastro-eosophageal reflux among severely retarded children. *J Pediatr.* 1979; **94:** 710–14.

Staiano A, Del Giudice E. Colonic transit and anorectal manometry in children with severe brain damage. *Pediatrics.* 1994; **94:** 169–73.

Stallings VA, Charney EB, Davies JC, *et al.* Nutrition related growth failure of children with quadriplegic cerebral palsy. *Dev Med Child Neurol.* 1993; **35:** 126–38.

Stoner JB, Bailey RL, Angell ME, *et al.* Perspectives of parents/guardians of children with feeding/swallowing problems. *J Dev Phys Disabil.* 2006; **18**(4): 333–53.

Sullivan PB. Gastrointestinal disorders in children with neurodevelopmental disabilities. *Dev Disabil Res Rev.* 2008; **14**(2): 128–36.

Sullivan PB, Juszczak E, Allison ME, *et al.* Impact of gastrostomy tube feeding on the quality of life of carers of children with cerebral palsy. *Dev Med Child Neurol.* 2004; **46**(12): 796–800.

Sullivan PB, Juszczak E, Bachlet AM, *et al.* Gastrostomy tube feeding in children with cerebral palsy: a prospective, longitudinal study. *Dev Med Child Neurol.* 2005; **47:** 77–85.

Sullivan PB, Morrice JS, Vernon-Roberts A, *et al.* Does gastrostomy tube feeding in children with cerebral palsy increase the risk of respiratory morbidity? *Arch Dis Child.* 2006; **91:** 478–2.

Thomas AP, Bax MCO, Smyth D. The health and social needs of young adults with physical disabilities. *Clin Dev Med. No. 106.* London: MacKeith Press; 1989.

Thommessan M, Heiberg A, Kase BF, *et al.* Feeding problems, height and weight in different groups of disabled children. *Acta Paediatr Scand.* 1991; **80:** 527–33.

Vanenplas Y, Ashkenazi A, Bellie D, *et al.* A proposition for the diagnosis and treatment of gastro-oesophageal reflux disease in children: a report from a working group on gastro-oesophageal reflux disease. *Eur J Pediatr.* 1993; **152:** 704–11.

Veness C, Reilly S. Mealtime interaction patterns between young children with cerebral palsy and their mothers: characteristics and relationship to feeding impairment. *Child Care Health Dev.* 2008; **43**(6): 815–24.

Williams KE, Riegel K, Gibbons B, *et al.* Intensive behavioral treatment for severe feeding problems: a cost-effective alternative to tube feeding? *J Dev Phys Disabil.* 2007; **19:** 227–35.

Wolf LS, Glass RP. *Feeding and Swallowing Disorders in Infancy: assessment and management.* Tuscon, Az: Therapy Skill Builders; 1992.

CHAPTER 11

Interventions with children who are tube fed

Mandy Bryon

INTRODUCTION

Feeding and eating difficulties in young children are common, with reports of more than 20% in infants with normal development and up to 90% in children with special needs (Clawson *et al.*, 2008; Reau *et al.*, 1996) – so common that it is more appropriate to differentiate between 'normal feeding difficulties' and 'severe feeding difficulties'. Children who are tube fed would appear to be at the severe end of the spectrum. However, infants and young children may require all or some of their nutrition delivered artificially via a tube for one basic reason – they are unable to consume sufficient calories orally to maintain adequate growth. The reason why these children cannot consume sufficient calories, of course, can vary widely, but the point is that tube feeding is a simple solution to a potentially serious problem. It is, therefore, likely to be an increasingly common phenomenon seen in local clinics, and not just in major paediatric centres. Although complex feeding difficulties ought to be treated by a multi-disciplinary specialist team, it is the case that increasingly primary care medical practitioners are developing skills to make thorough and complex assessment of feeding difficulties (Bernard-Bonnin, 2006).

Tube feeding is the delivery of a liquid nutritional formula to the infant or child by a tube. The place of entry of the tube varies according to the physical condition of the child and the length of time tube feeding is planned. The four different types of tube feeding are:

1 nasogastric (NG) tube-feeding where a tube is passed through the nose and into the stomach
2 nasojejunum (NJ) tube-feeding where a tube is passed through the nose into some other part of the gut, e.g. the jejunum

3   gastrostomy feeding where a tube is passed, surgically, into the stomach with the
    end protruding from the surface of the body
4   total parenteral nutrition (TPN) where a tube is passed directly into the blood
    stream.

A more inclusive medical description and rationale of tube feeding is described by
Milla (2007). The decision to feed a child via a tube is a medical decision and such
children often have a physical condition that makes oral feeding or absorption of
nutrition deficient or impossible.

Tube feeding can be prescribed in conjunction with a wide range of paediatric
organic conditions (Hans *et al.*, 2009; Linscheid *et al.*, 1995), and many chronic
diseases invariably require some form of tube feeding (Joffe *et al.*, 2009). Some, relatively common, gastroenterological conditions may require temporary tube feeding, e.g. gastroenteritis, recurrent vomiting and gastro-oesophageal reflux. Other
medical conditions result in tube feeding because the illness reduces appetite, and
good nutritional status is important to reduce the degenerative progress of the disease, e.g. cystic fibrosis. In some cases, the medical condition will prevent oral feeding from ever occurring, or from being the sole source of nutrition. For others, the
period of tube feeding is temporary, and oral feeding can begin following medical
go-ahead. Some children are tube fed for non-organic failure to thrive, and, in these
cases, oral introduction of food can begin immediately following accurate diagnosis. Although these children will not have physical incapacity for oral intake, their
restricted experience can result in difficulties accepting food orally.

When an infant or child has received nutrition via a tube for a period of time significant in relation to their age, the transfer to oral feeding appears to be problematic
in the majority of cases (Davis *et al.*, 2009). An evaluation of feeding dysfunction
following tube feeding in children with chronic renal failure was carried out by
Strologo *et al.* (1997). Persistent feeding problems identified were food refusal, difficulties chewing and swallowing and 'panic attacks' when swallowing.

Clinical experience also supports the descriptions in the literature of feeding difficulty following tube feeding. The feeding programme for young children at Great
Ormond Street Hospital for Children in London offers assessment and treatment
for a range of feeding difficulties. An attempt to classify feeding difficulties produced
some differentiation but no mutually exclusive categories indicating the complexity
of these problems. Types of feeding difficulty reported included inadequate quantity
eaten, selective eating, refusing to chew or swallow, slow eating and inappropriate
texture for age. One-third of all the children seen had experienced tube feeding in
the first six months of life, and many more had experienced a period of tube feeding
at some stage in their pre-school years (Douglas and Bryon, 1996). The indication
is that tube-feeding is prescribed for a wide range of feeding difficulties in children
with the corresponding implication that a proportion of these children will have
difficulties with consequent oral intake.

Despite the wide prevalence of tube feeding in the paediatric population and the difficulties of resuming oral feeding following medical decision to terminate tube nutrition, there is scant attention paid to this problem in the literature. There are no studies that lead to empirical hypotheses for food refusal following tube removal and few references to descriptions of the problems and treatment interventions. This chapter focuses on clinical experience of interventions following tube feeding for children and the treatment is described by case illustration.

WHY DO CHILDREN FOOD REFUSE FOLLOWING TUBE FEEDING?

Is it possible to speculate why children find acceptance of oral feeding difficult following a period of tube feeding? It is important that this question is explored as it allows more adequate understanding of the problem. Any valid areas can then form the basis of assessment for an individual child and family, which will inform appropriate intervention.

MISSED CRITICAL PERIOD

Tube feeding in infancy will restrict experience of oral feeding but to what extent is this disruption significant for the development of feeding skills? Theories of critical periods for the acquisition of skill have been mostly dispensed with as recent studies have thrown doubt on the stage model of development and demonstrated that child development is a complex process of physical, cognitive and experiential influences. There have been few studies that have examined the development of oral-motor function following periods of tube feeding in infants. However, research that has examined the development of sucking, swallowing and breathing in term and pre-term infants may throw some light on this area. Results of these studies indicate that adequate neuromuscular co-ordination is more a function of gestational maturity than of postnatal sucking experience (Roig-Quilis and Rodríguez-Palmero, 2008). Whilst not directly answering the question, the suggestion is that oral-motor capability is more strongly determined centrally (i.e. neurologically) than locally via oral experience.

The notion of critical period may not have a major bearing on the infants' refusal of oral intake following tube feeding but does the experience of tube feeding itself interfere with the child's developing expectations of feeding behaviour? There is some evidence that the type of feeding established in early infancy influences the child's demands for food at later stages (Vohr et al., 2006). It has been found that breast- versus bottle-fed babies differ in the amounts of feed taken at various times of the day with breast-fed babies being more likely than the bottle-fed babies to control the amount of feed taken themselves. Tube-fed babies have no control over their intake and as such, there may be subtle, yet pervasive, effects on the infant's experience of the success of their interactions with their environment.

EXPERIENCE OF HUNGER AND APPETITE REGULATION

Clinical experience suggests that parents frequently make the observation that their tube-fed infants never cry for food. Disinterest in food was reported in 63% of pre-school children referred for feeding difficulties (Douglas and Bryon, 1996). Non-tube-fed infants without feeding issues will attract carer attention by crying, exhibit restlessness and execute seeking movements toward the food (Delaney and Arvedson, 2008). As the nature of tube feeding is to ensure adequate nutrition for the infant's physical size, the infant has no control over the amount of the feed nor spacing between intake as have normal infants, although good practice tries to mimic natural regulation. It can be hypothesised therefore that tube-fed infants neither learn to identify the physical sensations of hunger nor do they develop a repertoire of behaviours to signal hunger cues to their carers. In turn, the carers cease to interpret behaviours in their infant that would normally signal hunger.

In many cases, tube feeds are given according to a regimen that does not match normal appetite patterns. Often tube feeds are prescribed to be given continuously as a drip overnight (pump-feeders for home use are widely available). The rationale here is to leave the day free for the possibility of normal appetite occurring. Some children and infants are prescribed feeds throughout the day in order to maintain adequate nutrition irrespective of natural appetite patterns. The overall result is that tube-fed babies and children do not have access to their body's physical regulation of hunger, they do not recognise the drive and they do not develop behaviours which indicate an active participation in feeding and appetite control.

FEAR OF FOOD AND AVERSIVE ASSOCIATIONS

All tube-fed children will have some physical disturbance of their normal alimentary processes. Many of these children would have had experience of pain and/or vomiting in association with feeding. Some would have undergone invasive medical intervention and may have chronic medical conditions for which such investigations will continue. On introduction of oral feeding, it has been reported that disturbances of chewing and swallowing are observed (Strologo *et al.*, 1997). It may be that these arise from a reluctance to accept oral food but, whatever the reason, it is almost inevitable that further failure to adequately ingest the food will maintain the aversive association.

> ### Paul
>
> Paul was referred by his nephrologist for refusal to eat orally. He was aged 3 years at referral and lived with both natural parents and an older sister aged 5 years. Paul was born with dysplastic kidneys; he had been exclusively tube-fed from birth and had received dialysis. He had received a kidney transplant at 2 years of age and following recovery from the operation oral feeding was attempted. Paul had refused any food and would cry and gag at the sight of food intended for him.

There are other aversive associations of the experience of tube-feeding itself, which are reported clinically though not in the literature. It may be that the position of a NG tube interferes with olfactory senses that affect appetite. Additionally, the experience of receiving a tube feed via both NG and gastrostomy tubes in some cases cause physical discomfort such as bloating, flatulence and hyperglycaemic symptoms. For these infants and children receiving nutrition via any source has strong aversive associations.

Megan

Megan was referred by her GP for refusal of oral solids and liquids. Megan was aged 19 months and lived with both her natural parents; she was an only child. Megan was born full-term, normal delivery but had meconium aspiration; she spent one week in SCBU where she was nasogastrically tube-fed. Megan was then discharged home on a mixture of breast- and bottle-feeding. She was slow to feed and did not gain weight. At 18 days, she began vomiting her feeds; investigations revealed pyloric stenosis, and she underwent corrective surgery. At 4 months of age, Megan was readmitted to hospital for food refusal and NG tube feeding recommenced. The ensuing months were marked by a constant attempt to introduce oral feeding to no avail. Mealtimes had become aversive for her parents and were more or less abandoned in favour of total tube feeding. Megan would refuse to open her mouth for the spoon.

BEHAVIOURAL AND EMOTIONAL 'BLOCKS'

Tube feeding as an infant's main source of nutrition renders the baby passive in all aspects of the experience of feeding. The child does not learn to recognise hunger or how to act on his or her environment to satisfy a natural drive. The child misses out on a learning experience not only of having needs met but in acquiring behaviours that have a cause-effect function, these are fundamentals of communication and enable experience of human interaction. Of course, there are other areas of the child's life whereby all these features can be expressed, but in respect of feeding, the child is very much 'mute'.

On a behavioural level, the child and parents have no need for a daily routine of feeding. Often in these families, the tube-fed infant or child is never required to sit at a dining table or high chair; there are no mealtime paraphernalia associated with that child. The parents are not used to shopping and preparing food for the tube-fed child. There must be a major behavioural shift for these families to begin to incorporate the tube-fed child in their normal mealtimes.

On an emotional level, the effects of being a tube-fed child and of caring for a tube-fed child are no less profound. Nutritional intake during the pre-school years can generally be described as a passive process, as the concept of 'feeding' or 'being fed' denotes, in comparison to the term 'eating', which implies more collaboration and choice. As mentioned, however, even neonates are not so passive in the process and learn to affect the behaviour of others in order to have their nutritional needs met. Tube feeding does not allow this freedom for control and it can be hypothesised that the tube-fed child's refusal of oral food is a means of initiating some control that is otherwise denied

An adult perspective may be that to be allowed oral intake following the discomfort of tube feeding can only be positive and pleasurable. A child's perspective may be very different. To consciously open one's mouth to receive a 'foreign-body' without the preparation of 'unconscious' neonatal experiences of taste, appetite regulation, drive satisfaction and trust in the mealtime behaviour and relationship of one's parents may be fraught with anxiety. Additionally, for the parents, the absence of feeding experience for their child may alter their emotional affect and competence. There is evidence that maternal sensitivity during mealtimes affects the likelihood of feeding problems in the child (Hagekull *et al.*, 1997; Sanders *et al.*, 1993). Thus, behaviourally and emotionally, both the child and parents may have failed to develop the appropriate routines and attitudes for satisfactory oral feeding.

EXPERIENCE OF TUBE FEEDING

The case of Alan illustrates the experience of families faced with the difficulty of a child refusing oral intake when there are no longer medical reasons for maintaining tube feeding.

Alan

Alan was referred by his gastroenterologist for refusal of oral intake. He was aged 11 months, lived with both birth parents and an older sister aged 3 years. Alan was born at 35 weeks gestation and was noted to have a poor suckle reflex. He refused the breast and so was bottle-fed but this was a slow process, he would cough and vomit throughout the feed. Each feed was a time-consuming process which became increasingly anxiety-provoking and aversive for Alan's parents as they feared he would vomit the feed. It can be suggested that feeding was also aversive for Alan with the bottle being associated with pain and vomiting. After 3 weeks, he was showing no progress in weight gain and a NG tube was sited. He was prescribed anti-reflux medication, which reduced the size and frequency of the vomits. At the appropriate age weaning to solid foods was commenced but this re-stimulated the vomiting and Alan began to cry at the sight of the spoon.

For all three families, though the reasons for commencement of tube feeding were different, the presenting problems were the same. The children had initial physical difficulties with food digestion and consequent adequate weight gain. There had been a history of vomiting with oral intake. Attempts to establish an effective oral feeding pattern had failed becoming aversive and anxiety-provoking for parents and child. Tube feeding had solved the weight gain problem and removed troublesome mealtimes from the households. For all three families, it had been a medical decision to start oral feeding, and it must be acknowledged that for the families tube feeding had its advantages.

MANAGEMENT OF CHANGE FROM TUBE TO ORAL FEEDING

Alan – initial assessment

A video-tape was made of a mealtime with Alan being offered age-appropriate solid foods by his mother, who was the major carer. It was noted that his mother chose appropriate food, texture, portion size and utensils for his developmental age. This indicated that she was aware of her son's level and of normal feeding expectations despite lack of feeding experience with him. She placed the bowl of food near to Alan and he touched the food tentatively. He held an empty spoon. His mother was wary of putting a spoon loaded with food to Alan's mouth in case it stimulated a vomit. She also kept control of the bowl. Alan gagged when his mother loaded a spoon with food even though she had not offered it to him.

It was clear that although Alan's mother was trying hard to maintain a friendly atmosphere, the interaction was strained and Alan showed increasing signs of distress the longer he sat near to the food. Same-age peers with no history of food refusal would have grabbed the bowl, touched the food, would have attempted to load a spoon by themselves and put it into their mouth; they may have been simultaneously gnawing on some finger foods too.

INTERVENTION I

The aims were to enable pleasurable mealtimes, to gain parent's trust and faith in the intervention and to instigate change to the current mealtimes. The initial goals were to support the friendly atmosphere seen in the video assessment. Alan's mother was given positive feedback, and discussions were around acknowledgement of the strain of mealtimes and reasons why they were not relaxed. The next step was to listen to and accept the parental need for a slow pace of change. They had to be allowed some jurisdiction in their position as Alan's parents and feel that the difficult feeding history they had experienced was acknowledged and appreciated. Behavioural changes took place that involved instigating regular family mealtimes, which included Alan. He was to be presented with food of a very runny texture. Parents were to play with the food, show him how they eat, utensils were to be present but no spoons should be loaded for Alan.

A programme of desensitisation to solid food was begun. Pureed food was first placed on mother's finger and dabbed around the plate and increasingly closer to Alan stopping at the moment of distress. Puree was then placed on a finger food and again placed nearer to him until he would hold the finger food himself. The parents' empty finger was then moved increasingly towards Alan's mouth in a playful manner but at a mealtime. Alan then began to accept an empty spoon to his mouth, held by himself, then an empty spoon held by his parents. These steps took several weeks and did not progress smoothly through a hierarchy but moved backwards and forwards depending on the emotional state of all concerned.

CHANGES TO MEALTIMES

Changes occurring during these initial interventions were as follows: Alan began to suck runny puree off his own fingers and finger foods. He was beginning to show interest in other people eating, particularly his sister. Alan then began accepting a spoon dipped in puree from his sister. He then began to accept a trainer beaker of water and would take about two sips per day. The range of food that his parents had thought to offer him increased. Alan was beginning to willingly taste a wider range of foods. The next breakthrough was that Alan allowed his mother to touch his lips with gravy on her finger. Overall, Alan's interest in food and mealtimes and his willingness to let his mother and sister offer food without stimulating distress or vomiting increased his mother's confidence and motivated her to offer more food. The atmosphere at mealtimes became less strained, and his parents even began to look forward to breakthroughs. Alan's parents had begun to change their perception of him from a non-eater (tube-reliant) to an eater.

INTERVENTION II

Alan had begun to accept minute amounts of food orally but still received all his nutrition via a tube. He had not experienced hunger or appetite though he was beginning to experience positive mealtimes. A goal now was to stimulate hunger and this would involve reducing tube feeds. At this stage, it was essential to consult with his gastroenterologist and dietician and to clarify a plan of action with agreement of all concerned.

The plan was first to establish that his weight was satisfactory and there was some weight to 'play with'. In some cases, it may be necessary to increase tube feeds to put up the child's weight before any reduction can begin. Tube feeds were then reduced by a small amount for two consecutive days then returned to their original amount. This pace satisfied his parent's need to maintain the weight gain that they had struggled for. Any changes in the quantity of oral food Alan consumed were noted. Tube feeds were then reduced for longer time periods. There was an initial weight loss that his parents had been warned to expect, and this predicted event was therefore easier to handle and accept. There was a slower but noticeable increase in Alan's oral intake of both solid foods and water. This pattern proceeded with gradually longer periods of time at reduced tube feeds. Alan's parents received regular support and his weight was monitored.

FINAL CHANGES

Alan began to accept thicker textures. Vomiting had occurred on occasions during this phase but this gradually reduced. He began eating more finger foods of bite-dissolve texture. The quantity of oral intake increased and eventually all tube feeds stopped. Weight gain was maintained without tube feeding. It took 12 months from referral to removal of the NG tube with fortnightly appointments for treatment intervention at the feeding clinic. Alan was then monitored much less frequently for another year.

SUMMARY OF INTERVENTION FOR CHILDREN WHO ARE TUBE FED
Mealtimes
- Regular mealtimes (with the family).
- Puree and bite-dissolve finger foods (irrespective of age of child) are within reach of the child.
- No pressure to eat.
- Mealtimes of short duration.
- Playful atmosphere.

Desensitisation
- To presence of food.
- To presence of utensils.
- To dipped utensils (in puree).
- To dipped finger foods.
- To dipped fingers.
- To approach of fingers to face.
- To approach of food to face.
- Encouragement of self-feeding.

Tube feeds

• Collaborate with other involved medical professionals.
• Ensure have weight to play with.
• Reduce tube feeds.
• There will be an initial weight loss.
• There will be an initial mismatch between hunger and eating.
• Then a gradual catch-up so oral intake increases.

This summary provides the skeleton of a behavioural intervention for introduction of oral feeding to pre-school children who are refusing food. It is important to remember that causes and maintenance of food refusal can be multi-factorial and a thorough assessment is essential with eventual interventions being tailored to the individual child and family (Harris, 1993).

CONCLUSION

Prolonged or significant tube feeding in the pre-school years can disrupt natural experiences of feeding for the child and parents to the extent that oral feeding cannot be successfully begun or resumed without professional intervention. Possible reasons why oral feeding may be refused in these children has been described and indicates the need for thorough assessment and multi-level intervention.

A typical behavioural intervention for food refusal following tube feeding was described which, in summary, incorporates three basic levels: (1) changes to the mealtime structure; (2) desensitisation of the child to the anxiety-provoking food; and (3) reduction of tube feeding. Similar behavioural interventions for feeding difficulties in pre-school children have also been successful (Clawson et al., 2006; Haywood and McCann, 2009). Benoit et al. (2000) compared a behavioural intervention similar to that described here with nutritional management alone and found the behavioural intervention to be significantly more effective in restoring oral food intake than nutritional advice. Prospective evaluation of such interventions will add greatly to clinical practice for food refusal in tube-fed young children.

REFERENCES

Benoit D, Wang EE, Zlotkin SH. Discontinuation of enterostomy tube feeding by behavioral treatment in early childhood: a randomized controlled trial. *J Pediatr.* 2000 Oct; **137**(4): 498–503.

Bernard-Bonnin A-C. Feeding problems of infants and toddlers. *Can Fam Physician.* 2006 Oct; **52**(10): 1247–51.

Clawson B, Selden M, Lacks M, *et al.* Complex pediatric feeding disorders: using teleconferencing technology to improve access to a treatment program. *Paediatr Nurs.* 2008; **34**(3): 213–16.

Clawson EP, Palinski KS, Elliott CA. Outcome of intensive oral motor and behavioural interventions for feeding difficulties in three children with Goldenhar Syndrome. *Pediatr Rehabil.* 2006 Jan–Mar; 9(1): 65–75.

Davis AM, Bruce AS, Mangiaracina C, *et al.* Moving from tube to oral feeding in medically fragile nonverbal toddlers. *J Paediatr Gastroenterol Nutr.* 2009 Aug; 49(2): 233–6.

Delaney AL, Arvedson JC. Development of swallowing and feeding: prenatal through first year of life. *Dev Disabil Res Rev.* 2008; 14(2): 105–17.

Douglas JE, Bryon M. Interview data on severe behavioural eating difficulties in young children. *Arch Dis Child.* 1996; 75: 304–8.

Hagekull B, Bohlin G, Rydell AM. Maternal sensitivity, infant temperament and the development of early feeding problems. *Inf Ment Health J.* 1997; 18(1): 92–106.

Hans DM, Pylipow M, Long JD, *et al.* Nutritional practices in the neonatal intensive care unit: analysis of a 2006 neonatal nutrition survey. *Pediatrics.* 2009; 123(1): 51–7.

Harris G. Feeding problems and their treatment. In: St James I, Harris G, Messer D, editors. *Infant Crying, Feeding and Sleeping: development, problems and treatments.* London, UK: Harvester Wheatsheaf; 1993. pp. 118–32.

Haywood P, McCann J. A brief group intervention for young children with feeding problems. *Clin Child Psychol Psychiat.* 2009 Jul; 14(3): 361–72.

Joffe A, Anton N, Lequier L, *et al.* Nutritional support for critically ill children. *Cochrane database Syst Rev.* 2009 Apr; 15(2): CD005144.

Linscheid TR, Budd KS, Rasnake LK. Pediatric feeding disorders. In: Roberts MC, editor. *Handbook of Pediatric Psychology.* 2nd ed. New York, NY: Guilford Press; 1995.

Milla PJ. Transition from parenteral to enteral nutrition. *Nestle Nutr Workshop Ser Pediatr Prog.* 2007; 59: 105–11.

Reau NR, Senturia YD, Lebailly SA, *et al.* Infant and toddler feeding patterns and problems: normative data and a new direction. *J Dev Behav Pediatr.* 1996; 17(3): 149–53.

Roig-Quilis M, Rodríguez-Palmero A. Oromotor disorders in a paediatric neurology unit: their classification and clinical course. *Rev Neurol.* 2008 Nov 16–30; 47(10): 509–16.

Sanders MR, Patel RK, le Grice B, *et al.* Children with persistent feeding difficulties: an observational analysis of the feeding interactions of problem and non-problem eaters. *Health Psychol.* 1993; 12(1): 64–73.

Strologo LD, Principato F, Sinibaldi D, *et al.* Feeding dysfunction in infants with severe chronic renal failure after long-term nasogastric tube feeding. *Pediatr Nephrol.* 1997; 11: 84–6.

Vohr BR, Poindexter BB, Dusick AM, *et al.* Beneficial effects of breast milk in the neonatal intensive care unit on the developmental outcome of extremely low birth weight infants at 18 months of age. *Pediatrics.* 2006 Jul; 118(1): 115–23.

CHAPTER 12

Management of feeding problems in children with a chronic illness

Anthony Schwartz and Zuzana Rothlingova

INTRODUCTION

Chronic illnesses affect the ability to have adequate nutrition as a result of structural, metabolic and mechanical difficulties, problems in absorption and the nature of the condition (Wolke and Skuse, 1992). Feeding problems are associated with underlying medical factors, the physical components of which are recognised. Over and above these factors, it is acknowledged that psychological components to feeding in children with chronic illnesses play an important role.

This chapter discusses feeding difficulties in the context of paediatric care, within the discipline of paediatric psychology. Paediatric chronic illness, feeding problems and their management require consideration at three levels: first, there are child influences (within and around the child); second, the family influences; and third, the interface of the child–professional system. Only once a clear and focused plan has been agreed, which takes into account interdisciplinary working, can clinical applications and techniques be implemented The aim of this chapter is to highlight this process, acknowledging the unique abilities and roles of all members of the treatment team, including the child, family and health professionals.

Psychological and social dimensions in both the course and treatment of a chronic illness are an important field of investigation. La Greca and Varni (1993) call for research to focus on psychosocial and developmental factors that contribute to the treatment of paediatric conditions. Issues for children with chronic diseases impact on the child, the family and the healthcarers often with multiple hospital admissions and numerous treatments. Unfortunately, Drotar (1997) points out that most psychological research on paediatric chronic illness has focused primarily on description of associated psychosocial problems rather than on interventions to reduce these. This criticism can be equally applied to feeding problems in children with chronic illness. The aim of this chapter is to consolidate some of the evidence on interventions so as to start redressing that imbalance.

The chapter outlines the psychological issues associated with and approaches to managing feeding problems in children with chronic illnesses. As such, it will look at both theoretical and practical applications of research in an attempt to provide a working definition of a feeding problem. Specific feeding issues are considered in children with a range of chronic conditions, along with factors associated with them. The chapter examines research evidence and the theoretical base informing assessment and interventions and brings into focus some specific problem areas of everyday practice, before making recommendations for intervention and good practice.

DESCRIPTIONS AND DEFINITIONS

What constitutes a feeding problem, and for whom it is a problem, is central to this review, as it helps to focus the research studies and interventions. A working definition of a feeding problem is proposed, where such a problem is secondary to chronic illness. This is to assist the process of assessment, facilitate decision-making with regard to the appropriateness of particular interventions and to plan the type of intervention required.

Research and writing point to discrepant systems of classification and diagnostic frameworks. Studies have used interview data, checklists and questionnaires to examine the prevalence of feeding problems (Lindberg *et al.*, 1991), yet the comparison of studies is hampered by lack of clear definitions. Useful definitions of feeding problems are represented in the literature that examines feeding behaviour, psychosocial functioning, physical skills, organic difficulties and the early experience of feeding and interaction. These descriptions and definitions are summarised in Table 12.1.

Lindberg *et al.* (1991) comments that feeding problems are defined solely on the basis of the feeding process (e.g. the inability or refusal to eat certain nutrients). Harris and Booth (1992) focus their attention primarily on feeding behaviours, irrespective of concurrent medical diagnoses. Limited case examples of feeding problems in children with chronic health problems are given, and brief acknowledgement of feeding problems secondary to organic disease is made. Behavioural factors are also central to most definitions of feeding problems (Douglas and Bryon, 1996; Sanders *et al.*, 1993). Feeding problems can be considered to be precipitated and maintained by organic or functional factors (e.g. motivational- or skill-based deficits), and may be characterised by an inability or refusal to eat certain foods due to neuromuscular, metabolic, skeletal and/or psychosocial functions (Babbitt *et al.*, 1994). Other studies (Budd *et al.*, 1992) distinguish between organic and non-organic characteristics of feeding, yet these authors acknowledge that there are

TABLE 12.1: Feeding problems: descriptions and definitions

Authors	Definitions or descriptions of feeding problems
Lindberg, Bohlin and Hagekull, 1991	Feeding problems defined on the basis of • The feeding process: inability or refusal to eat certain nutrients
Harris and Booth, 1992	Behaviours happening occurs separately or together in a particular child: • refusal to take in sufficient calories to enable expected growth velocity, • refusal to take in sufficiently wide range of foods to constitute a balanced diet
Budd et al., 1992	Classification of four diagnostic categories affecting feeding problems: • presence of only organic problems • presence of primarily organic problems • presence of primarily non-organic problems • presence of only non-organic problems
Sanders et al., 1993	Difficulties reported by parents considered to define feeding problems: • persistent food refusal • struggling or resisting during feeds • refusal to self-feed • eating very slowly • being a fussy eater • consuming small amounts of food • disruptive behaviour during meals
Babbitt et al., 1994	Inability or refusal to eat certain foods because of neuromuscular, metabolic, skeletal and/or psychosocial dysfunction (motivational or skill-based deficits), e.g. • refusal • selectivity • behavioural difficulty • tube dependence • rumination and vomiting • absence of self-feeding skills • excessive meal duration • adipsia and polydipsia

Hampton, 1995	In all cases of non-organic failure to thrive, underlying reasons can be: • carers not offering the child enough calories to meet their needs • unhelpful behaviour patterns/interactions between parents and child • unpleasant associations that the child has with feeding.
Douglas and Bryon, 1996	Inability to consume sufficient calories for adequate growth, with difficulties centred on: • inadequate quantity eaten • selective eating (i.e. restricted range of foods) • refusing to chew or swallow • slow eating • inappropriate texture for age
Kedesdy and Budd, 1998	Multidimensional classification of childhood feeding disorders includes: descriptive factors • eating too little/too much • eating the wrong things • feeding skills deficits background factors • diet • physical competence • appetite • illness (acute or chronic) • interaction/management • child constitution • caregiver competence • systemic features
Linscheid, 1998	Disorders which lead to the • lack of ingestion of nutritionally or developmentally appropriate diet in children who are not prevented from eating for medical reasons.

likely to be difficulties in the feeding situation, irrespective of cause. An overarching classification that incorporates behavioural and physiological features is also given (Kedesdy and Budd, 1998). Treatment approaches may differ despite similar presenting problems (Harris and Booth, 1992).

Early feeding problems can be seen as arising from an interaction of a number of factors: constitutional, physical, temperamental, learning and emotional (Skuse *et al.*, 1992). The original aetiology of the feeding problem (e.g. developmental, medical, motor or cultural factors) is important, but behavioural interactions between child, parent or caregiver usually become the target for intervention (Linscheid, 1998). In this sense, behaviour plays a role in all feeding problems.

Table 12.1 classifies feeding problems in terms of both descriptive characteristics (e.g. food refusal) and implied causes (e.g. underlying physical problems). The absence of a general consensus in the literature on what constitutes a feeding problem is likely to be attributable to a number of factors: (1) the heterogeneity of feeding problems; (2) varied theoretical perspectives on causation; (3) the number of professions involved in these problems; and (4) the fact that there are frequently other, more urgent, concerns (such as the diagnosis and treatment of concomitant underlying conditions), particularly where chronic illness is concerned. The following working definition follows research that suggests that feeding problems rarely fall into one category, but have 'mixed' aetiology (Budd *et al.*, 1992).

TOWARDS A WORKING DEFINITION OF A FEEDING PROBLEM

Drawing from the definitions already described, the following types of feeding problems could be expected to be referred to a specialist practitioner:

- problems with eating behaviour (e.g. refusal, selectivity or range of food)
- counter-productive patterns of interaction between care-giver and child (e.g. cajoling or punitive responses)
- heightened anxiety in parent, child or both.

This formulation leans more towards problem description than medical diagnosis. Medical criteria for a feeding disorder in infancy or childhood require that it 'generally involves refusal of food or extreme faddiness' (ICD-10, 1992). Archer *et al.* (1991) accept that the assessment and treatment of these problems has been highly variable. They recommend that eating and mealtime disorders be regarded as a separate clinical entity regardless of medical diagnosis. Researchers have begun to treat feeding problems as distinct from the syndrome 'failure to thrive' or malnutrition and based solely on the feeding process (Lindberg *et al.*, 1991), as many children with feeding problems do not reach this cut-off point. Linscheid (1992) supports this view and cites estimates suggesting that between 25% and 35% of children have recognised or reportable eating problems, whereas only 1%–2% have feeding problems that result in impaired growth.

CHRONIC ILLNESS AND FEEDING PROBLEMS

The total prevalence of children with chronic conditions is estimated at around 10%, and it is suggested that chronic illness can have a profound impact on the psychological wellbeing of the child and family (Fielding, 1985). Determining the incidence of feeding problems in children with chronic illnesses depends on problem definition as examined above. If there has been no co-ordinated data collection on feeding problems, one of the first tasks might be to list feeding problems most often associated with certain medical conditions. This approach (Baer, 1997) using data collated from a number of regions within the United States gives a between 10% and 42% of children with chronic illnesses having feeding problems (e.g. those with kidney conditions, liver disease, inflammatory bowel syndromes, human immunodeficiency virus infection, cystic fibrosis, diabetes, cancer, phenylketonuria, neurological problems and allergies).

If anxiety, depression and other emotional factors are considered to affect the feeding process of otherwise healthy children, how much more is this likely when a child has a chronic or life-threatening illness? Hence, the importance of management of emotional factors associated with feeding and chronic illness. It is necessary to be fully aware of the literature and to understand general child development with its transitions and emotional and behavioural concomitants from a number of theoretical perspectives as well as their critiques (Carey, 1985; Eriksen, 1980; Piaget, 1976). Although one needs to pay attention to the child's age and stage of development, research on developmental aspects will not be covered here other than to acknowledge these as important: these are covered in Chapter 5. Parental emotional issues have been discussed in some of the earlier chapters and so will be reviewed only briefly later in this chapter, in terms of how they affect the feeding process (*see also* Figure 12.1).

Medical sources affirm that chronic conditions such as cystic fibrosis, heart disease, lung disease, metabolic disorders (e.g. diabetes), neurological disorders and renal disease are often associated with problems of feeding and nutrition that contribute to poor growth and development (Harris and Booth, 1992; Jenkins and Milla, 1988; Martin and Shaw, 1997; Ruley et al., 1989; Stark et al., 1990). Wolke and Skuse (1992) comment that chronic illnesses and growth disturbances are closely linked and state that the process of feeding may be difficult (especially for infants). The psychological components associated with feeding behaviour in children with chronic health problems are increasingly being acknowledged. Douglas (1995) shows that behavioural eating problems are common in children with physical conditions, with referrals from particular medical specialities (e.g. gastroenterology, nephrology, cardiology, immunology, metabolic medicine, neurology, surgery and ear, nose and throat medicine).

Several studies identify feeding problems in children who have physical health problems (Douglas et al., 1998; Foreman and Chan, 1988; Ravelli, 1995; Rees et al., 1989; Ruley et al., 1989). The treatment of some childhood diseases may also result in iatrogenic effects, based on the medication used (e.g. in cancer), hospitalisation experience (e.g. procedural anxiety), or manner of induced feeding (e.g. naso-gastric feeding), which affects the feeding process (Cairns and Altman, 1979; Culbert *et al.*, 1996; Strologo *et al.*, 1997; Warady *et al.*, 1990).

Studies of feeding problems in children with chronic medical conditions are scarce and are usually focused on single or multiple case studies, with small sample sizes and with methodological problems due to the nature of the sample. Table 12.2 presents a brief summary of the types of feeding problems associated with chronic illness and gives the reported or perceived rates of incidence of feeding problems from selected studies. Unfortunately, very few studies give incidence figures. Despite the limitations of the studies, they serve to open the area to examination, beginning with anecdotal and descriptive data and small sample research that explores and tests hypotheses. It is suggested that these studies should be followed by examination in greater depth through more large-scale co-ordinated research work (Drotar, 1997; La Greca and Varni, 1993; Wallander, 1992).

SPECIFIC CATEGORIES OF ILLNESS

As suggested earlier, demarcating difficulties into 'medical' versus 'psychological' categories is not particularly helpful in the process of treatment. The need is for a holistic formulation of the child within the biological, psychological and social context, using ideas from health psychology and systemic theory (Bradford, 1997). However, one might suggest that there is practical use in retaining a 'medical condition' framework, since we frequently encounter this diagnostic division first when being presented with a feeding difficulty in a child with a concomitant illness. Research supports the contention that children with chronic illness are at greater risk for feeding problems (Culbert *et al.*, 1996). There is meagre information on percentages of children with feeding problems by selected medical diagnosis with only one author (Baer, 1997) quoting prevalence figures collated from a specific geographical region. What proceeds are descriptions of feeding issues in the most commonly presenting conditions in the paediatric psychology context. It is not meant to be an exhaustive exemplar of work in this field, but it is aimed at highlighting some pertinent management problems.

Cancer

Overt malnutrition is often found in children with cancer (Wardley *et al.*, 1997). The aetiology of this has been variously described, with descriptions ranging from children having a lack of appetite, psychological factors such as learned food aversions, malabsorption, excess nutrient loss and increased caloric demands as a result of tumours (van Eys, 1979). Early effects of treatment may affect adequate intake with disturbances in taste, changes in food preference, nausea and vomiting. Useful psychological interventions with learned food aversions are behavioural and cognitive strategies, which may include relaxation techniques to improve patients' intake.

Research has highlighted non-medical treatment for cancer-related anorexia (Cairns and Altman, 1979) through the use of positive reinforcement. Epston (1994) describes a case study from a family systems perspective using hypnosis for management of chemotherapy-related appetite loss. Zeltzer et al. (1996) in a seven-site study show that eating problems occur in siblings of children with cancer. Yet these authors confirm that healthcare interventions in siblings are reduced in comparison to other children. They recommend that the needs of siblings should not be forgotten, and questions should be asked about the other children and their eating habits when meeting with the family of children with chronic and life threatening conditions. This is additional to special work helping children whose siblings have cancer in oncology units at specialist children's hospitals (Balen et al., 1998).

Cystic fibrosis

As a result of the number of physical treatments required and the widely held belief that higher calorific intake and added weight may act as a buffer against infection, feeding issues are at the forefront when children have cystic fibrosis. Excessive focus on food, feeding and weight gain can lead to abnormal feeding patterns and negative feeding behaviour, with 37% of children over a year old with cystic fibrosis experiencing feeding difficulties (MacDonald, 1996). Pearson et al. (1991) found that youngsters aged 8–15 years were significantly more likely to have eating disturbances in the form of resisting food, being preoccupied with food and using food as a control issue than an older group aged 16–40 years. The latter groups were found to have more depressed and anxious symptoms. MacDonald (1996) indicates that problems may include prolonged mealtimes, vomiting and gagging, force feeding, constant parental nagging and food refusal and suggests help from a psychologist with an interest in feeding problems is invaluable. Parental anxiety about food, acute infections and frequent disruptions as a result of hospital admissions may all affect the home atmosphere and interactions. This may be manifest in tense and upsetting mealtimes with parents pressing food onto a child, giving increased attention through coaxing, or removal from the feeding situation all of which serve to maintain a child's avoidance (Singer et al., 1991). They also found that mothers verbalising their fear that their child would die affected their mealtime interactions with their child.

Sanders et al. (1997) found that parents of cystic fibrosis children reported more disruption, emphasised behaviour management problems and cited lower marital satisfaction. Problems associated with growth abnormalities were also in evidence. However, observational data did not indicate that these children were significantly different in mealtime behaviours. This has implications for psychological practice around mealtimes, which are pressured times for parents who are trying to ensure their child received adequate nutrition. They suggest that interventions would need to be at three levels: The first deals with how to promote dietary compliance (e.g. through learning non-aversive parental management strategies and having guidelines about optimal instruction giving). The second addresses parental feelings on inadequacy, helplessness and uncertainty about how to cope with their child's illness as well as expectations about the dietary intake needed. Third, programmes would need to focus on family distress and the interrelationships between the parents.

Diabetes

Emphasis on diet and eating in diabetes care, along with concerns about weight may be considered to make young people vulnerable to experiencing problems related to food and eating. Pollock *et al.* (1995) found that 11.4% had at some stage had a period of eating problems. However, in surveying the literature, we need to be cautious in considering the relationship between eating *problems* and eating *disorders*. In fact in this study, the most significant finding was that the diagnosis of eating disorder was linked to the youngster having other mental health problems. The authors recommend therefore that, if young people with diabetes have eating problems, it is necessary to check if they have any other psychological problems.

Human immunodeficiency virus (HIV)

There have been few studies on feeding problems in children with HIV, and yet there are often many physical signs associated with the condition (e.g. symptoms of diarrhoea, weight loss, poor growth and developmental weakness). Melvin *et al.* (1997) emphasise that poor underlying nutrition threatens physical and psychological development. In addition, dealing with feeding-related aspects places a burden of time and effort on carers who may have their own HIV-related problems. Developmental considerations to be taken into account include the difficult period in transition from milk to solid food, which requires more energy, as well as sophisticated chewing and swallowing movements. In their study, cultural issues were implicated with the group being of African background, where differences in weaning practices and conflicts over traditional foods versus western 'fast' foods were evident. Other aspects include parental pressure on the child to eat, which serves to enhance negative mealtime behaviours.

Renal failure

Types of feeding problems associated with chronic kidney disease include reduced appetite, gastro-oesophageal reflux, nausea, vomiting and anorexia (Ravelli, 1995; Sadowski *et al.*, 1993; Strologo *et al.*, 1997), all of which play a major role in growth failure often found in this group of young people. A recent study by Douglas *et al.* (1998) has shown that children's severe eating problems dramatically improved following kidney transplantation. Despite the small sample size and retrospective nature of the study, the conclusions are helpful. It also suggests that early nasogastric feeding does not affect transfer to total oral intake. The transition is likely to have been made easier by there having been less anxiety around feeding, which reinforces an earlier study (Douglas, 1995) that by not having been force-fed or made to eat, children had not experienced early aversive learning.

TABLE 12.2: Feeding problems associated with chronic illness

Chronic illness	Feeding problem	Studies	Type of study	Incidence*
Cancer	Conditioned anxiety	Culbert et al., 1996	Case study	NFG
	Cancer-related anorexia	Cairns and Altman, 1979	Case study	NFG: 'a frequent problem'
Renal disease	Dietary adherence	Magrab and Papadopoulou, 1977	Case study	NFG
	Eating anxiety	Strologo et al., 1997	Retrospective study	NFG
Cystic fibrosis	Behavioural	Crist et al., 1994	Cross-sectional	NFG
	Behaviour-interactional	McCollum and Gibson, 1970	Cross-sectional	37%
	Eating behaviour	Singer et al., 1991	Case study	NFG
Diabetes	Eating behaviour	Pollock, Kovacs and Charron-Prochownik, 1995	Longitudinal N = 79	11%
HIV	Parental concerns	Melvin, Wright and Goddard, 1997	Cross-sectional N = 42	50%

*Incidence rates: NFG = No figures are given. Quotations of frequency of problem outlined in the study are reported.

Table 12.2 indicates the presence of feeding problems associated with particular conditions. Since most of the work has been undertaken using case studies with methodological limitations, larger samples are suggested. Longitudinal studies exploring feeding problems that may occur at different times during the chronic illness process have not been undertaken. Obstacles in conducting research to examine feeding difficulties in this population include difficulties in recruiting samples of sufficient size, matching control groups, arranging ongoing assessments and ethical considerations (e.g. imposing further demands on children and families who are already under stress, to take part in additional evaluative procedures). As a result, the research base for examining evidence of co-existing feeding and chronic health problems is limited. Whilst there is evidence of a number of feeding-related problems in children with chronic illnesses, more rigorous research is needed to clarify the extent and range of the problems. The preceding discussion would suggest that the feeding problem classification also needs to be firmed up and applied consistently.

FAMILY FACTORS ASSOCIATED WITH FEEDING PROBLEMS

Feeding-related difficulties are linked with factors both within and outside of the child as shown in Figure 12.1. Douglas (1995) presents this model, based on children without health problems for examining factors that maintain the child's feeding problems. The focus is on 'child factors' and 'family factors'. These factors relating to the child and family are substantiated by the literature (Blissett and Harris, 2002; Harris, 1993; Werle *et al.*, 1993; Zeltzer *et al.*, 1984). The model can be adapted and extended to children with chronic illness who have feeding problems by adding an 'illness factors' dimension (e.g. illness requirements, the stress of chronic illness and treatment experiences).

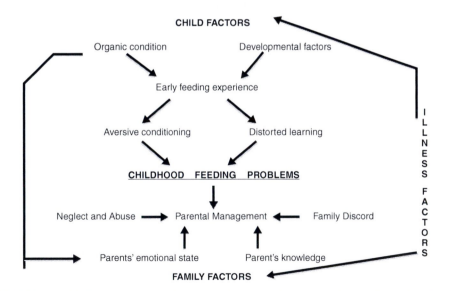

FIGURE 12.1: Multiple interacting factors linked with feeding problems (Douglas, 1995).

In children with chronic illness, reduced oral intake occurs as a result of feeding interaction problems, parental anxiety and stress of the long-standing condition (Kedesdy and Budd, 1998). Children with life-threatening conditions may be perceived by parents to be 'vulnerable'. This might also result in parents feeling unable to set limits on their children's behaviour. In the general population, behaviour problems have been associated with feeding problems (Linscheid, 1998). There is no evidence of the link between behaviour and feeding problems in chronic illness, although sick children may, by virtue of physical limitations, not be able to exhibit clear externalised behaviour problems.

Causative factors linked to feeding problems and which present for psychological management have been identified earlier (*see* Table 12.2). The assessment of these factors both within the child (e.g. conditioned anxiety), within the caregivers (e.g. parental anxiety) and across both (e.g. behavioural and interactional difficulties), needs further examination in the clinical assessment, through the use of feeding assessment scales, clinical interviews and other measures.

FEEDING ASSESSMENT

The assessment process is covered in earlier chapters and is generally undertaken with a view to determining whether the feeding problem is isolated or whether it is related to other problems the child may be having. Parental assessment may also be undertaken focusing on individual or family factors such as stress using, for example, the Parenting Stress Index (Abidin, 1986).

Although the assessment methods already described in this book apply equally to children with chronic illnesses, care must be taken as some measures do not apply well to this group. For example, the Child Behaviour Checklist (Achenbach, 1987) contains a number of items that relate to physical functioning and may negatively skew the results for children with a chronic health problem. Above all, the clinician will need to bear in mind this added dimension: the child has a chronic condition that impacts on feeding, just as the feeding may impact on the illness.

Apart from methodological problems relating to feeding assessment measures, flaws in research studies on feeding need to be acknowledged. The examination of 'child', 'parent' and 'interactional' factors contributing to feeding problems in chronic illness have been undertaken in small-scale studies usually directed at improving the child's feeding behaviour. Few studies use any control condition, and as such it is difficult to assess which component of the treatment package is effective. Problems also result from the arbitrary classification of feeding problems. The binary, medically based differentiation of problems as 'organic' versus 'non-organic' is considered an unhelpful distinction (Budd *et al.*, 1992). Comparing studies is further complicated by dissimilar inclusion criteria, discrepancies in the ages of children studied and the rate at which weight changes occurred.

INTERVENTION

In the literature examined, the main focus on feeding problems is on anxiety surrounding eating and feeding, individual behaviours and the process of interaction.
A number of studies have investigated feeding problems in chronic illnesses and
the treatment approaches to ameliorate the problems are described next. The link
between feeding problems and conditioned anxiety has been cited in the study by
Culbert *et al.* (1996). In this series of case studies, the authors describe the treatment
of maladaptive eating behaviours including the conditioned fear of eating. Using
a hypno-behavioural approach, the child is introduced to the concept of gradual
self-regulation as a way of counteracting anxiety about swallowing chemotherapy
medication to which he had a conditioned vomiting response. Key elements include
building rapport, providing information to relieve fears, enhancing mastery and
control through offering choices, using links between positive feelings associated
with favourite foods and imaging desired outcomes as if they had already been
accomplished. The work described in this study is exploratory in nature, but illustrates the need to define, identify and develop treatment protocols for children with
maladaptive feeding and swallowing problems.

Regarding psychosocial concomitants of children's feeding problems, Budd *et al.*
(1992) examined the interaction between biological and environmental variables.
In this study, high levels of parental emotional distress were related to:
(a) low levels of child feeding skills
(b) older children
(c) parents who used less positive disciplinary practices
(d) parents with higher educational or occupational status.

Since parental emotional welfare is implicated in children's feeding, clinicians need
to consider parents' emotional adjustment. Additionally, studies have made a link
between parental anxiety about their child's health and eating problems (Chase
et al., 1979; Crist *et al.*, 1994; Lindberg *et al.*, 1991; Melvin *et al.*, 1997; Singer *et al.*,
1991). A single-case study by Blissett and Harris (2002) illustrates the process of a
behavioural intervention in a child with Silver Russell Syndrome, a growth disorder,
and emphasises treatment focusing on reducing parental anxiety, returning a sense
of control to the child and the implementation of a feeding programme focusing on
positive reinforcement for feeding behaviour.

FAMILY ANXIETY

Hampton (1995) makes the point that problems are exacerbated when parents'
anxieties (e.g. regarding a child's refusal to eat) are not being taken seriously, or
when professionals fail to recognise the existence of a feeding problem. In a study of
normal children, the most worrying and challenging problem was of children's food
refusal (Lindberg *et al.*, 1991). Links are highlighted between parental concerns and

the origins of feeding problems. Although this is of some worth, it did not follow the children through over time for a sufficiently long period. They suggest that early feeding problems that have caused concerns for parents may contribute to an altered response to food and feeding on the part of the mother, the infant, or both.

Where the child has been diagnosed as having a clear organic condition, general child management and feeding can be affected. However, anxiety about feeding seems to 'go with the territory' of early child-rearing. Wardley *et al.* (1997) make the point that an array of symptoms occurs in babies, which are associated with or ascribed to feeding or digestive processes. These cause parents emotional concern and can lead to emotional disturbances and distort the parent–child relationship (*see* Chapter 4). Most practitioners only see children whose parents have sought help with general feeding problems. When feeding problems are of deeper concern, usually there is a referral from a healthcare professional who is worried about a child's condition. Assessment would normally occur following referral such as a health visitor, nurse, general practitioner or paediatrician. A good psychological and medical screening needs to be undertaken to differentiate between a feeding problem, an acute or chronic illness or when a child's refusal to eat is related to unrealistic parental expectations. Leung (1994) supports the provision of psychological input in all the above, beginning with reassurance and counselling and possibly later working at a deeper and more complex level if the assessment, formulation and therapy undertaken indicate this would be beneficial. Such considerations should take into account evidence-based practice.

Sanders *et al.* (1997) compared children with cystic fibrosis, children with feeding problems and a normal control group. Their finding concerned mealtime behaviours, with parents of cystic fibrosis children reporting more disruption, emphasising behaviour management problems and citing lower marital satisfaction. Problems associated with growth abnormalities were also in evidence. However, observational data did not indicate that these children were significantly different in mealtime behaviours to other children (i.e. those without feeding problems). This has implications for psychological practice: mealtimes are pressured times for parents who are trying to ensure their child receives adequate nutrition. They suggest that interventions would need to be at three levels: the first deals with how to promote dietary compliance (e.g. through learning non-aversive parental management strategies and having guidelines about optimal instruction giving); the second addresses parental feelings on inadequacy, helplessness and uncertainty about how to cope with their child's illness as well as expectations about the dietary intake needed; and the third suggests that the programmes would need to focus on family distress and the inter-relationships between the parents.

Behavioural and interactional factors implicated in feeding problems are illustrated by Clawson *et al.* (2006) and in the study by Stark *et al.* (1990) with children with cystic fibrosis. This research, using a multiple baseline design with five children and their families, provided further evidence of the usefulness of behavioural interventions with groups of both children and parents. Intervention included nutritional education and gradual increase of calorie goals, teaching parents management strategies and a reward system for clearly identified dietary goals for children. Children were aged between 5 and 12 years. The weight gain following the programme was maintained at a level comparable to that of a normal population. The application of a behavioural component is seen as critical in producing increased calorie consumption. Both studies are compromised by the small sample size, and further research is necessary: (a) to show treatment effectiveness across a larger sample of subjects; (b) to evaluate the specific treatment components; and (c) to examine the interface between physiological and environmental variables.

PSYCHOLOGICAL APPROACHES

There is a wide variety of psychological approaches to treating feeding problems in children with chronic illness. An example of a behavioural approach is that of Stark *et al.* (1990) who used a star chart as reinforcement for compliance with calorific intake in children with cystic fibrosis. (O'Brien *et al.*, 1991). Other methods include relaxation and cognitive coping skills to assist children to cope with anxiety aroused by eating foods that are feared (Singer *et al.*, 1991).

Besides the behavioural approaches to treating feeding problems, Culbert *et al.* (1996) in their study on self-management techniques for food refusal and food aversion use educational approaches, reassurance and hypnotherapy procedures in addition to cognitive-behavioural strategies to treat these problems. Their study used an approach, which was the first reported case series based on hypnotherapy and behavioural work; nevertheless, further research is recommended. The age range of children was between 6 and 13 years, and, as such, these strategies appear most likely to be applicable with children over the age of 6 years who have reasonable verbal skills.

Group work with parents of children with feeding problems has also been shown to be helpful, whether in the form of a support and management group (Chamberlin *et al.*, 1991) or as a parent training group (Sanders *et al.*, 1993; Werle *et al.*, 1993). The role of the parents in treating feeding problems is shown by these studies to be critical, and work on increasing desired behaviours generally includes parents as part of the management approach. The training of parents also establishes an important link between the natural environment and the therapeutic setting.

RECOMMENDATIONS FOR INTERVENTION AND GOOD PRACTICE

Implications for practice based on the research evidence from the studies described above relate to both application of psychological approaches and to skilled practitioner technique.

Whilst most research focuses on behavioural and interactional strategies to promote feeding, the key components to achieve change are less clear. It is acknowledged that a number of behavioural interventions form part of the management process. Examples of these effective interventions are given in Table 12.3, which outlines the major behaviour management principles (Kedesdy and Budd, 1998), and gives examples of the applications in addition to citing the research studies, which underline these approaches. Two major organising principles are distinguished:

1   increasing appropriate behaviour
2   decreasing maladaptive behaviour (Babbitt *et al.*, 1994).

GUIDELINES FOR GOOD PRACTICE

General issues common to chronic conditions, which have been raised earlier in the chapter, include anxiety and phobic responses, attachment, control and separation issues, listlessness, despair and depression. Throughout the chapter on feeding problems associated with chronic and life threatening illness, reference has been made to the significant role of psychological practice in the management and treatment of feeding problems overall.

The practitioner needs to understand medical interventions and common problems associated with the chronic and life threatening conditions as a whole, but more specifically and importantly should be au fait with particular medical conditions and their implications, both physically and psychologically. The need to consider the mutually influencing individual and system effects, with the impact that this has on collaboration and inter-professional working, has already been highlighted in Chapter 7.

Practice would indicate that psychological management of feeding problems should comprise both an 'individual perspective' and a 'meta-view'. Individual focus may encompass behavioural, cognitive and psychodynamic frameworks, and an overarching perspective can be taken by using systemic approaches. Kendall and Norton-Ford (1982) clearly set out the need for proper assessment, problem formulation, treatment and evaluation of the approach used.

The research studies above have focused on psychological components in treatment, although feeding problems present following investigations by other professionals. Increasingly inter-agency and multi-disciplinary work is undertaken, which may offer both benefits and challenges for the individual practitioner. Lefton-Greif and Arvedson (2008) also emphasise a 'whole child' approach by a team, including the educational environment, since interventions may impact on the child's education. Whilst research suggests that a multi-disciplinary approach to the management of complex feeding problems contributes to their successful management (Tawfik *et al.*, 1997; Wooster *et al.*, 1998), the challenges of working within a team can also be significant; they include working with different professionals with wide-ranging and possibly conflicting perspectives, role conflict, challenges to practice and the

TABLE 12.3: Outline of psychological interventions suggested in research studies for the management of feeding problems

Psychological principles and intervention approaches recommended in the literature

Research studies	Aimed at increasing desired behaviours					Aimed at decreasing undesired behaviours			
	Positive reinforcement	*Negative reinforcement*	*Discrimination*	*Shaping*	*Fading*	*Extinction*	*Satiation*	*Punishment*	*Desensitisation*
Babbitt et al., 1994	✔	✔	✔	✔		✔		✔	
Bernal, 1972	✔			✔	✔	✔			
Cairns and Altman, 1979	✔								✔
Hoch et al., 1994	✔	✔				✔			
O'Brien et al., 1991	✔	✔	✔						
Stark et al., 1990	✔		✔		✔	✔			
Werle et al., 1993	✔		✔	✔		✔		✔	

Principle	Positive Reinforcement	Negative Reinforcement	Discrimination	Shaping	Fading	Extinction	Satiation	Punishment	Desensitisation
Description	Provide positive consequences for desired behaviours	Terminate aversive stimulus contingent on desired behaviour	Reinforce target behaviour in presence of defined stimulus	Reinforce successive approximations towards desired response	Gradually remove assistance and reinforcement needed to maintain behaviour	Withhold rewarding stimulus contingent on target response	Continually present desired stimulus until it loses its reinforcing value	Present aversive stimulus or remove rewarding stimulus contingent on desired behaviour	Pair conditioned aversive stimulus with absence of aversive events or with presence of positive events
Example	Give praise, physical affection, preferred food or tangible rewards	Release physical restraint (for food expulsion) when the child accepts food	Praise the modelled behaviour of eating. Reward cooperation with feeding requests	Praise for: looking at food, allowing food to touch lips, opening of mouth and accepting food	Decrease extent of guidance and self-rewards as child gains self-feeding skills	Ignore mild inappropriate behaviour. Continue prompts during escape behaviour	Offer unlimited portions of food to reduce rumination	Use time-out, give verbal reprimand, restrict toys and use over-correction	Distract child during fearful procedure. Use gentle massage to promote acceptance of touch

Psychological principles/intervention approaches/recommendations from the literature practical problems of which professional takes a central role in the management of a particular child's problem (*see* Chapter 7).

In terms of time and cost effectiveness, little research has been undertaken despite the team approach having 'anecdotal champions' (Kedesdy and Budd, 1998). An alternative model is one of individual specialists who may be consulted whilst working alongside the team. In this situation, specific referrals can be made to a particular professional, and decisions on who to include in the management are based on the problem and its context. These authors offer examples of case studies, which show the advantages from using a transdisciplinary team in the evaluation and treatment of feeding problems. In their approach, they actively promote the inclusion and participation of the family as 'the most vital member of the team'.

EXAMPLES OF FEEDING DIFFICULTIES ASSOCIATED WITH CHRONIC ILLNESS

Studies of children in hospital with chronic illness have indicated a high prevalence of malnutrition (Wardley *et al.*, 1997). Malnutrition has effects on the child's resilience and has potentially serious consequences for all systems of the body. As a result, nutritional interventions are used in order to supplement calorific intake and alter the natural history of the disease. Linked with these specific treatments come anxieties about how and when to intervene, fears about invasive procedures, worry about whether the child is gaining sufficient weight, issues of control and problems in managing treatment; all of which have psychological relevance. Archer *et al.* (1991) clearly link elements in a vicious cycle by which professionals' therapeutic decisions to increase the frequency of feeding or provide special diets, results in parental worry or fear about nutritional intake, which makes for a functional feeding problem where feeding behaviours and management is affected.

ENTERAL NUTRITION IN CHRONIC ILLNESS

Artificial feeding reduces food to its barest essential, that of nourishing the patient, and excludes the social dimensions, cultural aspects and physical sensations that normally go with eating (Padilla and Grant, 1995).

Psychological considerations surrounding this method may be linked to the timing (i.e. when this form of feeding is instituted), to the treatment procedure itself (i.e. insertion or passing of the tube) and to the consequences of long-term use of this means (i.e. inability to take oral feeds subsequently). Decisions to institute naso-gastric feeding may be made where there have been unsuccessful attempts at providing sufficient nutrition orally (*see* Chapters 2, 10 and 11). Frustration on the part of parents when a child is not taking adequate food orally may lead to an aversive parent–child feeding milieu. Psychological involvement may support a medical intervention or might focus on management of the vicious cycle of anxiety and dysfunctional interaction. There is also often a need for support to be given to the parents regarding the benefits of this form of treatment. Some of these issues are critically psychological, as they affect management, adherence and emotional concerns for both individuals and families.

Invasive procedures have been shown to be some of the most feared aspects for children undergoing medical treatment (Ross and Ross, 1988). The management of distress, fear and pain in the paediatric setting has been cited as an area for specific psychological applications (Schwartz and Mercer, 1998). Practical psychological help is useful in the form of distraction, relaxation and reframing the experience of the naso-gastric tube insertion, as highlighted in the case below.

Nicky

Nicky, a 10-year-old girl with cystic fibrosis, was seen by individual nurses in the Paediatric Community Nursing Team to help pass her naso-gastric tube. Sessions often lasted for up to three hours. Nicky's mother was concerned about her daughter and often interrupted the process to ask how Nicky was feeling about the procedure. She also emphasised to the professionals how difficult it was to perform, and how worried Nicky was about the procedure. As a result, sessions were highly emotionally charged. Following discussion at a case management meeting, it was decided to focus on what had made interventions successful in the past. Assisting Nicky's mother to manage her anxiety was suggested. Following distraction for both Nicky and her mother (which included mother being asked to focus on another activity such as making coffee) the level of anxiety diminished, and a cycle of positive experiences was started. The major benefit from psychological formulation and management procedures meant that the passing of the tube took a few minutes rather than a few hours.

NAUSEA AND VOMITING AS A SIDE EFFECT OF TREATMENT

Medical treatment advances have led to the control of vomiting and nausea in patients undergoing cancer chemotherapy. However, with other conditions, there remain concerns about nausea as a side-effect of treatment (e.g. haemodialysis) or as a result of acute anxiety. Problems such as habitual reflex vomiting have been shown to benefit from psychological approaches (Sokel *et al.*, 1991), focusing on helping the young person to achieve gradual control over the symptom (e.g. using relaxation and guided imagery). These authors also mention shaping of behaviour by positive reinforcement of food retention, and 'time-out' for vomiting as alternative approaches to managing vomiting. An example of work which began with multi-disciplinary role confusion in managing a conditioned anxiety state is described below:

James

James was a 16-year-old young man who had a long history of feeding problems and had been hospitalised for a number of months on the paediatric ward. On the ward, he had been found to be very selective with his eating and frequently went to the toilet immediately following meals. He expressed feeling anxious and tense and was under pressure to 'eat properly', so that there was sufficient confidence in the medical staff to discharge him. There was continuing confusion about whether James had an 'eating disorder' and should be referred for a psychiatric assessment. The paediatric psychologist suggested a 'working definition' of a feeding problem be adopted and ongoing work was initiated. James was discharged after a graded programme to manage his anxiety and to re-integrate him into the home and school environments. Interventions were continued on an out-patient basis.

NUTRITIONAL DEFICITS

Medical management of nutritional deficits, absorption problems and anatomical changes such as anorexia in chronic conditions are usually through the use of nasal-oesophageal feeding tubes or hyperalimentation where nutrients are delivered directly into the blood. There is limited published research on behavioural treatments for anorexia (rather than anorexia nervosa) in children with chronic illness. One study (Cairns and Altman, 1979) describes the use of positive social reinforcement, access to play activities and token system to reverse weight loss in paediatric oncology. Other researchers comment on the importance of management of anorexia but fail to include any psychological frameworks (Ravelli, 1995). Emphasis appears to be on the usefulness of physical treatments to deal with these problems (Warady *et al.*, 1990), although where there are learned food aversions, behavioural strategies have been shown to be effective (Hoch *et al.*, 1994; O'Brien *et al.*, 1991) as have hypnobehavioural approaches (Culbert *et al.*, 1996). In addition, where there are high states of anxiety, for example, in swallowing disorders, use of biofeedback and psychophysiological methods can be usefully applied (Stroebel, personal communication, see www.ncbiofeedback.org/conference2006_presenters.htm).

CONCLUSION

In working with parents of chronically ill children, Knafl *et al.* (1992) consider essential professional skills to be the ability to provide technically competent services, communicate with families, participate as an effective team member, be sensitive to ethical issues and to conceptualise problems in ecological terms.

In their review on chronic illnesses, Elander and Midence (1997) comment on training and research implications in this specific field including training of other professionals, which is an effective way of stretching limited resources. However, the others involved need supervision and support from a psychological perspective, especially in complex conditions such as feeding problems in chronic illness populations.

Constant evaluation of practice is needed so as to build up a research literature on effective management in line with the current national focus on clinical effectiveness and evidence-based medicine. Evaluation of practice and committing the findings to paper for peer audit and review is one step to improving research output in this area.

In the application of psychological approaches to feeding problems, it has been demonstrated that a clear history and detailed assessment is required. This includes the use of validated measures such as the Children's Eating Behaviour Inventory (Archer *et al.*, 1991). Information pertaining to the context and interaction around feeding should also be included (Blissett and Harris, 2002).

From the literature it is evident that a number of strategies are used to manage feeding problems effectively. Implications for practice include suggestions that at least two different treatment components are needed, and indeed studies using behavioural reinforcement with parents, on closer reading also demonstrate the use of other methodologies. It is recommended that an approach is used that focuses concurrently on the targeted behaviour at the same time as establishing a positive environment (e.g. through decreasing anxiety), and which also gives evidence of incremental changes. Therefore, it is suggested that the consistent application of psychological principles, appropriate for the presenting client, whilst clearly focused should include clear baseline and intervention recording.

For maximum impact of individual practitioner's working it may be helpful to consider ways of improved training and awareness rising amongst professionals as well as parents, with the facilitation of parent training (Werle *et al.*, 1993). Periodic reviews, opportunities to summarise and reflect on the current situation and

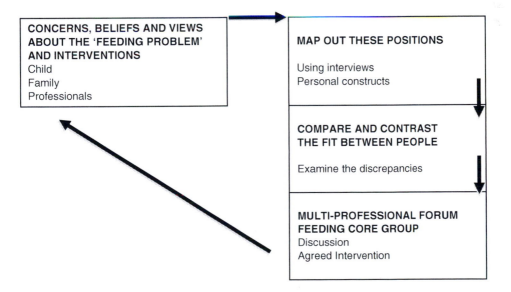

treatments all need time and require evaluation to see whether the aims of inter-ventions are being achieved. It may be considered helpful to 'map out' the position which the child, family and professionals find themselves with a long-term illness and feeding problems, and to take into consideration the beliefs and views of all concerned. A useful method of doing this arises from personal construct psychology (Kelly, 1955) and has been presented in the context of 'fit' between professionals where there are treatment adherence problems (Schwartz, 1998). This model can be applied quite easily in the feeding context.

Consideration of individual practitioner skills and acknowledgement of the boundaries to competence needs to be weighed up against the need to inter-vene to the best of one's ability based on experience and training. Puntis (2008) reaffirms that team working and good communication across different disci-plines and practitioners is crucial, and promotes the working of a specialist feeding team.

To conclude this chapter, it is anticipated that the outline of good practice will serve to consolidate the main themes and act as a mental checklist. Good practice would be underpinned, amongst other things, by:

- The awareness that the feeding problem does not 'stand alone' but is intricately associated with the contextual factors and the child's chronic condition.
- Communication and contact between professionals involved is essential to the assessment formulation and development of a comprehensive treatment plan.
- Interdisciplinary practices, applications and techniques need to be clear.
- Individual, family and systems-level consultation, liaison and practice should occur which may include local professionals and agencies (e.g. different direc-torates, trusts and voluntary bodies) and national networking (e.g. with tertiary referral centres).
- Acknowledgement that each professional's perspective, together with those of the family and child should be taken 'as parts which make up the whole picture'.
- Expect conflicting positions to be taken and make use of 'supervision' and opportunities for reflection and the adoption of a 'meta-stance' by someone not closely involved in the family professional system. Gain experience and practice in using a number of strategies and techniques for working with complex prob-lems (e.g. cognitive strategies such as 'reframing' and positive reinforcement) in addition to general 'tools of the trade'.
- Make certain that there is ongoing training and enthusiasm to develop new and creative approaches for work in this field (it can be 'infectious').
- Consider the needs of the family (e.g. for practical support and exploration of emotional issues for parents/relatives).
- Use of feedback cycles to assess interventions and consider the 'fit' of views and constructs between participants as regards the diverse inputs.
- Constant evaluation of practice is needed for so as to build up a research literature on effective management so as to add to current research in this important area.

It is hoped that, through this book as a whole, and this chapter specifically (in relation to children with chronic illness) we may begin to refute the early criticism by Wolke and Skuse (1992) that feeding problems are referred to a variety of specialists with few having adequate experience of the problem. Considering the collaborative working and shared research that has been undertaken since then, it is incumbent on those working in the field to examine the academic and clinical material and explore practice-based evidence so as to inform ongoing research and clinical practice.

REFERENCES

Abidin RR. *Parenting Stress Index*. Charlottesville: Pediatric Psychology Press; 1986.

Achenbach TM, Edelbrock C, *Manual for the Child Behaviour Checklist and Revised Child Behaviour Profile*. Burlington: University of Vermont; 1987.

Archer LA, Rosenbaum PL, Streiner DL. The children's eating behavior inventory: reliability and validity results. *J Pediatr Psychol*. 1991; **16**: 629–42.

Babbitt RL, Hoch TA, Coe DA, *et al*. Behavioral assessment and treatment of feeding disorders. *J Dev Behav Pediatr*. 1994; **15**: 278–91.

Baer MT. Nutrition services for children with disabilities and chronic illness. In: Wallace HM, Biehl RF, MacQueen JC, *et al*., editors. *Mosby's Resource Guide to Children with Disabilities and Chronic Illness*. St. Louis: Mosby; 1997.

Balen R, Fielding D, Lewis IJ. An activity week for children with cancer: who wants to go and why? *Child: Care, Health and Development*. 1998; **24**: 169–77.

Bernal ME. Behavioural treatment of a child's eating problem. *J Behav Ther Experi Psychiatr*. 1972; **3**: 43–50.

Blissett J, Harris G. A behavioural intervention in a child with feeding problems. *J Hum Nutr Diet*. 2002; **15**: 255–60.

Bradford R. *Children, Families and Chronic Disease*. London: Routledge; 1997.

Budd KS, McGraw TE, Farbisz R, *et al*. Psychosocial concomitants of children's feeding disorders. *J Pediatr Psychol*. 1992; **17**: 81–94.

Cairns GF, Altman K. Behavioral treatment of cancer-related anorexia. *J Behav Ther Exp Psychiatr*. 1979; **10**: 353–6.

Carey S. *Conceptual Change in Childhood*. Massachusetts: MIT; 1985.

Chamberlin JL, Henry MM, Roberts JD, *et al*. An infant and toddler feeding group program. *Am J Occup Ther*. 1991; **45**: 907–11.

Chase HP, Long MA, Lavin MH. Cystic fibrosis and malnutrition. *J Pediatr*. 1979; **95**: 337–47.

Clawson EP, Palinski KS, Elliott CA. Outcome of intensive oral motor and behavioural interventions for feeding difficulties in three children with Golden hair Syndrome. *Paediatr Rehabil*. 2006; **9**(1): 65–75.

Crist W, McDonnell P, Beck M, *et al*. Behavior at mealtimes and the young child with cystic fibrosis. *Dev Behav Pediatr*. 1994; **15**: 157–61.

Culbert AP, Kajander RL, Kohen DP, *et al*. Hypnobehavioral approaches for school-age children with dysphagia and food aversion: a case series. *Dev Behav Pediatr*. 1996; **17**: 335–41.

Drotar D. Intervention research: pushing back the frontiers of pediatric psychology. *J Pediatr Psychol*. 1997; **22**: 593–606.

Douglas J. Behavioural eating disorders in young children. *Curr Paediatr*. 1995; **5**: 39–42.

Douglas JE, Bryon M. Interview data on severe behavioural eating difficulties in young children. *Arch Dis Child*. 1996; **75**: 304–8.

Douglas JE, Hulson B, Trompeter RS. Psycho-social outcome of parents and young children after renal transplantation. *Child Care Hlth Dev*. 1998; **24**: 73–83.

Elander J, Midence K. Children with chronic illness. *The Psychologist*. 1997; **Mar**: 1–5.

Epston D. Strange and novel ways of addressing guilt. In: Epston D, White M, editors. *Experience, Contradiction, Narrative and Imagination*. Adelaide: Dulwich Centre Publications; 1994.

Eriksen E. *Identity and the Life Cycle*. New York: Norton; 1980.

Fielding D. Chronic illness in children. In: Watts FN, editor. *New Developments in Clinical Psychology*. Leicester: British Psychological Society Books; 1985.

Foreman JW, Chan JCM. Chronic renal failure in infants and children. *J Pediatr*. 1988; **113**: 793–800.

Hampton D. *Failure to Thrive*. London: The Grange Press; 1995.

Harris G. Feeding problems and their treatment. In: St James I, Harris G, Messer D, editors. *Infant Crying, Feeding and Sleeping: development, problems and treatments*. London: Harvester Wheatsheaf; 1993.

Harris G, Booth IW. The nature and management of eating problems in pre-school children. In: Cooper PJ, Stein A, editors. *Feeding Problems and Eating Disorders in Children and Adolescents*. Philadelphia: Harwood Academic Press; 1992.

Hoch TA, Babbitt RL, Coe DA, *et al*. Contingency contracting. *Behavior Modif*. 1994; **18**: 106–28.

Jenkins J, Milla P. Feeding problems and failure to thrive. In: Richman N, Lansdown R, editors. *Problems of Pre-school Children*. Chichester: Wiley; 1988.

Kedesdy JH, Budd KS. *Childhood Feeding Disorders*. Baltimore: Paul Brookes; 1998.

Kelly GA. *The Psychology of Personal Constructs*. New York: Norton; 1955.

Kendall PC, Norton-Ford JD. *Clinical Psychology: scientific and professional dimensions*. New York: Wiley and Sons; 1982.

Knafl K, Breitmeyer B, Gallo A, *et al*. Parents' views of healthcare providers: an exploration of the components of a positive working relationship. *Child Health Care*. 1992; **21**: 90–5.

La Greca AM, Varni JW. Editorial: Interventions in pediatric psychology: a look to the future. *J Pediatr Psychol*. 1993; **18**: 667–9.

Lefton-Greif MA, Arvedson JC. Schoolchildren with dysphagia associated with medically complex conditions. *Lang Speech Hear Ser*. 2008; **39**: 237–48.

Leung AK, Robson WL. The toddler who does not eat. *Am Fam Phys*. 1994; **49**: 1789–800.

Lindberg L, Bohlin G, Hagekull B. Early feeding problems in a normal population. *Int J Eating Disord*. 1991; **10**: 395–405.

Linscheid TR. Eating problems in children. In: Walker CE, Roberts MC, editors. *Handbook of Clinical Child Psychology*. New York, NY: Wiley; 1992.

Linscheid TR. Behavioral treatment of feeding disorders in children. In: Watson TS, Gresham FM, editors. *Handbook of Child Behavior Therapy*. New York, NY: Plenum Press; 1998.

MacDonald A. Nutritional management of cystic fibrosis. *Arch Dis Child*. 1996; **74**: 81–7.

Magrab PR, Papadapoulou ZL. The effect of a token economy on dietary compliance for children on hemodialysis. *J Applied Behavior Analysis*. 1977; **10**: 573–8.

Martin M, Shaw NJ. Feeding problems in infants and young children with chronic lung disease. *J Hum Nutr Diet*. 1997; **10**(5): 271–5.

McCollum AT, Gibson LE. Family adaptation to the child with cystic fibrosis. *J Pediatr*. 1970; **77**(4): 571–8.

Melvin D, Wright C, Goddard S. Incidence and nature of feeding problems in young children refereed to a paediatric HIV service in London: FEAD screening. *Child Care Hlth Dev*. 1997; **23**(4): 297–313.

O'Brien S, Repp AC, Williams GE, *et al*. Pediatric feeding disorders. *Behav Modif*. 1991; **15**: 394–418.

Padilla GV, Grant MM. Psychosocial aspects of artificial feeding. *Cancer*. 1995; **55**: 301–4.

Pearson DA, Pumariega AJ, Seilheimer DK. The development of psychiatric symptomatology in patients with cystic fibrosis. *J Am Acad Child Adoles Psychiatr*. 1991; **30**: 290–7.

Piaget J. *The Grasp of Consciousness*. Cambridge, MA: Harvard University Press; 1976.

Pollock M, Kovacs M, Charron-Prochownik D. Eating disorders and maladaptive dietary/insulin management among youths with childhood onset insulin dependent diabetes mellitus. *J Am Acad Child Adoles Psychiatr.* 1995; **34**: 291–6.

Puntis JW. Specialist feeding clinics. *Arch Dis Child.* 2008; **93**(2): 164–7.

Ravelli AM. Gastrointestinal function in chronic renal failure. *Pediatr Nephrol.* 1995; **9**: 756–62.

Rees L, Rigden SPA, Ward GM. Chronic renal failure and growth. *Arch Dis Child.* 1989; **64**: 573–7.

Ross DM, Ross SA. *Childhood Pain.* Baltimore, MD: Urban & Schwarzenberg; 1988.

Ruley EJ, Bock GH, Kerzner B, *et al.* Feeding disorders and gastroesophageal reflux in infants. *Pediatr Nephrol.* 1989; **3**: 424–9.

Sadowski RH, Allred EN, Jabs K. Sodium modelling ameliorates intradialytic and interdialytic symptoms in young haemodialysis patients. *J Am Soc Nephrol.* 1993; **4**: 1192–8.

Sanders MR, Patel RK, le Grice B, *et al.* Children with persistent feeding difficulties: an observational analysis of the feeding interactions of problem and non-problem eaters. *Hlth Psychol.* 1993; **12**: 64–73.

Sanders MR, Turner KMT, Wall CR, *et al.* Mealtime behavior and parent-child interaction: a comparison of children with cystic fibrosis, children with feeding problems, and nonclinic controls. *J Pediatr Psychol.* 1997; **22**: 881–900.

Schwartz AL. Adherence in children with renal disease. In: Myers LB, Midence K, editors. *Adherence to Treatment in Medical Conditions.* Amsterdam: Harwood Academic Press; 1998.

Schwartz AL, Mercer A. The role of the clinical psychologist. In: Twycross A, Moriarty A, Betts T, editors. *Paediatric Pain Management.* Oxford: Radcliffe Medical Press; 1998.

Singer LT, Nofer JA, Benson-Szekely LJ, *et al.* Behavioral assessment and management of food refusal in children with cystic fibrosis. *Dev Behav Pediatr.* 1991; **12**: 115–19.

Skuse D, Wolke D, Reilly S. Failure to thrive: clinical and developmental aspects. In: Reschmidt H, Schmidt, MH, editors. *Developmental Psychopathology.* New York, NY: Hofgrefe and Huber; 1992.

Sokel B, Devane S, Bentovim A, *et al.* Self hypnotherapeutic treatment of habitual reflex vomiting. *Arch Dis Child.* 1991; **65**: 626–7.

Stark LJ, Bowen AM, Tyc VL, *et al.* A behavioural approach to increasing calorie consumption in children with cystic fibrosis. *J Pediatr Psychol.* 1990; **15**: 309–26.

Strologo LD, Principato F, Sinibaldi D, *et al.* Feeding dysfunction in infants with severe chronic renal failure after long-term nasogastric tubefeeding. *Pediatr Nephrol.* 1997; **11**: 84–6.

Tawfik R, Dickson A, Clarke M, *et al.* Caregivers' perceptions following gastrostomy in severely disabled children with feeding problems. *Dev Med Child Neurol.* 1997; **39**: 746–51.

van Eys J. Malnutrition in children with cancer. *Cancer.* 1979; **43**: 2030–5.

Wallander JL. Theory driven research in pediatric psychology: a little bit on why and how. *J Pediatr Psychol.* 1992; **17**: 521–35.

Warady BA, Kriley M, Belden B, *et al.* Nutritional and behavioural aspects of nasogastric tube feeding in infants receiving chronic peritoneal dialysis. *Adv Perit D.* 1990; **6**: 265–8.

Wardley BL, Puntis JWL, Taitz LS. *Handbook of Child Nutrition.* Oxford: Oxford University Press; 1997.

Werle MA, Murphy TB, Budd KS. Treating chronic food refusal in young children: home based parent training. *J Appl Behav Anal.* 1993; **26**: 421–33.

Wolke D, Skuse D. The management of infant feeding problems. In: Cooper PJ, Stein A, editors. *Feeding Problems and Eating Disorders in Children and Adolescents.* Philadelphia, PA: Harwood Academic Press; 1992. pp. 27–60.

Wooster DM, Brady NR, Mitchell A, *et al.* Pediatric feeding: a transdisciplinary team's perspective. *Top Lang Disord.* 1998; **18**: 34–51.

Zeltzer L, LeBaron S, Zeltzer PM. The effectiveness of behavioural interventions for reduction of nausea and vomiting in children and adolescents receiving chemotherapy. *J Clin Oncol.* 1984; **2**: 683–90.

Zeltzer LK, Dolgin MJ, Sahler OJ, *et al.* Sibling adaptation to childhood cancer collaborative study: health outcomes of siblings of children with cancer. *Med Pediatr Oncol.* 1996; **27**: 98–107.

CHAPTER 13

An intensive coaching approach to the management of feeding problems

Monique Thomas-Holtus, Gerben Sinnema and Anthony P Messer

INTRODUCTION

The feeding counsellor is a relatively unique role in the Netherlands and links important aspects of psychology, dietetics and paediatrics through a long-term practical experience of feeding problems within a multi-disciplinary setting. She plays an important part in the initial assessment, exploring dietetic, behavioural and paediatric issues, all of which provide important information about the feeding problem. The specific role of the feeding counsellor is to integrate information from the assessment to facilitate a formulation of the feeding problem and then to co-ordinate and implement the multi-disciplinary intervention. The intervention is based on an intensive coaching system, which is implemented and co-ordinated by the feeding counsellor, who offers the parents remote access via telephone or email at fixed times. Thus, the feeding counsellor acts as an interface between the parents and the multi-disciplinary team, enabling progress to be monitored on a continuous basis. This can be invaluable when such things as new tastes are being introduced or oral feeding is initiated. Such a system ensures prompt feedback and continuous data collection and monitoring whilst also providing a source of support for parents.

This chapter introduces the feeding counsellor as a unique member of the multi-disciplinary team and describes how the intensive coaching protocol is used. The protocol may be used for children treated in hospitals either as in- or outpatients (i.e. community).

THE ROLE OF THE FEEDING COUNSELLOR

The role of the feeding counsellor has been developed over a period of more than 30 years of assessment and treatment of young children and their feeding problems. It has a specific remit to work towards optimal treatment and co-ordination of care in cases of severe and chronic food refusal in young children (aged 0–4 years) with medical conditions. The feeding counsellor's role is summarised below.

The role of the feeding counsellor

To treat severe and chronic food refusal with behavioural techniques aimed at the behavioural components that maintain the feeding problem by a combination of the following:

1 co-ordination of care during the treatment of the food refusal both in the in- and outpatient settings
2 advising on prevention by informing parents, caretakers and multi-disciplinary teams in various healthcare settings
3 coaching paediatricians, medical specialists inside and outside the hospital on how to develop new feeding coaching systems and protocols
4 implementing an intensive coaching system[1] for parents of young children with a feeding problem
5 preventing a waiting list of patients needing outpatient treatment.

THE SKILLS OF THE FEEDING COUNSELLOR

The feeding counsellor is a member of the Paediatric Psychology Department and is a graduate psychologist trained in behaviour therapy and supported and supervised by the Clinical Psychologist. It is essential that she is able to use her skills creatively, is open minded and calm. Additionally, she must be inspired by a team approach, which is an important feature of the work.

The skills of the feeding counsellor

- skilled in detailed history-taking pertaining to feeding problems
- has an ability to apply behaviour modification and child management techniques
- skilled in training others to understand the clinical aspects of feeding problems in young children

---

[1] The intensive coaching system uses multimedia to inform, advice and give feedback to parents and the multi-disciplinary team.

- has an understanding of the issues pertaining to young, sick children and their parents
- has an ability to work with multi-disciplinary teams and severe feeding problems
- is competent in co-ordinating the work of other disciplines involved
- is skilled at managing complexity demands and working under pressure.
- has the capacity to use skills creatively for individualised approaches to food refusal.

THE INTENSIVE COACHING SYSTEM

The intensive coaching system is used for both in- and outpatients, with the feeding counsellor acting as a personal coach for the parents and their child. Using multi-media techniques, email and telephone contact, the feeding counsellor can encourage both children and parents to progress through each stage of the intervention, whether it is the introduction and tasting of new foods or beginning the process of oral feeding and eliminating tube feeding. In turn, there is prompt feedback to the multi-disciplinary team on the family's progress as well as on any unexpected behavioural or medical problems that may occur. Speed of communication between family, feeding counsellor and team is a distinct advantage of this method.

Intensive coaching system protocol

- consultation by the feeding counsellor
- detailed history
- observation and video recording, in real time, in the family home
- analysis of all information leading to a working hypothesis
- multi-disciplinary consensus and strategy
- parents' debrief
- beginning feeding treatment in the in- or outpatient setting.

The intensive coaching system is used for as long as necessary.

The inpatient system

Children are generally admitted to hospital when their medical status is compromised as a result of their feeding problems. In these cases, the aetiology of the food refusal is mostly based on a medical history, chronic illness, immature oral functioning, breathing problems, vomiting without a clear diagnosis or a failure to thrive due to inadequate food intake (Nicholls and Bryant-Waugh, 2009).

Food refusal can be total, i.e. the child refuses all food that is offered at feeding time, or partial. In the case of partial refusal, feeding is often atypical for the child's age or developmental stage. Examples include the older child who will only breastfeed or those for whom weaning has failed. Other children may be selective for consistency, texture or taste, or only accept fluids. These children have been described in detail in the preceding chapters.

The protocol

The child is admitted to a general paediatric or gastroenterology ward. A multi-disciplinary trajectory then begins, including supplementary medical investigation as required. These take place in the context of multi-disciplinary assessment, which combines the skills of the feeding counsellor, dietician and speech and language therapist (SALT). Oral functions are screened by the SALT, and the dietician undertakes a dietary assessment. Assessment of family function may be undertaken by the social worker or psychologist.

The feeding counsellor is responsible for taking a detailed feeding history with the parents and observes several episodes of feeding in 'real time'. Video footage is also used to record feeding behaviours and the interaction between parents and children (and/or nurse and child) during the first 2 days of the inpatient stay. Assessment information is then shared within the multi-disciplinary team. If there is a multi-disciplinary consensus about the formulation of the feeding problem, the feeding counsellor discusses this with the parents and begins to co-ordinate all interventions. From now on, the intensive coaching system begins for the parents. During the inpatient phase, parents are able to telephone the Feeding Counsellor on all 7 days of the week at a fixed time in the evening to discuss their child's progress, their worries or concerns in relation to the inpatient programme. The feeding counsellor therefore acts as a personal adviser for the parents during this time. She also acts as a mediator in the case of any miscommunication between nurses, medical specialists and other professionals within the hospital.

The feeding counsellor gives detailed instructions and feedback to the parents and the multi-disciplinary team about behavioural conditions and techniques used during feeding times/meal times. Formulations and strategies may evolve, as a feeding problem is a dynamic process, and are updated every day and noted in the personal electronic patient record (EPR). The length of the inpatient stay depends on the nature of diagnosis and intervention possibilities; an average inpatient stay lasts between 2 and 3 weeks.

As soon as the child is ready to leave the hospital, the feeding counsellor begins to monitor and support the parents by means of the intensive coaching system. She continues to be on call every day at a pre-arranged hour in the evening. In addition, parents can use email to exchange updated information about the progress of their child. They can do this the day before their consultation call, so that the information can be discussed. This enables both the parents and feeding counsellor to make maximum use of the time available.

The feeding counsellor always provides here-and-now feedback to the parents on their management of their child's feeding behaviour. Other members of the team

can be informed immediately by email, or by updates in the personal EPR, thus
ensuring that a close communication is maintained.

Noortje

Noortje, aged 10 months with a diagnosis of congenital hip dysplasia and failure
to thrive, was admitted clinically for a second opinion by a paediatric referral
from a regional hospital. Noortje was vomiting every day from the moment tube
feeding commenced. The feeding scheme was 5 × 180 mL. This consisted of no
more than 60 mL by bottle at each feed, with the remainder supplied by tube,
using the siphon technique. Supplementary medical examination failed to provide an explanation for Noortje's vomiting problem.

The feeding counsellor was asked for consultation and took a detailed feeding history with the parents. They explained that growth had been a problem from birth.
Noortje had been fed with breast milk by bottle, because breastfeeding had not
been possible. During the first 6 months, the parents were feeding Noortje seven to
eight times a day, because she did not take enough feed. Between 4 and 6 months,
her poor feeding and low weight began to concern the parents but, at this stage,
their concerns were not shared by those professionals involved in Noortje's regular
care. A change from breast milk to high-calorie formula led to even greater refusal of
the bottle, though Noortje began to accept a few tiny spoons of fruit and vegetables.
Her growth began to fall away from the expected trajectory. Eventually, Noortje was
admitted to the regional hospital for an observation of her feeding problem. The
quantity of milk taken per feed remained low, leading to a decision to initiate tube
feeding; since then Noortje had vomited every day.

The paediatrician decided on following a 'wait and see' policy and so Noortje was
discharged from hospital. However, concerns remained. A second episode occurred
in hospital when the orthopaedic surgeon examined Noortje to review her hip dis-
plasia. By this time, she was 7 months of age. The vomiting problem had continued
and had become a major concern for the parents. Finally, Noortje was admitted to
the Wilhelmina Children's Hospital in Utrecht.

Noortje's feeding programme

After the assessment phase, which included several observations, the feeding
counsellor was able to hypothesise that the volume of the stomach was Noortje's
main problem. From birth onwards she had developed a feeding habit of a maximum of 60 mL at each feed; therefore the stomach was not used to accepting
more volume. Before the tube feeding commenced, Noortje had a daily feeding

scheme of more than six feeds a day and never vomited. The vomiting problem only began after the tube feeding was initiated. Vomiting is an unfavourable condition for oral feeding in general as it is a highly aversive experience, which can increase the risk for total feed refusal. The strategy was therefore to stop all oral feeding, stop the siphon technique and start feeding a high-calorie formula using the feeding pump five times a day at an amount and speed that was believed to be acceptable for Noortje's stomach. Within a day the vomiting stopped. Noortje accepted the speed of 145 mL in 60 minutes within a week and began to gain weight. By the third week, the speed was 145 mL in 45 minutes and the good news was that she was growing sufficiently.

During Noortje's inpatient period, the feeding counsellor co-ordinated the feeding programme with the multi-disciplinary team and worked closely with the parents every day. Noortje was discharged from hospital after the fifth week. The feeding counsellor supported the parents to develop their skills and confidence in a number of behavioural techniques (e.g. rehearsal and distraction) that would help them gradually re-start oral feeding (weaning) in tiny steps, with the idea of 'training' Noortje to accept solid food and start accepting different tastes and textures.

From the moment Noortje became an outpatient, intensive coaching by the feeding counsellor was initiated. Parents were able to telephone her for advice on speed and amount of Noortje's tube feed and also of Noortje's oral feeding experience. This approach enabled any behavioural or medical problems to be immediately addressed and, if necessary, to be passed on to the multi-disciplinary team. At follow-up at 15 months, Noortje was growing well and her general development was good. She was eating solid foods and was no longer dependent on tube feeding.

OUTPATIENT SYSTEM

The outpatient programme follows an assessment procedure by the same multi-disciplinary team, with the feeding counsellor observing and analysing the behavioural components of the feeding problem within the actual situation at home. Typical candidates for outpatient treatment are children whose previous medical history is no longer problematic but whose feeding problems persist. Some may have been treated in the community, without success.

Following the initial multi-disciplinary consultation and working hypothesis, the team is able to arrive at a formulation of the problem. The feeding counsellor contributes to this process by gathering data from interviews with the parents and through observations of feeding, using both video and 'live' observation in the parents' home. Home visits are used not only for analysis of the feeding problem but also for treatment sessions at home; this also has the advantage of avoiding any disruption to the children's feeding and sleeping routines.

A summary of the initial assessment period undertaken by the feeding counsellor is given below.

The feeding counsellor's role in gathering information
- Detailed history-taking at the hospital with the parents but without the presence of the child.
- Parent recording of feeding episodes at home.
- Home visit to observe a 'live' feeding episode with the family and to explore the possible options for therapeutic interventions.
- Multi-disciplinary evaluation.
- Second home visit for discussing the multi-disciplinary strategy with the parents.
- Introduction for the *Eat-Well* program for children.
- Start of the intensive coaching system.

After the history-taking with the parents and feedback by the feeding counsellor on the videotaped feeding episodes, a home visit is planned for a live observation of feeding at home. At the same time, possible options for therapeutic interventions are explored. After this home visit the multi-disciplinary team meets with the feeding counsellor to discuss the strategy for addressing the feeding problem. Occasionally, the feeding counsellor may raise a need for supplementary medical examinations, based on information revealed by her discussions and observations with the family. The intervention 'pathway' is summarised below. Once the strategy is agreed with both professionals and parents, the feeding counsellor visits the parents again to help them prepare; both the parents and the child are included in this process (Van Eijkelenborg and Thomas-Holtus, 2008).

TREATMENT PATHWAY
- In- or outpatient system.
- Selection of behavioural techniques to be used for solving the feeding problem.
- Introduction of intensive coaching system.
- Information about the intensive coaching system.
- Post-treatment award of child's personal feeding certificate.

Case study 2, Kees, describes a typical intervention, comprising a period of inpatient assessment, followed by intensive intervention in the community.

Kees

Kees, aged 5 months, known to have a cleft lip and palate, was admitted clinically to the Wilhelmina Children's Hospital in Utrecht 2 weeks after surgery to his palate because he was increasingly refusing his bottle. He was initially found to have a virus infection. However, once the virus infection had cleared Kees still had a minimum oral intake. His parents were very worried because he began to lose weight again and did not grow for several weeks. Kees was sent to the surgical department where he had been operated on two weeks ago. As this department is not specialised in feeding problems, they were slow to diagnose that there was a serious issue of feeding refusal. They only had focused on his palate and could not find any symptoms that explained his refusal to feed. Nursing staff had taken over a number of his feeds and even tried force-feeding to get Kees to take his bottle, after 4 days of which the feeding counsellor was contacted.

The feeding counsellor discovered a number of unfavourable feeding conditions, including low weight, a viral infection and a persistent fungal mouth infection, which was being treated by the application of a bitter-tasting ointment in Kees' mouth shortly before feeding commenced. After a summary history-taking, the feeding counsellor advised the medical and nursing staff to stop offering the bottle and to start a 'time out' of oral feeding for 3–4 weeks. The feeding counsellor discussed with the parents the reasons for stopping all oral feeding efforts because of the stress and negative associations it caused. Kees' parents were relieved not to have any responsibility for his daily intake by bottle. They remained in the hospital for two more days so that they could learn how to manage the tube-feeding system. Then, from the moment they left the hospital with Kees, they had intensive contact with the feeding counsellor.

Further detailed discussion with the feeding counsellor revealed that Kees had been hard to feed from birth due to recurrent fungal infections in his mouth. For a period of 4 months, he would only accept the bottle from his mother. Her feeding technique at home was to walk into a separate room where she could be alone with him. Every feed took more than an hour.

After 2 weeks the feeding counsellor made a house visit. Kees' parents were happy with the tube feeding because Kees was thriving and they could see some development of his motor skills. As a result of his progress, the feeding counsellor suggested restarting some oral feeding, beginning with a little solid food, just for an experience of taste. The feeding counsellor used a range of behavioural techniques (modelling, rehearsal and distraction) while the lightly loaded spoon was offered to Kees (Gillis, 2003). Over the next few weeks there were intensive telephone and email contacts between the parents and the feeding counsellor. Within 6 weeks the tube feeding was stopped completely (Gutentag and Hammer, 2000) and Kees was fed without any problem.

Geeske

Geeske aged 3 years was known to have a mild food allergy and was a selective eater. According to the feeding history provided by her parents, Geeske had evidenced feeding problems from birth. Her milk was changed several times in the first few months after birth because of severe colic and there were constant concerns about inadequate growth. The paediatrician referred to the feeding counsellor to analyse the behavioural components of Geeske's feeding problem when the parents indicated that they could no longer handle her feeding. Geeske accepted bread but refused all hot food. She had a preference for crunchy food, such as toasted bread instead of soft bread and a general taste preference for salty food but according to her parents she had always refused to eat hot food. Geeske's parents explained that their daughter was strong-willed.

The *Eat-Well* management program for learning to taste and to accept new food was introduced to Geeske during a home visit. An *Eat-Well* dinner set, designed and tested by the feeding counsellor[2] was used to explain the principle of positive reinforcement. This dinner set is based on behavioural techniques, such as reinforcement and distraction.

At the end of the history-taking, the feeding counsellor discussed with the parents elements of the *Eat-Well* management program that would be used to address Geeske's feeding problem. Once a consensus had been reached between the multidisciplinary team and parents, the programme began. From that point the parents were able to contact the feeding counsellor by telephone and/or email to discuss Geeske's progress with taste 'lessons'; if they felt it necessary, they could even contact every day at a fixed hour. If the parents had a lot of questions to ask, the feeding counsellor would advise them to email before telephoning, to give her time to reflect on their questions. The Feeding Counsellor also offered to visit the family at home as soon as possible to give live feed back on a taste lesson. These things seemed to help Geeske's parents feel that their concerns were taken seriously. The Feeding Counsellor was able to support the parents' own development of the practical techniques necessary to manage the behavioural components of Geeske's feeding and move her gradually to tasting, and eating, family meals after a period of 4 months.

---

[2] This feeding set was designed in cooperation with *Difrax*, a firm specialising in baby equipment.

How the *Eat-Well* dinner set works

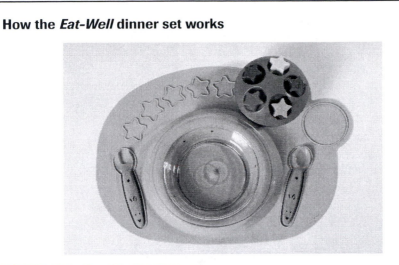

FIGURE 13.1: The *Eat-Well* dinner set.

The dinner set has been designed to make eating fun and to also provide concrete reinforcement for good eating behaviour. The stars on the placemat can be used for rewarding individual therapeutic steps, such as tasting or swallowing a particular food or trying food of a specific consistency or texture. The different colours of the stars can be used for different categories of food, for example, green for vegetables yellow for pasta or rice, red for fruit and so on. Also on the placemat there are two buttons. One button lights up the lamps inside the plate; every touch of the spoon on the plate illuminates the lights, thus stimulating the child to take more food. A second button activates lights and music and may be used when the child has finished a certain amount of food. There is a red 'toadstool' on the right-hand side of the plate where parents or caretakers can put a note with a surprise at the end of the mealtime. The toadstool can also be used for serving desert.

The average number of telephone coaching interventions during the treatment of a feeding problem such as the one described above is seven during the first two weeks. This tends to taper off, depending on the progress of the treatment. In general the introduction of cooked meals is always limited to a maximum of four different meals, the choice of which always involves the child in advance. The feeding counsellor monitors the introduction and progress of the child with cooked meals.

Extensive practical experience of medically related feeding problems in the Wilhelmina Childrens' Hospital has led to a publication of a practical guide with tips, hints and pitfalls for parents in managing feeding problems at home (Van Eijkelenborg and Thomas-Holtus, 2008). You can read a summary of this publication in Part III of this book.

SUMMARY

Since 2000, the diagnosis and treatment of young children with feeding problems at the Wilhelmina Children's Hospital in Utrecht has been by means of an intensive coaching system. Both this system and the role of the feeding counsellor are innovative developments in the field. The Utrecht experience has been encouraging. The feeding counsellor manages an average of 120 new patients a year, 60% of whom begin as inpatients and proceed to the outpatient system mode. The starting point depends on the medical complexity of the case and the pedagogical skills of the parents. Around 40% of feeding problems are treated exclusively by means of the outpatient system. Future development includes expansion of this approach into the community aiming at exporting the practical knowledge of how to deal with the first symptoms of a feeding problem in order to focus on early intervention and the prevention of feeding disorders in young children.

REFERENCES

Gillis L. Use of an interactive game to increase food acceptance – a pilot study. *Child Care Health Dev.* 2003 Sep; **29**(5): 373–5.

Gutentag S, Hammer D. Shaping oral feeding in a gastronomy tube-dependent child in natural settings. *Behav Modif.* 2000 Jul; **24**(3): 395–410.

Nicholls D, Bryant-Waugh R. Eating disorders of infancy and childhood: definition, symptomatology, epidemiology, and comorbidity [review]. *Child Adolesc Psychiatr Clin N Am.* 2009 Jan; **18**(1): 17–30.

Van Eijkelenborg V, Thomas-Holtus M. *Eat-Well.* 1st ed. Holland, Bilthoven: Difrax BV; 2008.

CHAPTER 14

Telehealth interventions for feeding problems

Alan Silverman

INTRODUCTION

This chapter considers the uses of telehealth technology, specifically videoconferencing, for the delivery of interdisciplinary treatment to children with feeding and nutrition problems. Families of children with feeding and nutrition problems frequently present to clinicians in primary care settings with significant concerns for their children's well-being (Linscheid *et al.*, 2003). Given the complexity of these disorders, inter-disciplinary treatment approaches including medicine, nutrition, speech and language therapy, and psychological interventions are considered to be optimal (Kedesdy and Budd, 1998). Unfortunately, there are relatively few experts who specialise in feeding problems and even fewer interdisciplinary feeding clinics. Telehealth may help to alleviate the effects of this shortage. Recent estimates show that families with children have a very high rate of computer ownership and that the vast majority of these families have online access (Kennedy *et al.*, 2008). Thus, for many families, effective telehealth services may be readily available and increased access to therapies not available in their local community.

Gage: a selective eater with severe food allergies

Gage was a 4-year-old boy who presented with a long history of food allergies and a highly selective diet. He was 108.9-cm tall (80th percentile) and weighed 17.9 kg (55th percentile). His body mass index was 15 (30th percentile) and he was 97% of his ideal body weight. His food allergies included wheat, oats,

---

egg, peanut, fish, tree nut and soy. He had a significant history of gagging, vomiting and diarrhoea after exposure to these foods. He took medication for management of his allergy symptoms and had an epinephrine pen for emergency use. Gage's parents also reported their own experiences of distress at each meal secondary to Gage's mealtime behaviour problems, which included frequent crying, gagging, retching and repeated attempts to flee from the table during meals. His food selectivity had caused micronutrient deficiencies, which required nutritional intervention. The family's goals were to expand his diet and help him to try new foods more willingly.

After his initial assessment, Gage's interdisciplinary treatment team determined that his feeding problems were likely to have resulted from aversive feeding events associated with feeding-related allergy exposures. Gage's initial food selectivity began when the family attempted a complete allergy elimination diet and was further strengthened by his parents who were concerned that negative feeding behaviours were stemming from allergy exposures. Gage's parents were informed that he would probably require a combination of behavioural interventions with nutritional and medical monitoring. Unfortunately, the family lived over 120 miles from the nearest feeding clinic. His parents reported their frustration at the lack of local feeding disorder experts. They were also frustrated that they had to choose between travelling great distances for care and managing a complex medical problem without access to appropriately trained specialists.

To increase the likelihood of a successful treatment outcome, the family opted to receive treatment by telehealth. The therapy model included real-time videoconferencing with store-and-forward clinical data (e.g. feeding records and behavioural scales) forwarded by email to the treatment team in advance of clinical sessions. The family completed six weekly telehealth sessions with a paediatric psychologist, a paediatric dietician and a paediatric gastroenterology nurse. By the end of treatment, Gage was eating at least three foods from each food group, he had significantly improved behaviours at meal times, he was taking a daily multivitamin and his parents reported significantly improved attitudes toward mealtimes. At the end of treatment, Gage's mother reported, 'I don't believe we would have been as successful if these sessions were not in our home. Videoconferencing allowed you to see exactly what happens in our home so that you could tell us exactly what to do'. Gage and his family have continued to make gains and were recently discharged from our clinical care. He now eats a wide variety of foods from all food groups, and his family reports looking forward to meals together. Gage continues to grow and develop well.

Many families experience dilemmas similar to those encountered by Gage's family and find themselves having to choose between seeking treatment from a distant provider or allowing their child's condition to remain untreated. Gage's family was fortunate to have a telehealth option that allowed the family to receive care in a manner that did not overwhelm the family's resources. Similar examples will be intermittently used to illustrate key concepts for the provision of telehealth services to treat feeding problems of childhood.

The primary objective of this chapter is to present telehealth technologies as an alternative treatment model that would increase access to feeding specialists and to interdisciplinary feeding clinics. To begin, first a brief overview of telehealth is presented, including a review of recent applications to paediatric populations. Second, uses of telehealth technologies in the treatment of feeding problems are discussed. Third, technical considerations for starting and maintaining a successful telehealth clinic are presented. Fourth, a study of an active telehealth feeding program including estimates of treatment efficacy and interpersonal/therapeutic alliance effects is described. Finally, considerations of potential barriers to optimal treatment by way of telehealth are considered.

INTRODUCTION TO TELEHEALTH AND ITS USE

In recent years, technological advances have provided a gateway for improving access to healthcare (Liss *et al.*, 2002). The term telehealth has been broadly defined as the use of modern telecommunications and information technologies for the provision of healthcare to individuals at a geographical distance (Jerome and Zaylor, 2000; Liss *et al.*, 2002). More precisely, telehealth is 'the use of telecommunications and information technology to provide access to health assessment, intervention, consultation, supervision, education and information across distance' (Nicklelson, 1998). The term 'telehealth' encompasses a wide variety of specific modalities including telephone-based interactions, internet-based information, still and live imaging, personal digital assistants (PDAs) and interactive two-way audio–video communication or television (i.e. point-to-point videoconferencing; Greeno *et al.*, 2000; Hilty *et al.*, 2002).

Telehealth advocates suggest that telehealth reduces barriers to care, enhances care relationships among providers, improves clinical outcomes and reduces costs. Telehealth points of service are theoretically limitless and have included patient's homes, outpatient clinics, inpatient facilities, hospital emergency rooms, schools, hospices, group and nursing homes, homeless shelters and forensic facilities (Capner, 2000; Rothchild, 1999). Videoconferencing has been specifically associated with a number of benefits including the expansion of services to families in remote locations where they would otherwise receive only sporadic access or no care at all (Dossetor *et al.*, 1999; Freir *et al.*, 1999). Videoconferencing also has the advantage of allowing the therapist to complete 'house calls' in which assessment of the home environment can be considered in a way that would not be possible through traditional office visits.

TABLE 14.1: Comparison of telehealth treatment models to traditional office-based services

Assessment/therapeutic intervention	Telehealth store and forward	Telehealth real-time connection	Traditional office visit
Medical Record Review	+ + +	-	-
Feeding Record Analysis	+ + +	+	+
Caregiver-Completed Questionnaires	+ + +	+	+
Clinical Interview	-	+ + +	+ + +
Behavioural Observation of the Child while being fed	+	+ +	+ +
Physical examination	-	-	+ + +
Behaviour management	-	+ +	+ + +
Parent training	-	+ +	+ + +
Consultation with specialists from other clinics	+	+ + +	-

- Not recommended: + May be useful: + + Likely to be useful: + + + Probably useful

The methodology

Telehealth technologies typically utilise 'store-and-forward' interventions (e.g. reviewing a previously recorded feeding or a previously recorded swallow study) or 'real-time' interventions (e.g. videoconferencing, directly receiving medical data through a web interface). Generally, both store-and-forward interventions and real-time interventions employ a 'hub and spoke' model in which one or more therapists located in a specialty feeding clinic (typically in a larger metropolitan area) consult directly with a distal treatment team, a patient's family, or both.

Store-and-forward interventions typically are less labour intensive for the treatment team and require little technical and/or administrative support. These sessions do not need to be scheduled, and the information is generally sent by electronic file transfers or as email attachments. Thus, sessions may be completed at the therapists' leisure and completed as the clinician's schedules allows, thus providing ample time for the materials to be reviewed before deciding on a course of treatment. Impressions and recommendations can be carefully considered and documented before feedback is sent to the distal site. One disadvantage of store-and-forward interventions is that contact with the patient and the patient's family is limited. Another disadvantage is that the clinician's questions cannot be directly asked and the clinician can only assess the materials sent in advance of a treatment session.

Store-and-forward techniques are therefore best suited to assessment techniques when no interaction between the client and the therapist is required. Examples include video swallow studies, video recorded feedings from families homes, nutritional analyses of feeding records, review of medical records and questionnaire data.

In contrast to store-and-forward techniques, real-time interactions allow clinicians to speak directly with a child's local treatment team and his or her family. This allows for a more flexible assessment during which the clinicians may set up a variety of situations they wish to assess. Additionally, clinicians are able to demonstrate techniques that they wish to model to the child's family and/or their local clinicians. Clinicians may also provide live teaching allowing for detailed discussions to occur and for questions to be answered directly. This style of interaction presumably grants opportunities for greater learning to occur. The disadvantages associated with real-time interactions are that they include greater needs for technical and administrative support, greater initial costs associated with purchases of hardware and software, and problems associated with adoption and comfort of use of the technology by the clinical staff.

Perceptions of service users and providers

Previous studies have generally shown that children and their parents who receive therapy services via videoconferencing generally report high levels of treatment satisfaction (Blackmon *et al.*, 1997; Liss *et al.*, 2002; Straker *et al.*, 1976; Wade *et al.*, 2005). The most commonly reported benefits of videoconferencing include improved accessibility of services and in some cases savings in time, money and travel (Elford *et al.*, 2000; Whitten *et al.*, 2002). Interestingly, providers' impressions of telehealth are mixed. While providers typically report that they are pleased by the increased access to care for their patients as a group, they also report concerns that the technology may make appointments more difficult to complete. Providers have also expressed concern that assessment and/or therapy will be inhibited because of a lack of physical contact with the patient. Some providers also report concerns that the therapeutic alliance with the patient will be negatively affected because the interactions are through electronic media. Interestingly, patients typically do share the concerns of a diminished therapeutic alliance with their providers. Finally, some investigators have suggested that cost-effectiveness of telehealth may be associated with heavier workloads (Bjørvig *et al.*, 2002; Stensland *et al..*, 1999), but others point out that videoconferencing may be cost effective even at low rates of utilisation if the distances are long and the costs of the lost working time are high (Mielonen *et al.*, 1998).

In summary, the available research suggests that telehealth is an effective low cost alternative to traditional therapy. Videoconferencing may specifically enhance the therapeutic efforts as services are delivered directly to a patient's home. Families benefit additionally as they will experience decreased travel time to and from appointments and reductions in time away from work. Families generally report satisfaction with telehealth services as well as satisfaction with other aspects of videoconferencing. Other possible benefits of telehealth include improved patient attendance rates (Zaylor, 1999), reduced time needed for follow-up appointments (Zaylor, 1999) and reduced appointment waiting time (Simpson *et al.*, 2001).

TELEHEALTH AND CHILDREN WITH FEEDING PROBLEMS

Feeding a child is one of the most fundamental and indispensable care-giving tasks associated with parenting. Unfortunately, feeding problems are all too common (Silverman and Tarbell, 2009). Feeding problems may include but are not limited to food refusal, disruptive mealtime behaviour, rigid food preferences, less than optimal growth and failure to master self-feeding skills consistent with the child's developmental level. Parents and caregivers frequently experience high levels of stress when children have feeding difficulties, which in turn negatively affects the parent–child relationship. Not surprisingly, approximately one-half to two-thirds of children with feeding disorders present with mixed aetiologies that include behavioural, physiological and developmental factors (Budd *et al.*, 1992; Rommel *et al.*, 2003). Often treatment is provided by a variety of healthcare professionals from medicine, psychology, speech and language therapy, dietetics and other specialties (Burklow *et al.*, 1998; Davies *et al.*, 2006). However, very few medical centres offer interdisciplinary clinics, which frequently results in difficulties in coordinating care and the child receiving suboptimal treatment.

Although services delivered via videoconferencing are not necessarily suitable for all paediatric populations, a number of factors support its use for the delivery of interdisciplinary treatments for feeding problems to children and their families.

1 Nutrition and behavioural interventions do not typically require physical examinations and are typically conducted via audiovisual communication, making videoconferencing a suitable mode of delivery.
2 Feeding therapy interventions generally involve several office visits as opposed to a single consultation; therefore, videoconferencing may reduce the need for significant travel for families (McGrath *et al.*, 2006).
3 Videoconferencing allows for greater transportability in the delivery of services. For instance, through videoconferencing, feeding therapy can be conducted in the family's home, which may provide clinicians the opportunity to identify and address aspects of the home environment, including patterns of interaction that may contribute to and/or maintain feeding problems.

Taken together, the available research supports the use of videoconferencing for the delivery of interdisciplinary interventions to children with feeding problems.

Applying a range of telehealth technologies

In the treatment of feeding problems, clinicians might take advantage of a variety of telehealth technologies in the provision of services to the family. For example, medical record reviews and diet diaries are easily reviewed by store-and-forward techniques (e.g. electronic files forwarded by the patient's primary providers). Questionnaires may also be completed online by a family and automatically scored in advance of an appointment. These data may also be collected for patient tracking purposes. Likewise, real-time technologies are well suited to conducting interviews and observations in the natural feeding environment. For example, some patients' willingness to enact certain feeding behaviours at an office visit may be very different than the typical feeding behaviours in the home.

Real-time telehealth assessments may be advantageous as clinicians are able to assess the home environment (e.g. child seating and mealtime structure) and make changes to the environment to evaluate effects on the feeding behaviour. Real-time observations may also enable the clinician to directly ask questions during the observation and grants the therapist the ability to manipulate specific elements of the feeding interaction for assessment and/or treatment reasons. Additionally, completing a feeding assessment in real-time presumably provides a more comprehensive assessment and allows the clinician to provide instant feedback to the family. To maximise the benefits of telehealth store-and-forward techniques may be combined with real-time techniques. For example, in preparation of an assessment session, a family may use store-and-forward techniques to record a video of a 'typical' meal at home and forward the video electronically to a feeding specialist in a distant feeding treatment centre. The family may follow up locally with a therapist who then consults in real-time with the specialty feeding clinic through videoconferencing. Continued use of telehealth may involve a family regularly obtaining height and weight measurements of the patient using telehealth peripherals (e.g. a telehealth compatible scale) which are automatically uploaded and sent to the family's various providers facilitating tracking and appropriate treatment follow-up.

A.J.: a gastrostomy tube-dependent child with cerebral palsy

A.J. was a 2½-year-old boy who presented with cerebral palsy, left-sided hemipaligia and gastrostomy tube (G-tube) dependence. A.J. had successfully completed an intensive inpatient behaviour therapy programme weaning him from G-tube dependence. Despite the fact that A.J. was completely weaned, his family remained worried that he would regress to his baseline behaviours upon returning home. After several weeks of driving over 100 miles each way to our outpatient clinic for routine follow-up appointments, the family decided that the burden of travel was too great. After approximately one month, they reported that he was beginning to show some dawdling behaviour at mealtimes, leading to increased meal duration and lower food intake. The family expressed concern that A.J. might return to his baseline behaviour. In response to these concerns they were invited to participate in videoconferencing, using a webcam, headset and encryption capable videoconferencing software. Weekly telehealth sessions were completed using the hub and spoke approach connecting the feeding clinic staff to the family's home. A.J.'s feeding behaviours rapidly improved and the treatment transition to the home environment was completed. Intermittent contact with A.J. and his family has continued via videoconferencing and through email updates. He now eats a wide variety food and continues to grow well.

HOW TO BUILD A TELEHEALTH SERVICE

The most essential element in the building of a telehealth program is not the hardware, software, or internet capabilities of a clinic. Although these elements are important to the success of the program, the critical components for building a telehealth program are the telehealth personnel who will drive the project forward (*see* Table 14.2). The telehealth development group should consist of enthusiastic individuals who are willing to develop and oversee the project despite the likelihood of encountering a variety of naysayers and technical setbacks. It is particularly advantageous to have an administration and organisational strategy that support the telehealth initiatives. These programs will also need the support of information technology specialists who are available not only to set up the initial system but to monitor and support the ongoing provision of services. Finally, the project will need support staff (e.g. clinical coordinator and providers who are willing to utilise new technologies) to manage the daily operation of the project. To ensure the success of a telehealth feeding program, there should be a telehealth clinic coordinator. Many of the traditional responsibilities of clinic coordination (e.g. scheduling patients, communication with families, ordering supplies for the clinic) will remain, but additional responsibilities will be added including electronic scheduling of appointments to allow connections through secure firewalls, coordination of multiple facilities including local and remote providers and room use (hub and spoke sites), distribution of equipment and helping families to establish their home telehealth setups and testing connections. If the project involves research, then the coordinator may also be asked to help with participant recruitment, data collection, tracking of patients and collecting longitudinal data. Without these core components telehealth is difficult to utilise and may not be a viable option for care.

Prior to starting a telehealth program, a plan for service delivery should be developed with a rationale for the telehealth technologies under consideration. The program plan should include the descriptions of the clinical population to receive services (diagnosis, medical needs, etc), general treatment plans, a rationale for why telehealth would be advantageous over traditional services for the patient population (e.g. reduces barriers to care associated with distance from clinic, reduces risk to immune compromised patient, facilitates medical monitoring, observations in the home environment facilitate care, etc). A detailed list of infrastructure needs should also be developed, including key personnel, hardware and software, dedicated internet resources including reliable and secure connection resources and dedicated bandwidth. A plan for tracking progress should also be considered, which might include tracking of clinical outcomes, tracking patient and provider treatment satisfaction, frequency and ease of use of telehealth technologies and economic benefits to families and the treatment facility.

TABLE 14.2: Essential components of a successful telehealth program

Key telehealth personnel	Responsibilities
Clinical Service Director	This individual spearheads the clinical practices of telehealth and works with practitioners to develop their clinical programs
Telehealth Administrator	This individual is an advocate for telehealth and helps to explain to the clinical/hospital staff why such programs should be supported
Information Technology Specialists	This individual or group of individuals consult with program in the selection of hardware and software selections and maintain equipment and connections to enable to program to exist
Clinical Coordinator	This individual is a liaison between the collaborating sites and the patient families. Duties include overseeing scheduling, helping patient families with questions, and collaborating closely with the Information Technology Specialists to ensure smooth daily operations

Organisational strategy	Issues to address
Rational for Telehealth Use	Reduces barriers to care associated with distance Reduces risk to immune compromised patients Facilitates medical monitoring Observations in the home environment
Descriptions of the Clinical Population	Diagnosis, medical needs, age, etc.
General Treatment Plans	Which services will be need? How will the services be used? What are the interventions? What are the expected treatment effects?

Infrastructure	Equipment considerations
Hardware	What are the main uses of the equipment? What resolution Camera? Purchase video integrated units or a personal computer with individual components (e.g. webcam and headset)? Cost?
Software	Is encrypted software needed? Does the software allow file transfer? Is the software readily available and does it interface with other programs? Cost?
Reliable and Secure Connections	Do you have a dedicated internet connection or are you using wireless connection
Dedicated Bandwidth	Greater bandwidth allows for more video and audio transmission Is the bandwidth shared with other uses which might degrade the sessions at times of high user traffic?

Potential telehealth start-up problems

Problem 1: technological difficulties. It is important to ensure that adequate band width is available. Bandwidth that is too low causes poor signal quality. Connections to patient homes may have more bandwidth difficulties secondary to dependence upon the public internet. Telehealth clinics will need to develop protocols in response to connection problems. Families should be provided with an alternative connection plan in case of technical difficulties.

Problem 2: scheduling/record keeping. As telehealth clinics are developed, confusion regarding responsibilities for scheduling patient records keeping is common. A dedicated support person from the telehealth clinic should reduce this problem. Prior to starting the clinical service, development of procedures for documentation should also be considered.

Problem 3: professional resources. To meet the additional demands on our professional staff (e.g. coordination across treatment sites, scheduling, etc.) additional personnel are typically needed.

Problem 4: training the professional staff. Clinicians will most probably avoid using telehealth technologies until they feel adequately trained and comfortable with the equipment and procedures. A special effort to invite personnel to observe telehealth sessions, completing training sessions with opportunities for staff to practice with equipment, and having support staff available for the first few sessions is advisable.

Once the decision has been made to proceed with a telehealth intervention, the appropriate technology should be purchased and maintained to meet the needs of the clinical service. Plans for connecting from the main clinical site to a distal site (hub and spoke model) should include protocols for satellite sites and/or patient's homes which include methods for managing firewall issues and maintaining encrypted connections (assuming treatment sessions are to remain confidential). Equipment should be chosen that will meet clinical needs of the service. For example, dermatology may need to purchase a very high resolution camera with store-and-forward capabilities, whereas mental health providers may only need basic video conferencing equipment that transmits real-time audio visual signals which can be transmitted at relatively low resolution (which also minimises demands on bandwidth). To ensure that providers and families adopt the new technologies, user-friendly equipment and ample support from an internet technologist are strongly encouraged.

In the treatment of feeding disorders, lower resolution equipment tends to be suitable and is readily available in stores that sell computers and computer accessories. This equipment may be purchased by a clinic or by a family at low cost. Individuals familiar with setting up home computer systems will likely have little difficulty setting up a telehealth system in their own home, but they may need additional support configuring connections to the 'hub' site. For many medical centres, navigating firewall protections while attempting to connect to distal sites can be particularly challenging. Therefore, having a dedicated information technology specialist to facilitate telehealth connections is strongly recommended.

Ethan: our first telehealth patient

Ethan was a 7½-year-old boy diagnosed with a feeding disorder with significant underlying anxiety characteristics including feeding phobia. Ethan's family lived approximately 90 miles from our outpatient clinic. Aside from his feeding difficulties, Ethan was a healthy boy who had reached all of his developmental milestones at or before the expected time and in the expected order. His family had expressed many concerns over his picky eating, noting particularly that his self-restrictive behaviours had become so severe that they were reluctant to eat outside of the home because of his disruptive behaviours at mealtimes. One of Ethan's personal interests was computers yet the family did not have videoconferencing capabilities in their home. However, they were willing to travel approximately 30 miles to the nearest satellite clinic for telehealth services. Prior to the first telehealth visit with Ethan, the remote site was visited and the videoconferencing equipment tested to ensure a reliable and secure connection. Ethan and his family had six sessions, three of which included problems with signal quality which required repeated attempts to re-establish the sessions. These problems were subsequently resolved by modifications to the system set-up. Fortunately, our pilot family was thankful that they did not need to travel far to get treatment, Ethan appeared to enjoy the videoconferencing aspects of treatment, and was very response to his behaviour plan. Since beginning our program with Ethan several years ago, we have solidified our procedures, upgraded our equipment, increased our dedicated bandwidth, and completed over 80 visits to our feeding centre via telehealth. Were it not for the hard work of the personnel and the interest and dedication of our patients, this program would have ended long ago and we certainly encountered our fair share of start up challenges.

EVALUATION OF A TELEHEALTH FEEDING CLINIC

Unfortunately, very few examples of feeding therapy delivered via videoconferencing have been reported (McGarth *et al.*, 2006). One exception is the recent work of Silverman and colleagues (2008, 2009), who have reported promising findings from their initial efforts using video conferencing for the treatment of children with feeding problems. Participants were randomly assigned to one of three groups as follows:

1 feeding therapy via videoconferencing to the patient's home
2 feeding therapy via videoconferencing to a satellite clinic nearest to the patient's home
3 feeding therapy via standard care in which the family was seen in an outpatient feeding clinic.

Primary outcome variables included patient satisfaction, clinician satisfaction, therapeutic alliance and treatment efficacy. The treatment intervention followed a standardised 6-week parent training treatment protocol with ongoing medical assessment and nutritional counselling. Twenty-two children diagnosed with feeding disorders of childhood were enrolled and to date 15 participants have completed the intervention (Silverman, 2009). Five of the program non-completers reported scheduling conflicts; one reported successfully reaching the treatment goals prior to the end of the sixth session; and one reported persistent internet connection problems. Aside from method of service delivery, all patients were treated using an identical interdisciplinary treatment protocol. The intervention consisted of an integration of specialty services involving a paediatric psychologist, a clinical nutritionist and a paediatric nurse.

Families assigned to home based telehealth were provided with desktop webcams (*see* Figure 14.1), universal serial bus (USB) headsets (*see* Figure 14.2) and Polycom® PVX™ video conferencing software. Once the software and hardware instillations were completed, families were able to establish encrypted connections with the hospital using the public internet. Technical support for setting up equipment in the family home was provided by the hospital information technologies staff. A test of the home connection was established prior to the first session to

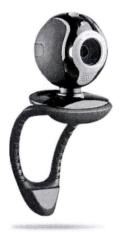

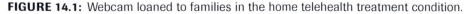

FIGURE 14.1: Webcam loaned to families in the home telehealth treatment condition.

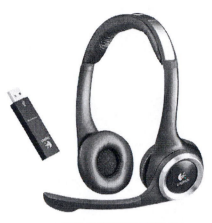

FIGURE 14.2: Headset loaned to families in the home telehealth treatment condition.

ensure the family was familiar with this technology and weekly telehealth sessions were scheduled with the clinical coordinator.

Families assigned to the telehealth intervention at a satellite clinic had their appointments at the satellite clinic which was nearest the family's home. Hospital videoconferencing equipment (*see* Figure 14.3) was provided by the satellite clinic and technical support was provided by the respective satellite clinics. Families assigned to standard care were seen in the feeding and swallowing centre at our medical centre's main campus. All families received weekly hour-long sessions with the interdisciplinary feeding team which included a psychologist, nurse and dietician.

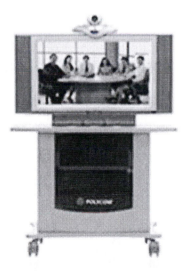

FIGURE 14.3: Videoconferencing equipment used at the 'hub' feeding clinic.

Telehealth treatment protocol (six weekly sessions)

Session 1. Appropriate mealtime structure and the effects of a positive mealtime environment.

Session 2. Reinforcement strategies to promote appropriate feeding behaviours (e.g. differential reinforcement, Premack principle).

Session 3. Strategies to decrease feeding problems (e.g. extinction, negative reinforcement, punishment).

Session 4. Additional reinforcement techniques (e.g. tangible rewards, behavioural contracting) and problem-solving obstacles to improvement.

Session 5. How to adapt and modify interventions to maintain optimal level of response to treatment.

Session 6. Review problem solving and generalisation techniques.

Findings from this research show that parents of children completing the intervention reported fewer mealtime behaviour problems and improvements in the caregiver–child feeding relationship. Many parents also qualitatively described benefits of telehealth sessions completed in the home, reporting that the treatment procedures were readily implemented because they were practiced in the home feeding environment. Families also reported high levels of treatment satisfaction, and families and providers alike reported strong therapeutic alliances suggesting that videoconferencing did not negatively affect the implementation of treatment or rapport building with families.

Utilizing our standardised protocol we have successfully completed over 80 telehealth appointments in the treatment of 15 children diagnosed with feeding disorder. Our preliminary data analyses have shown improvements on several clinical indices, including reductions in problem mealtime behaviours and improved nutritional and growth status. Furthermore, measures of treatment satisfaction and therapeutic alliance scores were moderately high and remained stable throughout treatment. These results show that families feel comfortable with telehealth technology and that videoconferencing does not appear to have a negative effect on the relationship between families and providers.

SUMMARY

A growing body of literature supports the use of interdisciplinary care in the treatment of paediatric feeding problems. Unfortunately, although interdisciplinary care is effective in the treatment of paediatric feeding disorders, the small number of specialised paediatric feeding centres may prevent many children from receiving treatment. This may be especially so for children living in remote, rural areas where providers may not be readily accessible or in underprivileged circumstances that make access to care difficult.

Telehealth interventions offer an alternative to traditional face-to-face treatment delivery and may aid in improving access to care for youth with feeding problems. However research in this area is relatively new; therefore outcome research involving telehealth should assess outcomes for both patients and providers in addition to investigating treatment efficacy (Amer, 2006). Efforts to expand this area of research can be promoted by the use of consistent and comparable assessment measures among investigators (Amer, 2006). While research studying feeding assessments and treatments via telehealth has been limited, pilot research results have been promising. In sum, earlier studies suggested that interdisciplinary feeding therapy can be successfully delivered via telemedicine, and that treatment satisfaction and therapeutic alliance were not negatively affected when compared with patients receiving standard care.

Many young families are affected by feeding problems, and the prevalence of feeding problems is on the rise. Young families also have the highest proportion of home computer ownership and access to the internet. Unfortunately, there simply are not enough clinicians with the appropriate training or resources to manage the growing number of children requiring treatment. Given the growing needs of families with feeding problems, and the many recent technological advances in recent years, it seems inevitable that telehealth technologies will play a significant role in the near future.

REFERENCES

Amer KS. Innovations in pediatric healthcare technology: a multidisciplinary conceptual framework for using and evaluating information systems. *Child Hlth Care*. 2006; **35**(1): 5–10.

Bjørvig S, Johansen MA, Fossen K. An economic analysis of screening for diabetic retinopathy. *J Telemed Telecare*. 2002; **8**(1): 32–5.

Blackmon LA, Kaak HO, Ranseen J. Consumer satisfaction with telemedicine child psychiatry consultation in rural Kentucky. *Psychiatr Ser*. 1997; **48**: 1464–6.

Budd KS, McGraw TE, Farbisz R, *et al*. Psychosocial concomitants of children's feeding disorders. *J Pediatr Psychol*. 1992; **17**: 81–94.

Burklow KA, Phelps AN, Schultz JR, *et al*. Classifying complex pediatric feeding disorders. *J Pediatr Gastroenterol Nutr*. 1998; **27**: 143–5.

Capner M. Videoconferencing in the provision of psychological services at a distance. *J Telemed Telecare*. 2000; **6**: 311–19.

Davies WH, Ackerman LK, Davies CM, *et al*. About Your Child's Eating: Factor structure and psychometric properties of a feeding relationship measure. *Eating Behaviors*. 2006; **8**: 457–63.

Dossetor DR, Nunn KP, Fairley M, *et al*. A child and adolescent psychiatric outreach service for rural New South Wales: a telemedicine pilot study. *J Paediatr Child Hlth*. 1999; **35**: 525–9.

Elford R, White H, Bowering R, *et al*. A randomized, controlled trial of child psychiatric assessments conducted using videoconferencing. *J Telemed Telecare*. 2000; **6**: 73–82.

Freir V, Kirkwood K, Peck D, *et al.* Telemedicine for clinical psychology in the Highlands of Scotland. *J Telemed Telecare.* 1999; **5**: 157–61.

Greeno CG, Wing RT, Shiffman S. Binge antecedents in obese women with and without binge eating disorder. *J Consul Clin Psychol.* 2000; **68**: 95–102.

Hilty DM, Luo JS, Morache C, *et al.* Telepsychiatry: an overview for psychiatrists. *CNS Drugs.* 2002; **16**: 527–48.

Jerome LW, Zaylor C. Cyberspace: creating a therapeutic environment for telehealth applications. *Prof Psychol: Res Pract.* 2000; **31**: 478–3.

Kedesdy JH, Budd KS. Environmental interventions in feeding: an overview. *Childhood Feeding Disorders: biobehavioral assessment and intervention.* Baltimore: Brookes; 1998. pp. 115–17.

Kennedy TLM, Smith A, Wells AT, *et al.* Networked families. Pew Internet and American Life Project; 2008. Retrieved March 3, 2010, from www.pewinternet.org/~/media//Files/Reports/2008/PIP_Networked_Family.pdf.pdf.

Linscheid TJ, Budd KS, Rasnake LK. Pediatric feeding problems. In: Roberts MC, editor. *Handbook of Pediatric Psychology.* New York, NJ: Gulford; 2003. pp. 481–98.

Liss HJ, Glueckauf RJ, Ecklund-Johnson EP. Research on telehealth and chronic medical conditions: critical review, key issues, and future directions. *Rehabil Psychol.* 2002; **47**: 8–30.

McGrath PJ, Watters C, Moon E. Technology in pediatric pain management. In: Finley GA, McGrath PJ, Chambers CT, editors. *Bringing Pain Relief to Children. Treatment Approaches.* Totowa, NJ: Humana; 2006. pp. 159–76.

Mielonen ML, Ohinmaa A, Moring J, *et al.* The use of videoconferencing for telepsychiatry in Finland. *J Telemed Telecare.* 1998; **4**: 125–31.

Nicklelson D. Telehealth and the evolving healthcare system: strategic opportunities of professional psychology. *Prof Psychol: Res Pract.* 1998; **29**: 527–35.

Rommel N, De Meyer AM, Feenstra L, and Veereman-Wauters G. (2003). The complexity of feeding problems in 700 infants and young children presenting to a tertiary care institution. *Journal of Pediatric Gastroenterology and Nutrition.* **37**: 75–84.

Rothchild E. Telepsychiatry: why do it? *Psychiatr Annal.* 1999; **29**: 394–401.

Silverman AH. *Telehealth Services: Treatment of Early Childhood Feeding Disorders.* Paper presented at the Children's Research Institute, Milwaukee, WI; 2009.

Silverman AH, Kirby M, Begotka A, *et al. Telehealth Delivery of a Behavioral Feeding Intervention in Pediatrics.* Poster session presented at the National Conference in Child Health Psychology, Miami, FL; 2008.

Silverman AH, Tarbell S. Pediatric feeding problems, undernutrition, and vomiting disorders. In: Roberts MC, Steele RG, editors. *Handbook of Pediatric Psychology.* 4th ed. New York, NY: Guilford Press; 2009. pp. 429–45.

Simpson J, Doze S, Urness D, *et al.* Telepsychiatry as a routine service: the perspective of the patient. *J Telemed Telecare.* 2001; **7**: 155–60.

Stensland J, Speedie SM, Ideker M, *et al.* The relative cost of outpatient telemedicine services. *Telemed J.* 1999; **5**: 245–56.

Straker N, Mostyn P, Marshall C. The use of two-way TV in bringing mental health services to the inner city. *Am J Psychiatr.* 1976; **133**: 1202–5.

Wade SL, Wolfe CR. Telehealth interventions in rehabilitation psychology: postcards from the edge. *Rehabil Psychol.* 2005; **50**: 323–4.

Whitten PS, Mair FS, Haycox A, *et al.* Systematic review of cost effectiveness studies of telemedicine interventions. *Br Med J.* 2002; **324**: 1434–7.

Zaylor C. Clinical outcomes in telepsychiatry. *J Telemed Telecare.* 1999; **5**(Suppl. 1): 59–60.

CHAPTER 15

Intensive intervention for childhood feeding disorders

Clarissa Martin and Terence M Dovey

INTRODUCTION

This chapter is dedicated to the difficult decision of when to admit children with feeding disorders (FDs) into in-patient (IP) intervention programmes. It will offer guidance on when to admit a child and discusses the potential benefits and consequences that may occur as a result of this course of action. To face this extremely difficult decision, multi-professional teams must be aware of the complexity of interrelated problems that both the child and family face as a result of the child's FD. Moreover, awareness, assessment and consideration of the potential repercussions of admitting the child to hospital must also be part of the clinicians' decision-making process. Paramount to the success of any intensive intervention must be the limitation of distress during the process, especially as the primary consequence of this regime requires the separation of the child from the family. Despite this separation, it is vitally important that the family is able to become an integral part of the treatment process in order to limit possible relapse upon successful completion of the program.

The primary variables that need to be considered when deciding on whether to admit a child into an IP programme involve distinct areas of the child's behaviour. First, practitioners must consider the complexity of the individual child's specific case beyond the simple criteria of failure to thrive (also termed growth faltering). Secondly, the child's mealtime behaviours must be observed and assessed to ensure that the problems cannot be rectified within the familial setting. Finally, one must consider the potential repercussions, both positive and negative, of removing the child from the family. Parental emotions are understandably strained during this time and practitioners will need to be aware of the perceptions of failure that may co-occur with admission to the IP centre. The overarching caveat to the decision of when and if to admit the child must be as a last resort, when all other avenues have been exhausted. Following the initial exploration of the pertinent factors, the chapter will move on to consider the primary question of how, when and where the admission to hospital should take place. The culmination of this chapter will consider the different IP programmes that are frequently employed internationally.

IP TREATMENT: TO ADMIT OR NOT TO ADMIT

The majority of children that present with feeding problems respond well to management strategies suggested by clinicians. Feeding clinics and hospital out-patient departments provide the most common settings where children with feeding problems are treated. However, there are a number of children whose difficulties are very resistant to intervention devised and offered within those settings. Severe and persistent problems may develop into a more complex FD. Long-term chronic feeding problems are also associated with increased health risks for the child (Berezin et al., 1986) and can easily jeopardise the child's quality-of-life.

Children with FDs may not respond to strategies that are commonly recommended for children with more transient problems (Piazza, 2008). Such children are likely to require intensive multi-disciplinary intervention that may necessitate admission to hospital. Interdisciplinary feeding programs that have included both caregiver and child variables across several feeding categories have been shown to be effective in the treatment of severe FDs (Greer et al., 2008).

THE CHILD WITH SEVERE FD

Feeding is a complex dynamic process that requires a well integrated development of biological systems effectively interacting with the environment (Kerwin, 1999). Any difficulty in one of the biological, psychological or environmental systems may create a 'domino effect' resulting in feeding problems or FDs. One such biological example is gastroesophageal reflux disease (GERD). This is typified in a study by Kerwin (2003) who showed that GERD was diagnosed in 56% of children with neurodevelopmental disabilities presenting with FDs. In addition, the rapid advances in medical techniques means that premature babies or those with severe medical complications in early infancy are fortunately surviving. These children represent a challenge to health professionals because they often exhibit feeding problems, either related to their medical conditions or induced iatrogenically as a result of medical treatment (Berezin et al., 1986; Dunitz-Scheer et al., 2009).

Several authors have commented that between 3%–10% of the children who experience severe and persistent feeding problems will also suffer from a general decline in health (Dahl and Sundelin, 1992; Lindberg et al., 1991; Reau et al., 1996).

Moreover, children with severe problems that develop into FDs can be at considerable risk of malnutrition and severe weight loss that may impact on their cognitive, emotional and physical development (Budd *et al.*, 1992; Riordan *et al.*, 1984).

This chapter uses the case study of one child, Stuart, throughout, with the aim of allowing the reader to follow the progress of his intensive intervention through its various stages. It begins below.

Stuart: a case for intensive intervention

Stuart was born at full term without complications after a 'normal' pregnancy. He was breastfed during the first 2 months, moved to bottle feeding when 3 months old and weaning started at 5 months of age without major difficulties. At 7 months he was urgently hospitalised after an episode of violent acidic vomiting. He was diagnosed as having GERD and given oral medication. GERD was inevitably reported as being painful and discomforting especially while eating. Stuart learned to avoid eating as he associated doing so with the symptoms of his disease (Pain, burning sensation and acidic vomit). Specifically and principally, he would refuse to eat from a spoon and expressed tantrums until he made himself physically sick. He completely refused any food offered orally and only accepted fluids, principally milk, from a bottle. Due to these behaviours, it was recommended by the medical team that Stuart be fitted with a temporary nasogastric tube (NG-tube) – a common treatment for GERD. This was recommended because of Stuart's persistent refusal to eat orally had led to him receiving the diagnosis of Failure to Thrive. Concurrent to Stuart's medical problems, he was also diagnosed with global developmental delay at 2 years old. As medical investigations and treatments for GERD were the clear priorities for professionals and parents alike, appropriate mealtime behaviour was never re-established. When he was 5 year old, he still was drinking milk from a bottle, systematically refusing any food offered orally and maintained his negative behaviours around mealtimes. At the time of referral to the clinic, Stuart was receiving all of his required daily nutrients through his NG-Tube.

ADVANTAGES AND DISADVANTAGES OF IP INTERVENTION

Hospitalisation as a potential treatment strategy for FD has history. Despite often at best having medical problems that would not require hospitalisation, many authors have advocated IP protocols. The use of hospitalisation for treating severe FDs was initially described by Linscheid *et al.* (1978) and since then, description of IP interventions for children that present with FDs associated with complex medical problems (spina bifida, short gut syndrome, cystic fibrosis, etc.) learning difficulties, cognitive delay and autism spectrum disorder (ASD) has grown in the literature (Ahearn *et al.*, 1996; Greer *et al.*, 2008; Hoch *et al.*, 1994; Linscheid *et al.*, 1987; Luiselli and Luiselli, 1994; Piazza *et al.*, 2003; Riordan *et al.*, 1984; Sisson and Dixon, 1986; Stark *et al.*, 1996).

Hospital admission can clearly be a benefit for high risk populations such as children who are severely malnourished, those who have life-threatening medical conditions (i.e. respiratory disorders such as bronchopulmonary dysplasia or swallowing dysfunction) or those whose parents cannot provide a safe environment for the intervention (Linscheid *et al.*, 2003). IP interventions allow professionals to deliver round-the-clock treatments that may produce more rapid behavioural change in a medically safe environment. This admission can be less emotionally distressing for parents in the medium to longer term, as they may experience a renewed hope for the treatment of their child's FD when trained professionals take the lead in the intervention. Further, re-establishing patterns of feeding behaviour in a child with a complex FD may require strict control of contextual factors and this may be better achieved through providing the child and the family with a completely new environment.

Several researchers (Blackman and Nelson, 1987; Byars *et al.*, 2003; Dunitz-Scheer *et al.*, 2009; Kerwin, 1999; Linscheid, 1978; Linscheid *et al.*, 2003; Piazza *et al.*, 2003) suggest other advantages and disadvantages of IP treatment and these are summarised in the sections to follow:

Advantages
- Medical intervention is readily available.
- It is possible to control and measure the child's intake of solids and liquids with precision.
- The child's weight and hydration status can be monitored and kept under strict control.
- Appetite manipulation can be professionally controlled.
- There is access to feeding specialists staff trained to implement behavioural treatment.
- Frequency of therapeutic feeding sessions can be controlled.
- Parents are free from other duties and can concentrate on learning behavioural techniques to improve their child's feeding.
- Children with long standing tube dependence respond more readily when an intensive weaning protocol is used.
- Rapid weaning promotes hunger.
- An appropriate context is provided for intensive weaning period that cannot be safely accomplished at home.
- Multiple daily treatments provide a consistent setting for diminishing negative mealtime behavioural resistance that cannot be provided in an outpatient setting.

Disadvantages

- Intensive interventions are high cost as they also requires extensive professional time investment.
- The artificial setting may mean that children can find it difficult to generalise the behaviour modifications achieved at hospital when returning home.
- Admission to hospital inevitably carries the risk of exposure to hospital acquired infections.
- IP admission disrupts the family's life and child's routine with consequent risk of trauma.

Stuart

At 6 years, Stuart was receiving his main nutrients via nasogastric tube feeds. In spite of all management strategies implemented to help him to eat orally at home and at school, he was observed eating only two tiny bites of a cheese sandwich at school on two occasions following an intensive coaching intervention. At school Stuart started to feel self-conscious because of his NG tube and this was impacting on his performance and behaviour. Mealtimes at home were even more strained with Stuart running around the house to avoid eating, which often escalated to the point that his family were chasing him to try to get him to eat. He also avoided the kitchen area of the house and when forced to go near it he would vomit. Vomiting was also evident when attempts were made to get him to eat. He also would wet himself, suggesting that his behaviours were as a result of fear rather than disobedience. His parents had also started to express some frustration, as they could not enjoy social activities as a family. They felt unable to accept invitations to attend barbecues in the neighbourhood or to have family meals at restaurants because of Stuart's disruptive behaviour in the presence of food or its associated surroundings. Subsequently, Stuart was placed on the surgical department's list for direct insertion of a gastrostomy tube (G-tube or PEG) with the aim of direct infusion of food into his stomach. His parents rejected this course of action as they believed that this was going to impact negatively on his quality-of-life. It had already been suggested by both Stuart and his parents that the tube-feeding was creating problems with his integration at school. His parents were very keen on an intensive IP treatment for Stuart, so that he could overcome his difficulties.

PRE-ADMISSION CRITERIA AND CONSIDERATIONS

Criteria for pre-admission to hospital for the treatment of a child's FD cannot be arbitrarily standardised, as it depends on the individual circumstances surrounding the case. Clinical decisions from the multi-professional team and from the many parties with a vested interest in the child's well-being have to include a careful consideration of resources at the hospital's disposal. It may be that whilst an IP intervention could be argued to be the better clinical decision it cannot be offered because of a lack of specialised hospital resources. Unfortunately, appropriate specialised FDs units are rare (Ahearn et al., 1996; Hoch et al., 1994). There is nevertheless a consensus in the literature that before admitting children to hospital for intensive intervention for their FD, it is imperative to maintain a multidisciplinary approach to carefully study the situation of the individual child and pre-assess total holistic suitability for such an intervention (Babbit et al., 1994; Byars et al., 2003; Warren and Fox, 1987). For example, aspects such as risk assessments to quantitatively assess the child's capacity to eat and swallow orally or how the child could respond to the intervention from a cognitive, emotional and social perspective will inform the decision-making and the development of an appropriate intervention.

Hospital admission can be necessary when the child's FD is resulting in excessive weight loss or poor nutritional status that interferes with adequate growth. Such determinants are usually derived from centile comparisons with the child's peer group, which determine whether he or she could be considered as failing to thrive. Particular emphasis should be given to comparisons with siblings and other related individuals in addition to growth centiles in order to avoid setting unrealistic goals from the outset. On other occasions the decision to admit may be based on the fact that all other efforts and strategies provided in other settings, such as home-based treatments, community, school-based intervention and out-patient hospital consultations have proven to be unsuccessful in helping the child to overcome their FD. In such serious situations, admission would be also required to avoid further health associated risks. The manifestation of these 'risks' may even become the primary reason for admission. It is this flexibility in the reason for admission that offers the clinician some flexibility in their decision-making, enabling the individual circumstances of each case and its associated features of chronicity and severity to be carefully considered.

FDs are not totally defined by the child's individual characteristics. Sometimes complex family and social dynamics have become difficult enough to make home-based intervention ineffective. In such cases, hospitalisation may be the only option for the child and their family. However, it is important to remember that an IP ward is an artificial setting where all elements impacting in the child's eating can be more easily controlled: there is no guarantee that any advances made within this setting are going to be transferred outside it. A focus must therefore be maintained on facilitating the reproduction of those behaviours learned within the hospital setting. In order to achieve this, it is necessary to explore parents' attitudes and willingness to participate with their child's IP treatment (Byars et al., 2003; Greer et al., 2008; Kerwin, 1999; Linscheid et al., 2003). By involving and considering the parents in the process, the clinician may further evaluate and provide rudimentary interventions for precipitating, maintaining and exacerbating factors coming from the home environment. However, it should be acknowledged that the main emphasis should be the child and their recovery from their FD. Moreover, the primary focus of any parent-led intervention should be education and empowerment to ensure stability in the child's behavioural change unless the parents' themselves ask for additional psychological provision.

There are some examples of interdisciplinary teams that offer IP intervention, such as the FDs Program at the Kennedy Krieger Institute (KKI-USA), the Munroe Meyer Institute (MMI-USA) and the Graz Hospital in Austria (EU). The interdisciplinary teams that participate in those programs include professionals from Gastroenterology, Developmental Paediatrics, Nutrition, Psychology, Occupational Therapy and Social Work. (Byars *et al.*, 2003; Dunitz-Scheer *et al.*, 2009; Greer *et al.*, 2008; Piazza *et al.*, 2003). Such multi-disciplinary teams appear to have large successes in treating FD and may be considered the gold standard in IP service provision.

Typically, once the child is admitted to the hospital the multi-professional assessment continues with more in depth investigations. Monitoring the child's weight and hydration status is necessary to control and maintain his or her physical stability for the rest of the specialist intervention. Dietetic assessment of child's daily nutritional requirements is undertaken through monitoring quantity and quality of food intake. This information can then be used to adjust the hospital's child-friendly menus to ensure adequate caloric intake to maintain positive energy balance. This ensures that the clinician is aware how much food the child must eat at every meal in order to gain weight. Programs to improve the child's feeding behaviour at mealtimes and parent training sessions can then be designed and implemented by psychologists and/or behavioural therapists. Where appropriate and available, occupational therapists, play specialist and speech and language therapists can also be consulted to devise programs to help the child in the development of specific skills needed for improving feeding (i.e. oral motor development, desensitisation to different textures) depending on the individual child and the characteristics of the FD.

The length of admission for treatment of a child's FD varies significantly in the literature across the different hospitals and programs. This situation can be understood by differences not only in patient's characteristics but in resources and distribution of services provided across geographical locations within and between countries. For example, the average regime for a child treated at the KKI (USA) has been reported to be 61 days (Babbit *et al.*, 1994). Graz Hospital (Austria) offers a 21-day program for helping children weaning from tube dependence (Dunitz-Scheer *et al.*, 2009) and at Columbus Children's Hospital (USA) a follow up study revealed that children were admitted and treated in less than 10 days (Cook *et al.*, 2000). It is not clear if differences in length of admission can be attributable only to child characteristics: contextual factors, such as differences in resource distribution may also be a pertinent factor in duration of intervention. Nevertheless, it is clear that research on children that require IP intervention for FD is very much needed, especially with regard to aspects of treatment efficacy.

Examples of criteria
Pre-admission clinical criteria
- Comprehensive evaluation by interdisciplinary team (paediatric gastroenterologist, dietician, etc.)
- Resolution or stability of the medical problem.
- Absence of anatomical or functional impairment precluding safe oral eating.
- Absence of oral motor problems (e.g. apraxia).
- Maintenance of adequate weight on tube feeding.
- Primary caregiver/parents characteristics: receptivity, motivation, willingness and capacity to actively participate in treatment.
- Child's cognitive and developmental status adequate to allow a response to behaviour therapy (i.e. >12 months age equivalent).

(Babbit et al., 1994; Blackman and Nelson, 1987; Byars, et al., 2003)

Criteria for exclusion of IP
- Child with poor motor control (Nelson et al., 1975).
- Child with structural or organic problem underlying the FP (Riordan et al., 1984).
- Parental and/or child non-compliance with verbal request (Luiselli, 1988).

Assessment at admission
- Medical fitness: tests aspiration, swallowing endoscope, blood tests, etc.
- Dietetic: calories, food diaries, hospital menus, etc.
- Child's general and cognitive development, oral motor skills, etc.
- Behaviour: classical and operant conditioning patterns exhibited at meal times,
- Parental willingness, attitude and stress.

(Babbit et al., 1994; Byars, et al., 2003; Linscheid et al., 2003)

Treatment duration
- Relatively brief (4–17 sessions).
- Moderately long (27–62).
- Long (88 sessions).

INTENSIVE TREATMENT IN AN IP SETTING
Research results indicate that IP treatment of children's FD should focus on all the components (biological, oral motor, cognitive and behavioural) that contribute to

the problem and should be multi-disciplinary in nature (Linscheid *et al.*, 2003; Piazza and Carroll, 2004). Existing IP interventions are provided in treatment packages that combine behavioural techniques, psychosocial or interactional intervention and parent training (Babbit *et al.*, 1994; Byars *et al.*, 2003; Martin *et al.*, 2008; Ramsay and Zelazo, 1988). The majority of treatment packages suggested by the literature include:

1 appetite manipulation
2 behavioural intervention
3 parent training.

These are discussed in the following sections.

Appetite manipulation

Appetite manipulation is defined as aiding the child to re-establish the association between psychobiological hunger sensations, which are essential drivers for eating, with the initiation of eating behaviour. Appetite manipulation through stimulating appetite drive is an important part of IP intervention for FD and needs to be carefully considered in the planning of the treatment (Byars *et al.*, 2003; Dunitz-Scheer *et al.*, 2009; Linscheid *et al.*, 2003). The ability to induce feelings of hunger, while ensuring that the child is medically safe, is often one of the strongest argued reasons for treating within a hospital setting.

For children who are tube-fed or have a tube-dependence, a frequent practice during IP intervention is to progressively reduce artificial feeding to the minimum daily nutritional needs and to deliver those calories at night during the child's sleep. This ensures the (re)establishment of daytime hunger. For example, Byars *et al.* (2003) treated nine children with dependence on gastrostomy tube (G-Tube) feeds in an IP setting. They reduced the G-tube feeds by 50% of the pre-admission levels and restricted children's access to food to the three daily treatment sessions. All fluids were also restricted 60 minutes prior to treatment sessions with the aim to maximise the children's subjective feelings associated with appetite. Dunitz-Scheer *et al.* (2009) have also adopted a similar protocol for children who are tube-dependent based on the statement that 'tube weaning is not possible without the presence of hunger'. In this instance, they treated 221 children with their protocol and have successfully reduced tube-feed volumes by 100%. They propose that the best way to do this is gradually, over a 72-hour period, until tube-feeding is terminated at the end of the third day of admission. In general, the percentage of daily calories needed and fluids delivered artificially can be adjusted to balance daytime hunger against weight loss and hydration status on an individual basis. Concurrently, the restriction of snacks ensures the child begins the intervention treatment strategies feeling hungry.

Stuart: an example of a meal intake schedule

Before Stuart's admission and to minimize the time he was at hospital, his diurnal and nocturnal tube feds were gradually reduced. At the second day of admission Stuart's Nasogastric tube was removed with his consent and participation. The frequency of his meals was established every 2 hours with snacks offered at 10:30 a.m., 11:30 a.m., 2:00 p.m., 4:00 p.m. and 7:00 p.m. during the treatment phase, as he had a tendency to vomit when a large amount of food was presented. The snacks consisted of a chocolate bar and a small quantity of liquid nutritional supplement. The nutritional supplement drink was also gradually increased from 10 mL/5 times during the first day to 40 mL/5 times by the fourth day. This gradual increase helped him to tolerate larger quantities of food without vomiting. One of the objectives of the program was for the child to be able to drink a whole pack of 200 mL of the nutritional supplement before being discharged. This aspect of the program was included at Stuart's parents' request. The duration of the main meals was established at the beginning of the treatment, which was 1 hour – considerable longer than what is generally recommended in the literature. Most of the meal time was dedicated to increasing the length of time Stuart was able to remain seated at the table and in front of a gradually increasing amount of food. The quantity desentisation process also included the addition of different types of food. This was to ensure that Stuart was exposed to as many different types of food to widen his food acceptance. It was agreed that Stuart should be allowed to eat at his own pace to begin with. Stuart's treatment goals included being able to increase the variety and amount of foods he could tolerate in front of him and a posteriori eaten without vomiting.

Behavioural intervention

Although FDs are particularly common in children with a variety of illnesses and growth problems, the behaviours indicative of organically derived feeding problems are the same as those observed in children where no organic cause has been identified (Harris *et al.*, 2000). Problematic mealtime behaviours can occur both in children who take food orally and for those who are tube fed (Burklow *et al.*, 2002). Crist and Nappier-Phillips (2001) suggest that the basic patterns of behaviour around mealtimes are quite similar in healthy, normally developed children and in a group of children with underlying medical conditions. The differences can be appreciated not in the type of behaviour the children exhibit (i.e. all children spit the food out) but in the frequency and intensity of those behaviours. Problematic mealtime behaviour may be exacerbated in children with severe FD because of their constant negative experience and association with food and eating that seems to perpetuate circular patterns of classical and operant conditioning. It is precisely their extremely conditioned behaviour that interferes at mealtimes that seem to be in need of a completely new environmental context. Behavioural interventions either used in isolation or with other treatment components are frequently cited in the literature as empirically supported treatments for FD in children (Douglas and Harris, 2001; Kerwin, 1999; Linscheid *et al.*, 1978) and researchers agree that behavioural interventions are a critical component in the treatment of FD (Ahearn *et al.*, 1996; Kerwin, 1999; Riordan *et al.*, 1984).

Behavioural interventions consist of the largest proportion (76%) of eligible studies reviewed by Kerwin (1999). This approach applied in IP setting requires highly specialised training in behavioural analysis and therapy with children (Kerwin, 2003). Intensive interdisciplinary programs that use behaviour-based treatments produce successful outcomes for the majority of patients treated and these outcomes are maintained at follow-up. Several studies have described behavioural operant-based techniques that have been designed to help children to increase the variety and quantity of food consumed, to decrease their feeding aversion, to progress beyond a limited diet denoted by specific textures and/or to overcome their holistic food refusal (Babbit *et al.*, 1994; Byars *et al.*, 2003; Piazza *et al.*, 2003).

Stuart: dietary considerations

A list of preferred food and developmentally age appropriate menus were discussed and created collaboratively with Stuart, his mother, the paediatric psychologist and the hospital senior dietician.

Food was classified into the following different categories:

1 Food that Stuart was able to eat such as chips, crisps, butter, toast, butter sandwiches, sausages, fish fingers, yoghurt and ice cream. This food would be used to increase the oral intake after a baseline measure.

2 Foods that the Stuart had tried once but to which he had developed negative associations (e.g. banana) were chosen for play and tactile experience with the aim of providing him with new positive associations. This food was used for working towards establishing new operant conditioning.

3 New food and food that Stuart generally rejected was used for the repeated exposure technique to increase his receptivity to and acceptance of new foods. For example, there were several choices for breakfast (cereals, milk, biscuits, cakes, toast, jam, butter, etc.) in a buffet-type presentation and Stuart was encouraged to taste as much as he wished.

Parent training

Parents are the natural link between the therapeutic IP setting and the child's natural environment. Training parents to manage their child's FD is one of the most important aims for intensive intervention, as it will allow them to master the necessary skills to provide continuity at home once the child is discharged from hospital. To what extent they accurately implement and follow the treatment started in the hospital will always be the measure of a successful IP intervention. Establishing continuity between the ward and home environments, to maintain the behavioural change, can be a daunting task. Several authors have stressed the vital importance of including parents in the treatment process to facilitate this transition. Generalisation of new feeding behaviours is therefore one of the biggest challenges for professionals (Babbit *et al.*, 1994; Luiselli and Luiselli, 1994; Werle *et al.*, 1993).

Training for parents to effectively manage their child's feeding may include several components such as training in behavioural approaches, nutritional education and supportive counselling, and may be devised through different training models and packages. Essentially, and in the preliminary phase, parents start learning theoretical principles through didactic sessions and having supportive counselling mainly to deal with the stress they experience from their participation in the intensive intervention. Afterwards, they move through a process of observing feeding therapists to mastering the necessary skills to create and maintain the new feeding behaviours, gradually taking full control of their child's feeding. Several authors (Ahearn *et al.*, 1996; Babbit *et al.*, 1994; Byars *et al.*, 2003; Linscheid *et al.*, 1987; Martin *et al.*, 2008) agree that training parents requires organised treatment in transitional stages with established targeted outcomes.

- Parents learn behavioural techniques and become familiar with the feeding behavioural protocol.
- Parents observe the feeding therapist in action using audiovisual material (i.e. video observation) or observing the session through unidirectional mirrors.
- Parents practice and rehearsal using role play techniques (i.e. with a doll, with the therapist playing a child, etc.) until they demonstrate proficiency skills.
- Parents continue observation and rehearsal until therapist achieves established and stable outcomes (i.e. child eats consistently; tantrums have disappeared, etc.).
- Parents are introduced to the session in an observatory role and therapist continues feeding the child.
- Parents feed the child with feeding therapist guidance.
- Feeding therapist moves on to an observatory role while parents feed the child.
- Parents feed the child and feeding therapist is not in the room but able to communicate with them through an electronic devises (e.g. bug-in-the-ear).

Parents have to have the constant support and feedback of therapists at every stage of their training. They are finally included in the different stages once the targeted child's behaviours at meal times have been achieved.

Parent training procedures in the case of Stuart
Stuart: the intervention begins

At the time of Stuart's admission to the hospital his parents were encouraged to express their fears. Through a problem solving strategy task those fears were listed and solutions to overcome each of them were discussed and included as a part of the treatment. All aspects of the intensive protocol were discussed with them and a flow chart was used as a visual aid. The protocol included systematic parent training. From the beginning, Stuart's parents were highlighted as part of the solution to their child's FD. They were told that they were 'in-charge' and they would make the final decisions at every stage of the treatment. Towards that end, feedback regarding aspects of the feeding treatment was provided everyday and training time for them to learn behavioural management at meal times was scheduled. Video observation of Stuart at feeding times was used for feedback and training. Parents were encouraged to practice and to discuss their difficulties with the paediatric psychologist. Modelling and behavioural rehearsal techniques were also discussed and training offered where appropriate. Stuart's parents were concerned about the maintenance of his feeding behaviour once they returned home and asked for the possibility of having a nutritional supplement to help him and for them to have peace of mind about him having most of the required nutrients to thrive accordingly. They participated in the multi-disciplinary team discussion during Stuart's admission and their suggestions were respected and included. This aspect provided them with a recovered sense of control that increased their self-confidence in managing Stuart's feeding behaviour

A MULTI-DIMENSIONAL AND MULTI-SYSTEMIC PERSPECTIVE

Intensive treatment of childhood FD varies across centres and countries as practice has not been standardised. The majority of research studies where behavioural management has proved to be successful (Linscheid *et al.*, 1987, 2003; Piazza *et al.*, 2003, 2004) come from the United States. European studies are mainly centred on weaning from tube feeding through appetite manipulation, family support and counselling (Dunitz-Scheer *et al.*, 2009; Van Dijk *et al.*, 2008). In the United Kingdom, Martin *et al.*, (2008) has offered a description of a multi-dimensional intervention that included an integration of evidence-based techniques such as cognitive behavioural therapy (CBT) and family systems therapy and where the focus on the different systems contributed towards effective maintenance of feeding behaviours across contexts such as the home and nursery school environments.

Clinical evidence suggests that when it is necessary to admit children with FDs to hospitals that do not have a specific FDs unit, it is important that the hospital adopts a multi-faceted approach. This will necessitate a multi-component and disciplinary treatment strategy that will assess the child's physiological, behavioral, parent–child interaction, emotional difficulty, and family functioning. It is common to find marked discrepancies in the perception of the etiology of the child's FD between and within the two subsystems (healthcare professionals like physicians, doctors, nurses, etc. on one side, versus the child's family on the other side) and this may disrupt clinical management and intervention (Ayour and Milner, 1985; Evans *et al.*, 1972). Focusing on maintaining harmonious continuity among the systems may help to facilitate the generalisation processes. If the total holistic environment and significant individuals within it are involved (i.e. family, school, etc.) share a similar understanding and perception of the child's problem, it will provide for the best prognosis and allow a supportive and coherent environment where the feeding behaviours learned during an intensive intervention can be generalised.

Stuart: intensive multi-disciplinary intervention

Stuart was admitted to a paediatric ward at a District General Hospital. A timetable for the whole day at hospital was devised with the aim to provide a meaningful structure for the various clinical components of his treatment:

- *CBT*: Stuart was having school time with the ward school teacher at the ward school room. The ward teacher helped him not only with his school work but she also helped to devise a health education program that was the baseline for a CBT therapy. Stuart was encouraged to develop a fascination with discovering the simplistic physiology of eating. From here, he was able to understand the meaning of eating from a cognitive perspective. For example he believed that the food was going straight down to his tummy to hurt him. The psychoeducational programme helped him understood the importance of eating and the meaning of the digestion of food from a nutritional needs perspective and therefore was able to participate more in the treatment. The programme changed the association of eating with pain to positive associations with health and social outcomes, e.g. 'growing', 'going to parties', etc.
- *Play therapy*: play therapy was included to allow Stuart to be in contact with phobic elements in food-related play situations and to facilitate the expression of his anxieties in a free environment through representational motor play (e.g. using chocolate as face paint).
- *Bio-behavioural therapy*: behavioural techniques (shaping, discrimination, etc.) were applied at meal times and activities pre- and post-meal times (e.g. watching videos after meals, etc.) were also included.
- *Parent training procedures*: constant feedback to parents and systematic training procedures made use of video observation and modelling techniques.

- *Systemic intervention at the mesosystem level*: a school based post-intervention program was designed to facilitate the generalisation of new feeding behaviours at Stuart's school.
- *Health promotion and education*: as Stuart was admitted to a general paediatric ward it was necessary to train ward staff and doctors in the feeding programme and in psychosocial aspect of paediatrics to create a consistent environment.

Timetable used for Stuart in the paediatric ward

- 9:00 a.m.–10:00 a.m.: breakfast. Behavioural techniques.
- 9:00 a.m.–11:00 a.m.: education in psychosocial aspects of paediatrics through diary feedback to the medical team (ward rounds) and ward staff regarding the psychological intervention.
- 10:00 a.m.–11:a.m.: school time. School work, health education and CBT.
- 11:00 a.m.–12:00 noon: play therapy.
- 12:00 noon–12.30 p.m.: activities pre-meals. To help the child to identify body signals using physical exercises as the mean (e.g. trampoline and bicycle exercises) and from there to help them to identify the hunger sensation.
- 12:30 p.m.–1:30 p.m.: bio-behavioural therapy applied at meal times.
- 2:00 p.m.–3.00 p.m.: post-meal time activities.
- 2:00 p.m.–4:00 p.m.: parent training procedures.
- 4:00 p.m.–5:00 p.m.: systemic intervention at mesosystem level. School-based post-intervention.
- 5:00 p.m.–6:00 p.m.: tea time. Generalisation of behavioural principles applied at meal times during family time.

SUMMARY

This chapter has focused on important factors to consider when admitting a child with FDs to hospital for intensive intervention. It has outlined advantages and disadvantages of these types of approaches, as well as highlighted the multi-disciplinary perspective that prevails. In keeping with the literature, the importance of including parents within the process has been emphasised. Although specialist FDs units are rare and intensive treatments for children's FDs vary across centres and countries, the evidence suggests they can achieve positive results where community treatment has failed. This chapter has offered a summary of their approaches.

REFERENCES

Ahearn WH, Kerwin M, Eicher PS, *et al*. An alternating treatments comparison of two intensive interventions for food refusal. *J Appl Behav Anal*. 1996; **29**: 321–32.

Ayour CC, Milner JS. Failure to thrive: parental indicators, types and outcomes. *Child Abuse Negl.* 1985; **9**: 491–9.

Babbit RL, Hoch TA, Coe DA, *et al.* Behavioral assessment and treatment of pediatric feeding disorders. *Dev Behav Paediatr.* 1994; **15**: 278–91.

Berezin S, Schwarz SM, Halata MS, *et al.* Gastroesophageal reflux secondary to gastrostomy tube placement. *Am J Dis Child.* 1986; **140**(7): 699–701.

Blackman JA, Nelson CLA. Rapid introduction of oral feedings in children to tube-fed patients. *J Dev Behav Pediatr.* 1987; **8**: 63–7.

Budd KS, McGraw TE, Farbisz R. Psychosocial concomitants of children's feeding disorders. *J Pediatr Psychol.* 1992; **17**: 81–94.

Burklow AK, McGrath AM, Allred KE, *et al.* Parent perception of mealtime behaviors in children fed enterally. *NutrClin Pract.* 2002; **17**: 291–5.

Byars KC, Burklow S, Kathleen A, *et al.* A multicomponent behavioral program for oral aversion in children dependent on gastrostomy feedings. *J Pediatr Gastroenterol Nutr.* 2003; **37**(4): 473–80.

Cook C, Linscheid TR, Rasnake LK, *et al.* Long term follow up of patients treated for feeding problems. *Paper presented at the Millenium Conference of the Great Lakes Society of Pediatric Psychology*, 2000; Cleveland, Ohio.

Crist W, Nappier-Phillips BA. Mealtime behaviors of young children: a comparison of normative and clinical data. *Dev Behav Pediatr.* 2001 Oct; **22**(5): 279–86.

Dahl M, Sundelin C. Feeding problems in an affluent society. Follow-up at four years of age in children with early refusal to eat. *Acta Pediatr.* 1992; **81**(8): 575–9.

Douglas J, Harris B. Description and evaluation of a day-centre-based behavioural feeding programme for young children and their parents. *Clin Child Psychol.* 2001; **6**: 241–56.

Dunitz-Scheer M, Levine A, Roth Y, *et al.* Prevention and treatment of tube dependency in infancy and early childhood. *ICAN.* 2009; **1**: 73.

Greer AJ, Gulotta CS, Masler AE, *et al.* Caregiver stress and outcomes of children with pediatric feeding disorders treated in an intensive interdisciplinary program. *Pediatr Psychol.* 2008; **33**(6): 614–20.

Harris G, Blisset J, Johnson R. Food refusal associated with illness. *Child Psychol Psychiat Rev.* 2000; **5**(4): 148–56.

Hoch TA, Babbit RL, Coe DA, *et al.* Contingency contracting: combining positive reinforcement and escape extinction procedures to treat persistent food refusal. *Behav Mod.* 1994; **18**: 106–28.

Kerwin ME. Empirically supported treatments in pediatric psychology: severe feeding problems. *J Pediatr Psychol.* 1999; **24**: 193–214.

Kerwin ME. Pediatric feeding problems: a behavior analytic approach to the assessment and treatment. *Behavr Anal Today.* 2003; **4**(2): 162–76.

Linscheid L, Bohlin G, Hagekull B. Early feeding problems in a normal sample. *Int J Eat Disorder.* 1991; **10**: 395–405.

Linscheid TR, Budd K, Rasnake LK. Pediatric feeding problems. In: Roberts M, editor. *Handbook of Pediatric Psychology*, 3rd ed. New York, NY: Guilford Press; 2003. pp. 481–97.

Linscheid TR, Oliver J, Blyer E, *et al.* Brief hospitalization for the behavioral treatment of feeding problems in the developmentally disabled. *J Pediatr Psychol.* 1978; **3**: 72–6.

Linscheid TR, Tarnowsy TJ, Rasnake LK, *et al.* Behavioural treatment of food refusal in a child with short gut syndrome. *J Pediatr Psychol.* 1987; **12**: 451–60.

Luiselli JK. Behavioral feeding intervention with deaf-blind, multihandicapped children. *Child Family Behav Ther.* 1988; **10**: 49–62.

Luiselli JK, Luiselli TE. Oral feeding treatment of children with chronic food refusal and multiple developmental disabilities. *Am J Ment Retard.* 1994; **98**(5): 646–55.

Martin C, Southall A, Shea E, *et al.* The importance of a multifaceted approach in the assessment and treatment of childhood feeding disorders. *Clin Case S.* 2008; **7**(2): 79–99.

Nelson GL, Cone JD, Hanson CR. Training correct utensil in retarded children: modelling vs. physical guidance. *Am J Ment Def.* 1975; **80**: 114–22.

Piazza CC. Feeding disorders and behavior: what have we learned? *Dev Disabil Res Rev.* 2008; **14**: 174–81.

Piazza CC, Carroll-Hernandez TA. Assessment and treatment of pediatric feeding disorders. In: Trembly RE, Barr RG, DeV Peters R, editors. *Centre of Excellence for Early Childhood Development*; 2004. Available at: www.child-encyclopedia.com/pages/PDF/Piazza-Carroll-HernandezANGxp.pdf (retrieved 18 May 2009).

Piazza CC, Fisher WF, Brown KA, *et al.* Functional analysis of inappropriate mealtime behaviors. *J ApplBehav Anal.* 2003; **36**: 187–204.

Ramsay M, Zelazo P. Food refusal in failure to thrive infants: naso-gastric feeding combined with interactive-behavioral approach. *J Pediatr Psychol.* 1988; **13**: 329–47.

Reau NR, Senturia YD, Lebailly SA, *et al.* Infant and toddler feeding patterns and problems: normative data and a new direction. *J Dev Behav Pediatr.* 1996; **17**: 149–53.

Riordan MM, Iwata BA, Finney JW, *et al.* Behavioral assessment and treatment of chronic food refusal in handicapped children. *J Appl Behav Anal.* 1984; **17**: 327–41.

Sisson LA, Dixon MJ. Improving mealtime behaviors through token reinforcement. *Behav Mod.* 1986; **10**: 333–54.

Stark LJ, Mulvihill MM, Powers SW, *et al.* Behavioral intervention to improve caloric intake of children with cystic fibrosis. Treatment versus waiting list control. *J Pediatr Gastroenterol Nutr.* 1996; **22**: 240–53.

Van Dijk EM, Kneepkens CF, Hartdoff CM, *et al.* Hunger provocation in young children with pathological food refusal. *Poster Presentation at the National Conference on Child Health Psychology, Society of Pediatric Psychology*, APA Div 54, 2008 April 10–12; Miami Beach, Florida; 2008. pp. 36 (67).

Warren LR, Fox CA. The use of video fluoroscopy in the evaluation and treatment of children with swallowing disorders. In: Pehoski C, editor. *Problems with Eating: Intervention for Children and Adults with Developmental Disabilities.* Rockville, MD: The American Occupational Therapy Association, Inc; 1987. pp. 9–14.

Werle MA, Murphy TB, Budd KS. Treating chronic food refusal in young children: Home-based parent training. *J ApplBehav Anal.* 1993; **26**: 421–33.

PART III

The Clinical Practice Toolkit

This section introduces examples of clinical practice tools for experienced clinicians to inspire clinical practice. The materials are organised according to a 'stepwise' progression which follows the stages of assessment, problem formulation and intervention with a child with feeding problems. The individual tools can also be downloaded for use from: www.radcliffepublishing.com/feedingproblems

ASSESSMENT PHASE

1. The assessment chart[1]

This is a flow chart of the different steps from assessment to intervention and follow-up phases. It may be used during parent interview as a visual prompt to help the parents gain an understanding of the different stages of the process. It contains the following.

- *Multi-professional assessment.* It is important to collect information from different professionals so as to be able to rule out unexplored medical, dietetic, oral-motor or language problems.
- *Consent form.* To inform parents about the stages of the procedure and obtain their consent and to help them to be involved in the decision-making process. Consent may be obtained for the whole process or for specific aspects of assessment, such as filming the family or the child at meal times or visiting the child's school for observation at lunch time, etc.
- *Assessment of the child's feeding behaviour.* This can be done through gathering information from the parents at the clinical assessment interview (i.e. the assessment form from the Munroe–Meyer Institute), specific assessment questionnaires completed by parents relate to the child's behaviour at mealtimes (i.e. the behavioural paediatric assessment scale), record charts and food diaries provided by parents, etc.
- *Direct observation.* If possible, the child's feeding behaviour should be observed within the natural environment where this behaviour happens (i.e. at home, at

---

[1]Adapted from Dovey *et al.* (2010).

school, etc.). This direct observation can be recorded using record sheets and/ or video recordings.

- *Multi-professional meeting.* Collating reports from other professionals will help develop a *whole child* picture of the current problems, which will, in turn, inform the action plan. A final multi-professional report is ideal.
- *Feedback to parents.* Parents should receive a verbal or written final report of the main presenting feeding problems with the professional formulation and the suggested plan of action.

2. The multi-professional assessment checklist[2]

This list is designed to help check whether information from other professionals has been sought/received. It could be used to explore whether the parents already have this information (i.e. letters or evidence of diagnoses from doctors, etc.) or it needs to be obtained from other sources. It is not an exhaustive list but a guide to collecting relevant information. It can be expanded as needed.

3. An example of an assessment form

This is the assessment form employed at the Munroe-Meyer Institute, kindly provided by Professor Cathleen Piazza (*see* Chapter 3). It is an example of the kind of information gathering used to draw together essential information pertinent to the child's feeding/eating behaviour.

4. Individual checklist

This individual checklist can be used at the clinical interview with parents to explore the different factors that are impacting in the child's feeding problem. It complements the parent's clinical interview and assessment form.

DECISION MAKING

5. Decision-making model

This algorithm makes it possible to clearly see the factors that need to be explored during the assessment and to find out which are significant at each moment. It also helps to specify different types of food refusal and to devise tailored management strategies[3].

6. Specific types of food refusal

Once completed, the algorithm leads to different types of food refusal and then to facilitate the development of specific action plans.

---

[2]Adapted from Dovey *et al.* (2010)
[3]Dovey *et al.*, 2009.

IDEAS AND RECORD CHARTS FOR INTERVENTION (SOME EXAMPLES)

7. Foods I have touched[4]

This is an example of a record chart for children to document the food they have touched during a week. This activity can be done in groups, such as children's desensitisation groups, or as family activities or simply as individual tasks for children with sensitivity but without ASD traits.

A similar chart can be created for children and families to taste new foods (i.e. foods I have tasted).

8. Next steps: moving on to chewing[5]

This is an example of a guideline created for parents. It provides ideas for parents to help their children to develop chewing skills.

9. Next steps: moving on to spoon feeding

This is another example of a guideline for parents and is part of a series entitled *Next Steps* for parents to help their children develop feeding skills.

10A and B. Play activity programme and report: example[6]

This is an example of play activities for a child admitted to hospital for treatment of a feeding disorder. It includes different interrelated activities designed to help the child to develop tactile experiences. This approach was part of a desensitisation process for the child designed to help him accept different textures and to decrease his tactile defensiveness. The second part of the play (Soft Play) had the secondary aim of creating a physical activity scenario before mealtimes. The child's experience of physical sensations and signals was designed to help him attune to his body and learn to identify the hunger sensation. The report narrates the plan of activities and outlines how the child engaged with them.

11. Feeding group[7]

This is an example of a group activity for children with feeding problems and tactile defensiveness. Their parents can choose either to be involved or to observe the child's activity behind a double mirror.

12. Supporting parents: eaters come in all sorts[8]

It is important to include parents in the assessment process and also to include them in the treatment team as experts on their own children. This handout provides ideas for parents to support their children in overcoming their feeding problems.

---

[4]Provided by Elaine Isherwood, Dietician.
[5]Provided by Elaine Isherwood, Dietitian & Lisa Brown, SALT.
[6]Provided by Julie Milestone, Hospital Play Specialist.
[7]Provided by Elaine Isherwood, Dietician, & Play Specialists at CDC centre.
[8]Provided by Monique Thomas-Holtus and colleagues at the Wilhelmina Children's Hospital, Utrecht.

13. Sharing knowledge: a dietician's perspective on assessment and intervention[9]

An overview on assessment and intervention from the dietician completes the toolkit.

REFERENCES

Dovey TM, Farrow CV, Martin CI, *et al*. When does food refusal requires professional intervention? *Curr Nutr Food Sci*. 2009; 5(3): 160–71.

Dovey TM, Isherwood E, Aldridge V, *et al*. Typology of feeding disorders based on a single assessment system: formulation of a clinical decision-making model. *ICAN*. 2010.

Dovey TM, Isherwood E, Aldridge V, *et al*. Typology of feeding disorders based on a single assessment system: case study evidence. *ICAN*. 2010.

FEEDING LINKS

http://scholar.google.com/scholar?q=%22author%3AA.+author%3ANapier-Phillips%22
www.mayoclinic.com/health/nutrition-and-healthy-eating/MY00431
www.kennedykrieger.org/kki_diag.jsp?pid=1084

---

[9]Dorthe Wiuf Nielsen, Klinisk Diætist, Copenhagen, Denmark.

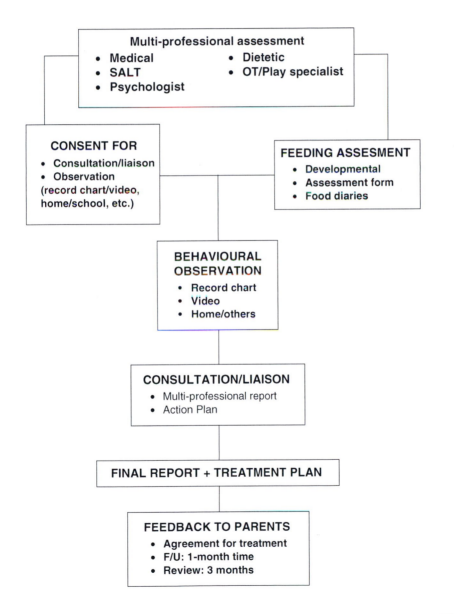

The assessment chart

Multi-professional assessment
- Medical
- SALT
- Psychologist
- Dietetic
- OT/Play specialist

CONSENT FOR
- Consultation/liaison
- Observation
(record chart/video,
home/school, etc.)

FEEDING ASSESMENT
- Developmental
- Assessment form
- Food diaries

BEHAVIOURAL OBSERVATION
- Record chart
- Video
- Home/others

CONSULTATION/LIAISON
- Multi-professional report
- Action Plan

FINAL REPORT + TREATMENT PLAN

FEEDBACK TO PARENTS
- Agreement for treatment
- F/U: 1-month time
- Review: 3 months

The multi-professional assessment checklist (adapted from Dovey *et al.*, 2010)

MEDICAL
- Is there evidence of any medical report?
- Is access to the child's medical notes feasible?
- Has the child any current medical diagnosis/illness, etc.?
- Are there any medical test results (i.e. blood tests, etc.)
- Has the child been seen by a GP, paediatrician in the last 3 months?
- Has the child an NG or PEG tube?
- Has the child been admitted to hospital?

DIETETIC
- Is there any dietetic report about this child we could have access to?
- Do we have the child's growth chart?
- Is the child taking supplement, vitamins, minerals, etc.?
- Do we have the child's food diaries?
- Does the child have any food intolerances?

SPEECH AND LANGUAGE (SALT)
- Has the child been seen by SALT?
- Do we have any SALT report?
- Is there any report about the child' safety during eating (aspiration problems, etc.)?
- Does the child present any oral motor-related problems (i.e. difficulties in chewing, etc.)?

OT/PLAY SPECIALIST

- Has the child been seen by these specialists?
- Is there any report about child' style of playing/socialising, etc.?
- Is the child easily engaged in messy play?
- How are the child' social communication skills?
- How is the child reacting to the nearest environment and new places (i.e. exploring, etc.)?

PSYCHOLOGIST

- Has the child been seen by a child psychologist specialised in Paediatrics?
- How is the child's development?
- Is there any report about the child's behaviour at mealtimes?
- Is there any report about family routines at mealtime?
- Is there any information about parental behaviour, attitudes, cultural issues, etc. regarding eating?

3

An example of an assessment form

TABLE 1: Sample evaluation form

Munroe-Meyer Institute			**UNH#:**	
University of Nebraska Medical Centre			**Patient:**	
Paediatric Feeding Disorders Program			**DOB:**	
Initial Evaluation and Treatment Plan			**DOE:**	
			Address:	
Weekly Outpatient:	☐ Recommended	☐ Not Recommended		
Day Treatment:	☐ Recommended	☐ Not Recommended	**Phone:**	(h)
Other	☐ Recommended	☐ Not Recommended		(c)

REFERRAL

_____ **(list contact information)** referred child's name to the Munroe–Meyer Institute's Paediatric Feeding Disorders Program. **Caregivers' chief complaint/ reason for referral is**_____.

BRIEF BACKGROUND INFORMATION

During the initial evaluation on _____ present were: _____ (clinical specialist), Cathleen Piazza, Ph. D. (licensed psychologist), and _____.
Primary caretaker is (name and relation to child). Caregiver's name is (list occupation). Child's name has _____ siblings and currently lives with _____.
Per caregiver report, child's name is diagnosed with (describe cognitive functioning level). Child's name's provisional diagnosis is 307.59 (Feeding Disorder of Infancy and Childhood).

CHIEF COMPLAINT/ REASON FOR REFERRAL

The chief complaint/reason for referral is _____. Caregiver's name reports that this behavior includes _____. This occurs during _____ meals _____ times a day. Prior to the meal, caregiver's name _____. When presented with food, child's name _____. When child's name engages in the inappropriate behaviors, caregiver's name _____. Child's name then _____. Caregiver's name reports that _____ management strategies have worked.

Caregiver's name's goal for child's name _____.

Direct observations indicate _____.

Secondary complaint/reason for referral is _____. Caregiver's name reports that this behavior includes _____. This occurs during _____ meals _____ times a day. Prior to the meal, caregiver's name _____. When presented with food, child's name_____. When child's name engages in the inappropriate behaviors, caregiver's name _____. Child's name then _____. Caregiver's name reports that _____ management strategies have worked.

Caregiver's name's goal for child's name _____.
Direct observations indicate _____.

All data are reported as a mean per session: 5 seconds = Number of bites accepted within 5 seconds of presentation/number of bites presented × 100%; Exp = Number of bites expelled per minute; MC = Number of bites not present in the child's mouth 30 seconds after acceptance/number of bites accepted × 100%; Pack = Number of bites in child's mouth 30 seconds after acceptance/ number of bites accepted × 100%; Gag = Number of gags per minute; CI = Number of inappropriate behaviour per minute; NV = Duration of negative vocalizations/duration of meal in seconds × 100%; Grams = Pre- minus post-meal weights in g (without vomit); G Emesis = Vomit in grams

SESSION 5 sec Exp MC Pack Gag CI NV Grams G Emesis
home baseline (n=1)
(Please list by condition)

CURRENT MEDICAL PROVIDERS

SCHOOL

PRIOR PROFESSIONAL CONTACTS TO RESOLVE REPORTED PROBLEMS

Service	Start/ End Date (month/ year)	How often?	Length of each therapy session	Did therapy focus on feeding?	Effect of therapy for feeding problem	Therapist information (name, address, telephone)
		☐ 1×/month ☐ 2×/month ☐ 1×/week ☐ 2×/week ☐ 3×/week ☐ _____	☐ 15 min ☐ 30 min ☐ 45 min ☐ 1 hr ☐ 1.5 hr ☐ _____	☐ Yes ☐ No	☐ Worse ☐ No change ☐ Improved	
		☐ 1×/month ☐ 2×/month ☐ 1×/week ☐ 2×/week ☐ 3×/week ☐ _____	☐ 15 min ☐ 30 min ☐ 45 min ☐ 1 hr ☐ 1.5 hr ☐ _____	☐ Yes ☐ No	☐ Worse ☐ No change ☐ Improved	

MEDICAL HISTORY

Medical history includes _____. Current medications include _____.

NUTRITION

Supplemental feedings (☐ NG tube, ☐ G-tube, ☐ J-tube) ☐ have ☐ have not been used in the past. Currently, child's name ☐ does ☐ does not receive supplemental feedings. Supplemental feedings

Formula type: _____

Tube feeding schedule:

Time	Amount	Method (Pump, Gravity, Bolus)	Rate

Caregiver's name reports that to the best of his/her knowledge, child's name ☐ does ☐ does not have food allergies. Child's name's diet ☐ is ☐ is not restricted in other ways _____. Caregiver's name reports that child's name expresses hunger by _____.

Child's name's feeding patterns is as follows:

Meal	Time	Location	Food and Approximate Amount
Breakfast			
AM Snack			
Lunch			
PM Snack			
Dinner			
HS Snack			

Anthropometric Parameters:

We used the Paediatric growth charts from the National Centre for Health Statistics in collaboration with the National Centre for Chronic Disease Prevention and Health Promotion (2000) to assess the growth patterns and rates of infants and children.

When plotted on the growth chart, child's name's growth pattern was as follows:

Weight: _____ kg (_____ lb)
Weight-for-Age: _____
☐ <3rd Percentile   ☐ 10th to 25th Percentile   ☐ 90th to 95th Percentile
☐ 3rd to 5th Percentile   ☐ 50th to 75th Percentile   ☐ 95th to 97th Percentile
☐ 5th to 10th Percentile ☐ 75th to 90th Percentile   ☐ >97th Percentile

Height: _____ cm (_____ inches)
Height-for-Age: _____
☐ <3rd Percentile   ☐ 10th to 25th Percentile   ☐ 90th to 95th Percentile
☐ 3rd to 5th Percentile   ☐ 50th to 75th Percentile   ☐ 95th to 97th Percentile
☐ 5th to 10th Percentile ☐ 75th to 90th Percentile   ☐ >97th Percentile

Standard height for age: _____ cm
Height-for-age as a % of standard: _____ %

Weight-for-Height:_____
☐ <3rd Percentile   ☐ 10th to 25th Percentile   ☐ 90th to 95th Percentile
☐ 3rd to 5th Percentile   ☐ 50th to 75th Percentile   ☐ 95th to 97th Percentile
☐ 5th to 10th Percentile ☐ 75th to 90th Percentile   ☐ >97th Percentile

Estimated Ideal Body Weight (IBW): _____kg
Weight-for-height as a percent of standard (IBW): _____%

Classification of Malnutrition Based on Growth Parameters:

Acute Malnutrition:

Weight-for Height as a % of Standard:

☐ ≥90% – Normal;   ☐ 80–90% – Mild ;   ☐ 70–80% – Moderate;
☐ 70% or less – Severe

Chronic Malnutrition (Stunting):

Height-for-Age as a % of Standard:

☐ >95% – Normal;   ☐ 90–95% – Mild;   ☐ 85–90% – Moderate;
☐ 85% or less – Severe

Child's name ☐ has ☐ does not currently have a diagnosis of failure to thrive. Child's name ☐ has ☐ has not previously had a diagnosis of failure to thrive.

FEEDING HISTORY

Caregiver's name attempted to ☐ bottle feed, ☐ breast feed, ☐ both, ☐ neither from _____ (age) to _____ (age). Child's name:

☐ drank very little,
☐ drank about half of what he/she was supposed to,
☐ drank most of what he/she was supposed to.
☐ had difficulty drinking – aspiration a concern

CHILD'S AGE	TYPE OF FOOD	CHECK ONE	
	Cereals	☐ REFUSED	☐ ACCEPTED
	Baby food	☐ REFUSED	☐ ACCEPTED
	Pureed food	☐ REFUSED	☐ ACCEPTED
	Table food	☐ REFUSED	☐ ACCEPTED

CURRENT FEEDING PRACTICES

Currently, child's name eats in a
☐ regular chair,
☐ booster seat,
☐ high chair,
☐ caregiver's lap,
☐ _____. Describe any additional support needed/received to maintain an upright posture.

During meals, child's name
☐ eats with the rest of the family.
☐ does not eat with the rest of the family.

Meals last:

☐ less than 10 minutes   ☐ 20–30 minutes   ☐ 40–60 minutes
☐ 10–20 minutes   ☐ 30–40 minutes   ☐ more than 60 minutes

CURRENT FEEDING SKILLS

☐ Drinks from bottle
☐ Fed by caregivers
☐ Feeds self with fingers
☐ Feeds self with spoon
☐ Feeds self with fork
☐ Uses knife

☐ Drinks from cup/glass controlled by caregiver
☐ Drinks independently from cup/glass
☐ Drinks from straw
☐ Pours own drink
☐ Prepares own snack

ORAL AND SENSORY MOTOR STATUS

Behavior/Demeanor: *Child's affect during evaluation.*
Neuromuscular/Developmental status: *Milestones, sitting ability etc.*

PROBLEM	HX of	HAS (PARENTAL REPORT)	OBSERVED
Poor suck (initiation; sustaining; able to pause and restart) Describe:	☐	☐	☐
Difficulty with tongue control (forward thrust, mobility limitations not expected at developmental level) Describe:	☐	☐	☐
Difficulty swallowing (initiation; needs multiple tries to clear oral cavity and pharynx) Describe:	☐	☐	☐
Difficulty with lip/jaw control (tone in oral-facial musculature; graded jaw opening/closing) Describe:	☐	☐	☐
Difficulty chewing (organization; sustaining long enough to ensure safety) Describe:	☐	☐	☐
Coughing with certain foods/liquids Describe:	☐	☐	☐
Gagging with certain foods/drinks, Describe:	☐	☐	☐
Can't bite off pieces of food	☐	☐	☐
Teeth Grinding	☐	☐	☐
Drooling (difficulty managing secretions)	☐	☐	☐
Vomiting/Rumination	☐	☐	☐
Grunting	☐	☐	☐
Profuse perspiration (diaphoresis)	☐	☐	☐
Oral defensiveness	☐	☐	☐
Other _____	☐	☐	☐

Sensitivity to food textures: ☐ smooth, ☐ crunchy, ☐ combined, ☐ none

SWALLOW SAFETY

☐ Date of last swallow study _____

Where?_____

Outcome of the study:

☐ Oral Dysphagia   ☐ Pharyngeal Dysphagia   ☐ Both   ☐ WNL

_____ If aspiration was noted – on what consistencies?:

_____ liquids; _____puree; _____ solids; _____ mixed

Diet Recommendations: ☐ Regular   ☐ Soft   ☐ Puree   ☐ Thickened Liquids

Fatigue Impact on swallow safety?: ☐ YES   ☐ NO

☐ Safe feeder/eater   ☐ have MBS reports   ☐ need MBS reports   ☐ no MBS needed

☐ Need follow up swallow study   ☐ needs MBS prior to admission   ☐ can be admitted in preparation for MBS

NOTES:

COMMUNICATION

Does the child have a functional way to communicate?   ☐ YES   ☐ NO

How does the child communicate?
☐ VERBALLY   ☐ GESTURALY   ☐ SIGN   ☐ OTHER: Crying and facial expressions

Can the child follow instructions?   ☐ YES   ☐ NO

OTHER BEHAVIORS

Caregiver's name reports that child's name goes to bed at _____, wakes at _____, and naps during the day at _____. Caregiver's name reports that child's name ☐ does ☐ does not have problems sleeping.

Caregiver's name reports that child's name exhibits other behavior problems such as _____.

CAREGIVER INFORMATION

Family's ability to follow through with treatment and other stresses on family.

RECOMMENDATION

Child's name is a _____ -year-old child diagnosed with _____. He/she would benefit from:

☐ Weekly outpatient therapy in the Paediatric Feeding Disorders Program at the Munroe–Meyer Institute

☐ Weekly outpatient therapy in the Paediatric Feeding Disorders Program at the Munroe–Meyer Institute pending further medical testing

☐ Intensive therapy in the day treatment program in the Paediatric Feeding Disorders Program at the Munroe–Meyer Institute

☐ Intensive therapy in the day treatment program in the Paediatric Feeding Disorders Program at the Munroe–Meyer Institute pending further medical testing

☐ Other.

This information was relayed to caregiver's name. Child's name was placed on the waiting list for the Paediatric Feeding Disorders Program. Caregiver's name was asked to send child's name's medical records to the support services coordinator at the Munroe–Meyer Institute to facilitate child's name's admission to the program. The support services coordinator will contact caregiver's name regarding child's name's insurance status and approximate admission date.

Physician

Certified Behavior Analyst

Nutritionist

OTR/L
Occupational Therapist

SLP
Speech Pathologist

LCSW
Clinical Social Worker

Support service instructions:
☐ The family received an information packet prior to the evaluation.
☐ The family received an information packet during the evaluation.
☐ Please send the family an information packet.
☐ Please call family and schedule a screening with the social worker.
☐ Family received recommendations (attached).

TABLE 2: Sample of an abbreviated goal sheet

Child: Date of Admission:

☐ **Increase Total P.O.** (from_____kcal to_____kcal)

    Please circle range

    90%–100%   80%–90%   70%–80%   60%–70%

    40%–50%   30%–40%   20%–30%   10%–20%

  1 ☐ *clinic – 3 out of the 5 last treatment days at the clinic (including meals at home using the final treatment protocol)*

  2 ☐ *home – 1 day in the home using the final treatment protocol*

☐ **Increase Liquid P.O.** (from_____g fl to_____g fl)

    Please circle range

    90%–100%   80%–90%   70%–80%   60%–70%

    40%–50%   30%–40%   20%–30%   10%–20%

  3 ☐ *clinic – 3 out of the 5 last treatment days at the clinic (including meals at home using the final treatment protocol)*

  4 ☐ *home – 1 day in the home using the final treatment protocol*

☐ **Increase Texture** (from _____ to _____)

  5 ☐ *clinic – 3 out of the 5 last treatment days at the clinic using the final treatment protocol with mean 5-s/independent/verbal acceptance and mouth cleans at 80% or greater*

  6 ☐ *home – 1 day in the home using the final treatment protocol with mean 5-s/independent/verbal acceptance and mouth cleans at 80% or greater*

☐ **Increase Weight** (from_____ kg to_____ kg)

  7 ☐ *day 1 of admission to the last day in the clinic*

☐ **Decrease Tube Feeding** (from_____% to _____%)

  8 ☐ *clinic – decrease by the last treatment day at the clinic*

  9 ☐ *home – decrease by the last day in the home*

☐ **Decrease Bottle Feeds** (from_____% to_____ %)

10 ☐ *clinic – decrease by the last treatment day in the clinic*

11 ☐ *home – decrease by the last day in the home*

☐ **Increase Self-feeding**

12 ☐ *clinic – 3 out of the 5 last treatment days at the clinic using the final treatment protocol with mean independent/verbal acceptance at 80% or greater*

13 ☐ *home – 1 day in the home using the final treatment protocol with mean independent/verbal acceptance at 80% or greater*

Chewing

☐ **Skill development (non-food items)**

14 ☐ *clinic – 3 out of the 5 last treatment days at the clinic using the final treatment protocol with mean chews between 8 and 15 per bite*

15 ☐ *home – 1 day in the home using the final treatment protocol with mean chews between 8 and 15 per bite*

☐ **Increase chewing (food items)**

16 ☐ *clinic – 3 out of the 5 last treatment days at the clinic using the final treatment protocol with mean chews between 8 and 15 per bite*

17 ☐ *home – 1 day in the home using the final treatment protocol with mean chews between 8 and 15 per bite*

☐ **Increase Variety**

From _____foods/liquids to _____foods/liquids

22 ☐ *clinic – 3 out of the 5 last treatment days at the clinic using the final treatment protocol with mean 5-s/independent/verbal acceptance of new foods/liquids at 80%or greater(___ foods should be presented during the last week at the clinic)*

23 ☐ *home – implementation of final treatment protocol with mean 5-s/independent/ verbal acceptance of new foods/liquids at 80%or greater (___foods/liquids should be presented during home visits) for all sessions conducted during home visits*

☐ **Decrease Inappropriate Mealtime Behaviours**(from ___ rpm to ___ rpm)

26 *clinic – 3 out of the 5 last treatment days in the clinic with mean rate of problem behaviour (i.e. head turns and disruptions) at 1 or below*

27 *home – 1 day in the home with mean rate of problem behaviour (i.e. head turns and disruptions) at 1 or below*

28 *clinic – 3 out of the 5 last treatment days in the clinic with mean 80% or greater reduction in problem behaviour – i.e, head turns and disruptions(mean standard baseline rate of problem behaviour should be used to calculate reductions)*

29 *home – 1 day in the home with mean 80% or greater reduction in problem behaviour - i.e., head turns and disruptions(mean standard baseline rate of problem behaviour should be used to calculate reductions)*

☐ **Training**

30 ☐ Primary caregiver

31 ☐ School

32 ☐ Other:_____

mean of 90% or greater accuracy for all sessions conducted by caregivers independently at the clinic and in the home using the final treatment protocol

33 ☐ **Generalisation** *(sessions to be fed in settings other than the session room at least 3 times within the last 10 days of admission)*

Comments:

_____   _____
Primary Caregiver Signature   Primary Therapist Signature

_____   _____
Date   Case Manager Signature

4

Individual checklist
(adapted from Dovey *et al.*, 2010)

MEDICAL/PHYSIOLOGICAL

- Has the child a current diagnosed chronic illness?
- Has the child had any acute illnesses?
- Has the child any physical reason which has prevented him/her from feeding?
- Has the child been hospitalised?
- Has the child suffered pain/vomiting associated with feeding/eating?
- What do you think the impact of these factors in the child's feeding pattern has been?
- What is their general appetite regulation like (hunger, fullness, etc.)?

SENSORY SENSITIVITIES/DEFENSIVENESS

- Does the child have any skin sensitivity?
- Does the child enjoy 'messy' play?
- Is the child refusing to touch certain textures?
- Has the child any problems with smells?
- What about tastes?
- Does the child have any problems with different temperatures?
- Do you have any problems when brushing the child's teeth?
- How is the child's reaction to the taste of the tooth paste?
- Is the child reluctant to accept any touch on his/her face?
- Does the child have any specific sensitivity to sounds?

DEVELOPMENTAL

- Has the child any oral-motor problems?
- Is there normal development of oral-motor skills (sucking, chewing, etc.)?

- Is overall development progressing normally (fine-gross motors, social, language, etc.)?
- Have feeding milestones been completed appropriately (weaning process, finger foods, etc.)?

ENVIRONMENTAL

- What is the usual scenario for mealtime (mealtime's habits)?
- What is the usual family mealtime's environment?
- What are the mealtime's schedules and routines?
- What are the parents' habitual feeding techniques and practices?
- What are the parental perceptions, beliefs and strategies about food and eating?
- What are the parental attitudes about food and cultural beliefs about food and eating?

Decision-making model (adapted from Dovey *et al.,* 2010)

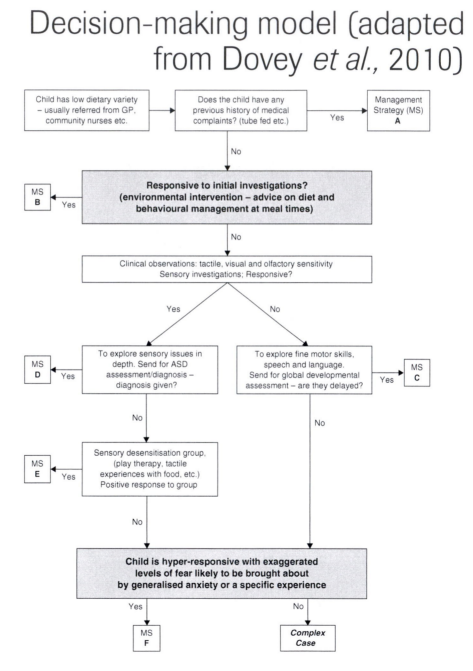

Specific types of food refusal (adapted from Dovey *et al.*, 2009)

Category A **Medical**	Children who have an underlying medical problem that has contributed significantly to the feeding problem (i.e. cardio-pulmonary conditions, renal diseases, anatomical anomalies, neurological disorders and NG-Tube fed).
Category B **Learning dependent**	Characteristics components are neophobia, exposure and learning. Children with an history of classical and operant conditioning and with lack of experience towards novelty food as a consequence.
Category C **Developmental**	Children that have some kind of developmental delay to which their feeding problem is or can be associated.
Category D **ASD**	Food refusal associated to ASD traits and/or diagnosis.
Category E **Selective**	Children with a tendency to over react to sensations; it could be expressed by being tactile-defensive and with sensory sensitivity (smells, noises, etc.).
Category F **Food Phobia**	Children having a fear-based (phobic) response to food. Often resulting in an extremely restricted diet. Other anxiety or affective disorder can be also associated as part of their profile.

Foods I have touched!

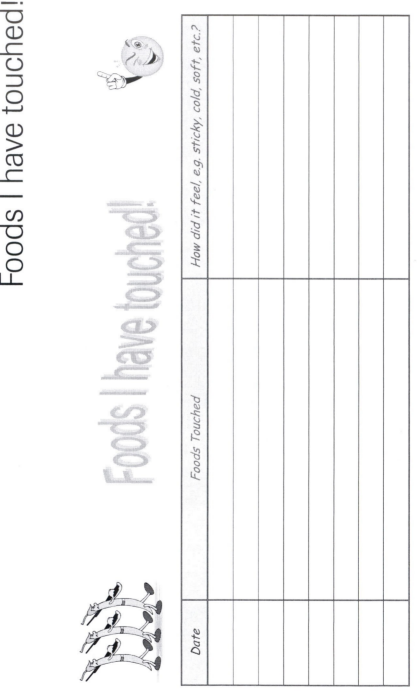

Foods I have touched!

Date	Foods Touched	How did it feel, e.g. sticky, cold, soft, etc.?

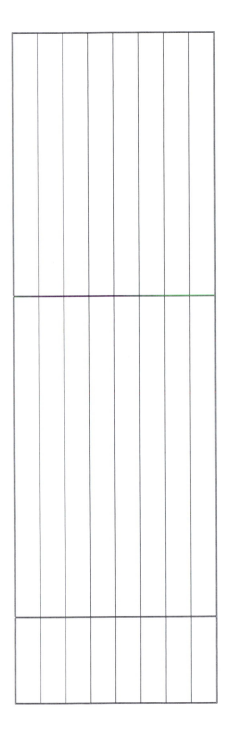

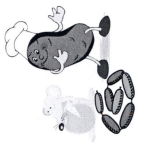

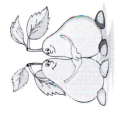

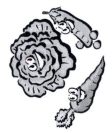

8

Next steps: moving on to chewing

Most children should be ready to start chewing at around 6 months of age. However, your child may only now be ready for this.

STARTING STEPS

- The earliest stage of chewing is munching. This is where your child's mouth will move up and down in order to break up the food. Foods given to your child to help them start munching are peeled fresh (or tinned) ripe pears, peaches or nectarines, soft boiled root vegetables (carrots, potatoes, etc.), pasta (without sauce), pieces of corned beef and small cubes of cheese.
- It is important to give foods of an even texture and to keep the food dry. Offer foods to both sides of the mouth.
- If your child finds this difficult you can help by:
  - Placing your finger on the front of their tongue, moving it up and down, tapping it on their tongue every second. This can also be done with food on your finger (e.g. thick pureed foods).
  - Placing chewable foods at the side of the mouth between the gums and teeth – a small piece of food the size of your thumbnail is ideal.
  - Rubbing their cheeks gently but firmly with two fingers.
  - Wrap the food you will use in a thin cotton handkerchief and tie it with a string. Place this between the back teeth or gums.
- Foods best avoided at this stage are bread, toffee, foods with shells (e.g. peas and sweet corn), foods of mixed textures (e.g. casseroles, tinned fruit and custard) and stage 2 baby jars.

IMPROVING CHEWING

- When children are able to munch (moving their tongue up and down), they need to move on to the next step, where their tongues will move left and right.
- It is best to start with rubber teething toys and foods that will not break up, e.g. dried fruit, strips of cooked beef, dehydrated fruit bars and liquorice sticks

(found in health food shops). Offer foods to both sides of the mouth.
- Try wrapping the food in an handkerchief (as mentioned above).
- Explore salty, sour and tart foods, e.g. lemon mousse or sorbet, lemon curd and beetroot in vinegar.
- Place the food on the teeth at one side of the mouth. Encourage the child to bite several times on the food. Try this on the other side and then keep repeating. This will help your child to learn to chew on each side of the mouth.
- Once your child is happy to chew food on each side of their mouth, encourage them to push the foods from the side to the middle of their mouth with their tongue. As this improves, use long thin foods, e.g. cheese strips, chips, bread sticks, partially cooked carrots or potatoes.
- To build up your child's skills of tongue movement and chewing together, try using raisins and dried fruits as well.
- As chewing matures (normally at 18–24 months of age) children will be able to move the food across their mouth from left and right, chewing and biting together. They should now be able to cope with most foods.

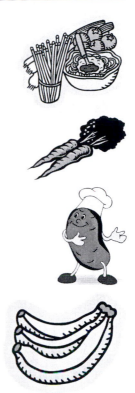

FINGER FOODS

By the age of 1 year most children should be trying to feed themselves. However, your child may only now be ready for this. Feeding using fingers is usually the first step towards self-feeding.

Be prepared for messy meal times. To start with your child may throw the food – on the floor, walls and themselves! Be patient and try not to become annoyed if your child is messy – this is normal. Have a cloth ready to clean-up when your child has finished.

Before you start
- Put a plastic tablecloth or shower curtain under your child's chair.
- If you want to use a bowl, make sure it is unbreakable!
- Make sure your child feels safe. If your child sits in a high chair ensure they are sitting at the correct height for the tray – use cushions behind and underneath your child if they are too small.
- If your child does not have a high chair, make sure they are at the right height for the table. Use a booster seat or cushions to help. A child's table and chair is also very useful.

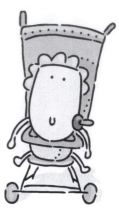

- Always stay near your child when they are finger feeding to make sure they do not choke.
- Try some of your child's food so they are not eating alone. Offer your child a small amount of finger food on their tray or in a bowl.
- Have a small drink available as this will help.

Here are some examples of finger foods you might like to try with your child.
- Small cubes of cheese.
- Small chunks of banana.
- Fingers of toast.
- Cooked pieces of carrot.
- Miniatures sandwiches with a soft filling, e.g. tuna.

Ask for a copy of the leaflet 'finger food fun' for more ideas.

If your child finds finger feeding difficult, you can help by:
- Making sure the food can be easily picked up. Usually children first start to pick things up using their whole hand at about 12 months of age. Later they have a grip using their thumb and first finger.

If children do not use two fingers they may find it difficult to pick up small foods, e.g. rice krispies, peas, etc. If you are concerned about this ask to see an Occupational Therapist.
- Try putting the food in your child's hand. If this does not lead to the food being put to the mouth, try moving his or her hand up to the mouth, but then let the food be placed into the mouth without help. Slowly, over time, reduce the amount of help until the child is able to do this alone.

Once your child places food in his or her mouth, then move their empty hand towards food on the tray or bowl and encourage them to touch and pick-up.

Children need your attention while eating: this means praising them when they eat well – ignore any naughty behaviour as your child will only repeat it if they get a reaction! Try to be relaxed and happy when eating with your child.

Remember feeding should always be fun

Next steps: moving on to spoon feeding

Your child may have difficulty using a spoon on their own. These difficulties may be for many reasons including:

- a delay in their development
- physical difficulties
- previously being fed by a tube.

This leaflet explains how to help your child to start using a spoon.

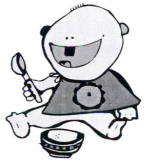

BEFORE YOU START

- Put a plastic tablecloth or shower curtain under your chair.
- Make sure your child feels safe. If your child sits in a high chair ensure they are at the correct height for the tray, use cushions behind and underneath your child if they are too small.
- If your child does not have a high chair, make sure they are at the right height for the table. Use a booster seat or cushions to help. A child's chair and table is also very useful.
- Never leave your child alone when spoon-feeding because of the risk of choking.
- Have a small drink available as this will help.
- Use a hard flat plastic child's spoon (ideally with a short handle). Using a large deep spoon may make it more difficult for your child to remove the food.
- Use a child's plastic unbreakable bowl. This will be easier than a plate as your child can get food by pushing their spoon against the sides.

STARTING STEPS

- At first your child may show interest in their spoon as another toy. They may bang, throw it and put it in their mouth. This usually starts at 9–12 months of age. However, your child may only now be ready for this.

- From the age of 12 months your child may show interest in bringing the spoon to their mouth. They will not have full control and may turn the spoon and tip over the food.

PRACTICAL TIPS

- Use foods your child likes and of a smooth texture (no lumps) that will stick to the spoon, e.g. mashed potatoes, fromage frais, ice cream, weetabix, puree meat and vegetables.
- Your child may try to hold your hand or grab your spoon. This is a good way of practising.
- Try giving your child their own spoon while you are feeding them. They may show interest in copying you.
- Start with a small amount of food on the end of the spoon. A large spoonful may cause your child to choke, or make it difficult for them to remove all of the food.
- The speed at which you help put the spoon in and take it out of your child's mouth should not be too fast. Your child needs time to see the spoon, feel it in their mouth, remove the food using their lips and swallow the food. Place the spoon in the middle of your child's tongue and press down lightly. Wait for their lips to close around the spoon. Do not scrape the spoon against your child's teeth as this does not allow your child to control or help with their own feeding.
- Make sure food is not too hot or cold for your child – they may refuse food or it may make it difficult for them to develop new skills.

If your child is finding it difficult to start spoon-feeding themselves, there are other ways in which you can help them.

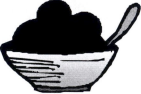

- You may need to try a special bowl or spoon (ask your Occupational Therapist for advice).
- Encourage your child to bear weight on his elbow on the table, while you help him to hold the spoon and move it from bowl to mouth.
- You may need to teach your child to use a spoon in small steps. The easiest way to do this is to teach them the last step first, i.e. putting the spoon to their mouth.

To do this:

Step 1. Stand behind your child while your child is holding the spoon; place your hand on top. Guide your child's hand to scoop up food from the bowl and move the spoon towards their mouth – at first you may need to place the

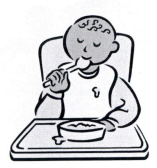

spoon in your child's mouth but let them remove food with their lips.

Step 2. Guide your child's hand to scoop up food from the bowel and move the spoon towards their mouth. Let your child place the spoon in their mouth.

Step 3. Guide your child's hand to scoop up food from their bowl – allow them to move the spoon towards their mouth. You may still need to give some help by holding lower down their arm or under their elbow.

Step 4. Allow your child to scoop up food from their bowl – you may still need to give some help by holding lower down their arm or under their elbow.

This process may take a long time and you should encourage and praise your child when they try hard (*even if they haven't succeeded!*).

When children are learning to feed they often throw food, spoons and even their whole bowl of food! They can also make a lot of mess. Do not give any attention to your child and if you need to clean up try to leave this until the end of feeding.

Remember meal times should be enjoyable and social times for all the family,
even if your child is eating very little!

Play activity program (example)

Week 1 – Day	Activity 1	Activity 2 (soft play)
One (arrival)	Paint	Building/knocking down towers
Two	Play dough	Hunting dinosaurs
Three	Finger painting	Building castles and fighting dragons
Four	Face painting (chocolate)	Playing Indians chasing buffaloes
Five	Jelly contest	Chasing for tickles

Weekend

Week 2 – Day	Activity 1	Activity 2 (soft play)
One	Cutting and gluing	Mini assault course
Two	Sand outside	Introducing new playmates
Three	Colouring	Walking outside – touching nature (plants, sand, etc.)
Four	Shopping for the party	Walking outside for sensorial experiences
Five	Creating biscuit faces (using sticky sugar ice as glue)	To organize a party for playmates (eating as a social experience)

Play report example

The role of the hospital play team was discussed at the multi-professional team meeting prior to admitting the child at the hospital for feeding disorder treatment. The child would spend 1 h with the hospital play specialist before mealtimes. The first half of the hour would be employed for decreasing child tactile defensiveness and to increase acceptance of different textures through messy play activities. In the second half energetic and boisterous play will be employed to help the child have strong physical sensations for him/her to learn to elaborate body signals.

The first day's session was a 'getting to know each other' time. We enjoyed doing activities that the child was familiar with. Paints were accessible. He/she was reluctant to start this activity and needed encouragement. He/she did not use hands but a paint brush being extremely cautious about splitting paint or moving outside limits of the paper. This activity lasted only 15 minutes as he/she wanted to stop and move on to soft play. He/she built towers and knocked them down and also jumped from high places and showed a forward flip.

The child showed interest in dinosaurs, therefore it was decided to do a walk display of them. The child was enthusiastic and participated fully. This facilitated the next session of messy play with play dough. There were lots of different dinosaur shapes and moulds and several colours and types of paints. This went well with the child using hands to shape the dough and press it into moulds. Still execution was clean with careful consideration to not mix colours as suggested by the child. Dinosaurs were lined up after being made. This naturally led to dinosaurs fighting each other and the transition to the soft play was smooth. The child suggested to build dinosaur caves and to hunt the dinosaurs all over the soft play.

The next session, painting, was tried again. Dinosaurs' pictures were already there for the child to paint. There were no brushes, only finger paint. The child dipped one finger carefully into the paint pot and used the finger to spread it on the picture but would not use the whole hand. After a while, the child asked for the hands to be washed. He/she was feeling anxiety and moved to the soft play were a lot of aggression was released playing fighting dragons and destroying castles.

The following day, I joined the child's breakfast where jam and chocolate sauce was put at the tip of the child's nose at breakfast time with the child laughing. This was discussed as in need to be built for the child to continue this experience. The messy play session was about playing buffaloes, cowboys and Indians. Faces were painted with chocolate and the session flowed very well with the child asking for the child's face to be painted and tasted the chocolate for the first time. The chocolate face was not washed up as we needed to play Indians. This session seemed a real breakdown in the child's treatment. After this session the child was engaged in touching and did not avoid messy play. The next session, the jelly context, was a real battle that created a big mess in the play room.

The rest of the sessions were to build this up and to maintain the level of contact the child had achieved. In sessions 3 and 4 of the second week the child was adamant to explore the exterior gardens and engaged in collecting plant, sand and looking for insects. This helped in integrating the tactile sensations into a natural accepted environment as this was one of the school activities that the child had to participate but was reluctant to do so.

The last two days were aimed at integrating eating and food with social activities. The child enjoyed shopping for a party we organised and creating surprise biscuits. This last activity was filmed and we could observe the child asking to taste the ice sugar voluntarily, sticking fingers on it and tasting naturally. We could also observe the child laughing in spite of having the hands completely 'dirty' with sticky ice sugar. The desensitisation program worked very well for the child and the soft play helped to release anxieties related to food and contact with sticky and messy elements.

11

The feeding group

SESSION 1

- Introduction to the group
- Ground rules of the group (check about drinks and snacks)
- Pre-group questionnaires and food diaries collected

Brainstorm with parents:
- Specific aims for each child
- Discussion of specific difficulties with food/drink
- Discussion of meal times.
- 10 minutes to share ideas.

ACTIVITIES

1 Home corner – free play
   - Cooker, sink, table and chair, plates and cups, play food.
   - Imaginary play.
   - Puzzles, colouring if needed
   - 15 minutes.
2 Glueing (on paper plates)
   - Glue, paper, pasta, lentils and spaghetti (all dry).
   - Creative picture with food.
   - 15 minutes.
   - Clean tables and wash hands.
3 Snacktime
   - Choice of cup, juice, banana, apple, grapes.
   - Chopping banana, grapes and apple, pulling banana skin.
   - 10 minutes.

4   Brushing teeth – 5 minutes
5   Water play – 10 minutes
6   Songs/stories/bubbles
    • Sitting on a mat, stories and songs about food – 5 minutes
7   Homework
    • Make a picture/collage using foods or materials at home.

12

Supporting parents: eaters come in all sorts

Monique Thomas-Holtus, Gerben Sinnema and Anthony P Messer

Eaters come in all sorts. There are slow eaters, children who play with their food, children who nibble little bits, downright picky eaters and those who will eat anything. Most parents would like their children to be in the last category. But is that realistic? (Dovey, 2007). Problematic eating behaviour in children can make you feel insecure as parents, especially if your friend's children really will eat anything – from garlicky olives to sushi and from herrings to beetroot salad. What you should realise then is that every child is unique and your approach to food needs to be geared to the individual child. General rules do not apply and not every child can manage to eat from the same pot as the rest of the family.

Food is a basic need for people and animals. A cub panics if its mother does not have any food for it. It is the same with children. If you put something in front of children that they think is horrible, they will panic. You recognise the resistance at once – turning aside the head, pushing away the spoon, pulling faces and so on. With children it is all about responding to the signals in the right way, and especially not allowing it to become a battle.

It is more important to respond to your intuition and to use it to get to know the individual preferences of each child in the family. One child may like soft bread, another may like crusty bread or toast. Bread is still bread, but the form in which children eat it sometimes makes a big difference. While peace and quiet, cleanliness and routine are back in fashion in child-rearing, the three basic concepts for eating and drinking are: intuition, responsiveness and individuality.

PREFERENCE OR AVERSION

Listen to what your child is trying to tell you – whether he does that in words or through his behaviour. You will notice that the signals that you interpreted as defiance at first are really to do with an aversion. Some children, for instance, will not eat pieces of tomato. That may be because they have an aversion to the texture of tomato. Some children get a tingling sensation in their mouths from tomato. Certain fruit, such as melon, can give the same tingling sensation. Children, just like adults, have preferences for, and aversions to, certain food products, such as soft fruit or seeds in bread.

What the three basic concepts mean for you in this case is that you should first ask yourself why your child does not want to eat tomato. Intuition: does he also object to other vegetables that are similar to tomato? Yes, that's right – he dislikes peppers too. In that case you can do something about it – respond to what he is telling you. Instead of offering pieces of tomato, you can liquidise or sieve peeled tomatoes to make a smooth purée. That way you are making an allowance for your child as an individual. And he can still eat healthy food together with the rest of the family.

THE EATING PHASES
From breast-feeding to solid food

Every child goes through different eating phases, usually without any problems worth mentioning. A little one learns a lot of new things in a relatively short time, especially in the first year of life. The child starts with breastfeeding or bottle-feeding and gradually moves on to spoon-feeding (O'Connor and Szekely, 2001). The first food given on a spoon is very smooth, such as puréed fruit and vegetables and baby cereal. In the next phase, the consistency of the food progresses to thick and smooth, to smooth with bits, to roughly mashed and finally to more solid food.

What many parents do not know is that there are children who never learn to accept one of the intermediate phases like smooth food with more solid bits in it. It is important to accept that as a fact before you go any further. It is also good to realise that there are also quite a few adults who have an aversion to smooth food with bits in it. They would be just as inclined to feel sick if you presented them with lumpy porridge.

After the first birthday, which is a milestone in more ways than one, parents often breathe a sigh of relief: 'Phew, what a relief, now my child can eat with the rest of the family!' But it seems that this cannot always be taken for granted. This is because it is not only in his or her eating behaviour that your child makes great strides in the first three years, but in other areas too. For instance, your child is very obviously developing her own will. The Dutch have an expression for this 'I am two, so I say no', and the English talk about the 'terrible twos'. There are good reasons for these common sayings!

EATING AND DRINKING BEFORE THE FIRST BIRTHDAY
Extra sensitive to stimuli

Children go through several phases in the development of their eating and drinking in the first year. These phases are characterised by the acquisition of new techniques and flavours, for example, moving on from breast or bottle to spoon and from liquid food to solid food. Most children progress through these different phases without difficulty. Some children are more sensitive to stimuli in their mouths and find a new flavour a more extreme experience. Children like this need a bit more time to get used to new flavours and methods of eating. Each child responds to change in his own way.

Your baby and a new skill

There are infants who find it difficult to adopt new skills, such as moving on from the breast to bottle-feeding or spoon-feeding. Always give your baby plenty of time to get used to something new. If you are breastfeeding and are planning to go back to work in a couple of weeks, use your maternity leave to gradually get your baby used to a combination of breast and bottle.

Your baby and a new flavour

If your baby is having difficulty accepting the first new flavours, try this step-by-step approach.

Step 1: on the lip

Do not give the new food on a spoon yet. Let your baby taste the first new foods as follows: smear a little fruit or vegetable purée on his or her lip with your finger and, at the same time, mime and make lip-smacking noises. Once this has gone well a few times, you can move on to the spoon.

Step 2: distract your baby

Sometimes, when you first try spoon-feeding, it is a good idea to distract your baby with a brightly coloured toy which has light effects or makes noises. Then your baby will gain the experience of new flavours without noticing. Stick to the same flavour for a week or two before trying a new one.

Step 3: be patient and keep it up

Modern parents tend to make allowances for their children's individual taste preferences while they are still too young, sometimes even as young as seven months old. After trying it a couple of times, the parents say that their child does not like this or that food. They stop trying new flavours too soon and that is not advisable. Experience has taught us that it is before the first birthday that a child learns to accept new flavours most readily. So you should familiarise them gradually. And be patient. Trust your own instincts. When a baby passively lets food run out of his mouth, the parents think that he does not want to eat or drink. But children only develop their own will after the first birthday. Having difficulty accepting new flavours may look like 'not wanting', but it is really something very different.

EATING AND DRINKING BETWEEN AGES ONE AND TWO

Be aware that broadening tastes and developing new skills is a very individual process. No child is the same in this respect – not even within the same family. Children all proceed at their own pace, have their own preferences, and have their own dislikes of certain flavours and ways of eating. One child, for instance, is really fond of his bottle, while another cannot wait to start eating cereal from a spoon. It is not that one method of feeding is better than the other. What is important is that the child is thriving on it.

It is a good idea to introduce as many flavours as possible before the first birthday. Research has shown that children have less trouble accepting different flavours in the first year of life. After that, you also have to deal with behavioural factors, the most familiar of which is the child's own will, which can play havoc with what should be an easy introduction to a new flavour. Your child may then suddenly start refusing things he has been eating up until then.

A lot changes for a child begin between his first and second birthday. He is already sitting in a high chair and is developing his own will. This behavioural factor can seriously thwart the eating pattern. In other words – rows at mealtimes. What is more, appetite decreases between the ages of one and two. That is completely normal and is certainly not something to worry about.

Once your child is over the age of 1 year, you can get into a daily routine of regular meals and drinks. Simply put, there are three main meals: breakfast, lunch and dinner. The rest can best be described as snack times – morning coffee, afternoon tea and pre-dinner drinks. It is best to keep the main meals predictable. That will give a naturally picky child a sense of security. Serve a dish that your child likes quite frequently; this is one way to avoid a battle over the main meals. Of course, you can make something different for yourself. At snack times, on the other hand, you can let your child experiment to his heart's content.

This is the way to avoid your child snacking and drinking all day long, which is not desirable in any case – it is certainly bad for your child's teeth. Teeth need time to repair themselves between meals!

In this way you challenge your child to imitate. The desire to imitate is very strong in the toddler phase. Let your child decide for himself what to try. Talk loudly to your partner about how delicious everything is, without interfering with your child. By not looking at him directly and not putting pressure on him you are teaching him that tasting is part of life and a very normal thing to do. If you stress it too much, you undo this effect. If your child asks for more, respond with a compliment: 'Clever boy! Of course you can have a bit more. But only when you've finished the first bit!'

Use the snack times (morning coffee, afternoon tea, evening drinks) for these tasting lessons. Just give your child a tiny speck to taste at first. If he asks for more, you can systematically increase the size of the pieces. It is important that the child eats up a piece before you give him another bit. It is also important that your child himself tells you that he wants to try something – either by pointing or asking.

It is not surprising that parents are sometimes at a complete loss when their toddler refuses to eat. One day your child is eating with relish and the next day she has no appetite at all for her favourite food. All of a sudden the sandwich that she could never get enough of is rejected with a sour face. Why does your toddler refuse something for apparently no reason? And how do you deal with that?

You will have learned what types of foods your child likes best by now – savoury, sweet or sour. Or perhaps she is a child who will eat anything. The arbitrary refusal of food we have just described is a kind of temporary 'madness'. Your child does not know what she wants and refuses food and drink for no reason. You take the plate away and then she says 'I want to eat it.' There is really only one answer to this – it is her age. 'Don't want it' is a behaviour that will regularly crop up at mealtimes. The eating pattern can be naturally capricious at this age.

There is very little you can do about this arbitrary wilfulness. What you can do is to make allowances for your child's individual preferences at mealtimes. Remember that you, as an adult, also like certain dishes more than others. If your child refuses to eat, give her 10 minutes to change her mind. If she continues to refuse, then ask 'Have you finished?' If she says 'yes', then take the plate away but do not give her anything else.

It is important to remain consistent in your approach immediately afterwards. Do not give your child anything to eat until the next meal. This means no snacks between meals, even if your child says she is hungry. Try to let your child build up sufficient appetite between the main meals and only offer something to eat again after 3 hours.

Parents have a coaching role in teaching their children to enjoy food. That means that you do not impose your own tastes or try to achieve results by force. If there is one golden rule with regard to enjoying food, it is that you accept that you can never force a child to learn to like something. As a parent you are embarking on a creative quest. There is no universal law that determines that your children will have the same tastes as you. After all, there are certain products that you, as parent, dislike. To put yourself in your child's place, imagine a dish that you find horrible. Now you can see what we mean! Just thinking about it makes you feel sick.

Genetic and other individual factors play a role in extreme pickiness. What that role is exactly is still unclear. Knowledge about extreme pickiness is spread across different fields, including physiology, biology and the behavioural sciences. More research is needed into this complex area. A moderate form of pickiness, also known as neophobia (fear of the new), is actually relatively normal in young children. Research has shown that children will only accept a new flavour after tasting it 10–15 (!) times.

Meals are a time of the day when the family comes together. So focus on this togetherness by creating a good atmosphere at the table. The younger children experience this, the better. The time will come soon enough when they have to eat separately from the family because of school or sporting commitments or because they have gone to play with a friend. Children can also experience eating with others at the crèche, where they will eat at the table with other children. It is also important to have regular mealtimes. We cannot overemphasise the importance of eating together. The social factor is extremely important: in addition to eating together, you can also share feelings, emotions and experiences of the day with each other during the meal.

EATING AND DRINKING BETWEEN THE AGES OF TWO AND THREE
No battles at the table

Between the second and third birthday very different issues suddenly come into play. Your child gets bigger, more independent and more articulate. Arguments at the table about what he does and does not have to eat become more and more frequent. Anticipate these arguments and set a number of basic rules for your family. After a while, everyone will know the rules and then you can simply refer to them briefly and clearly. Once again, do not invite battles at the table.

EXAMPLES OF BASIC RULES
- You have to taste.
- Stay seated at the table for 20 minutes.
- Food is not for playing with.

Give and take

Some children go through all the eating phases up to now with relative ease. But there are children aged 2 or 3 years who continue to be extremely picky and so become selective eaters, often to the great dismay of their parents. This is where your ability to give and take comes in. Be flexible, show give and take and be prepared to compromise – these are all ways to avoid conflict. Some children are extremely fussy eaters; that is just the way it is.

How much do you dish up?

Do not put a huge plate of food in front of them at this age, but dish up small portions at every meal – preferably on a small plate. It is a big reward for your child to sometimes be the first to finish his plate. It is nice too if he can sometimes ask for more instead of always hearing 'finish what's on your plate'. If your child does ask for more, serve up a small amount again.

It's possible to 'not like'...

Your child has to learn to taste before she can learn to enjoy food. It is important that she does this, because at this age she is going to go and stay with other children or with grandparents more and more often. It is nice then if she has already learned how to deal with learning to both taste and enjoy unfamiliar foods at home.

...but it's also possible to 'learn to like'!

Learning to enjoy food goes like this. Talk to your child beforehand about what she wants to learn to like. Explain to your child that learning to like something starts with learning to taste it. Anyone can learn to taste. Explain that it is just like learning to ride a bike, to run, to jump or to swing. And explain that if you want to learn something you can learn it.

In the example we are going to learn to taste apple. But you could, of course, start with any other kind of food. The instructions are written in such a way that you can explain to your child what he or she has to do. When learning to taste a meal consisting of meat, potato and vegetables always get your child to try one product per step. So let her try a tiny speck of vegetable first. Once she has licked that, then comes a speck of potato and after that a speck of meat. Only then does she get the reward star. Make an agreement with your child about what she is going to try. You decide together what she wants to learn to taste and enjoy eating. If your child is extremely picky, you should also decide beforehand how the food is to be prepared. For example, whether the potatoes will be boiled or baked, and whether the vegetable will be boiled or stir-fried. Some children prefer meat, fish and vegetarian products to have a crispy crust. Make allowances for this.

THE FIRST TASTING LESSON

Step 1
- Touch your lip with the speck of apple and count to three.
- Wipe your mouth with a serviette.
- Well done. You have earned the first reward star.
- We'll put that on the place mat.

Step 2
- Touch your tongue with the speck of apple.
- Take it out of your mouth again and wipe your mouth with a serviette.
- Well done. You have earned the second reward star.
- We'll put that on the place mat.

Step 3
- Put the speck of apple on your tongue and count to five with your mouth closed.
- Take it out of your mouth again and wipe your mouth with a serviette.

- Well done. You have earned the third reward star.
- We'll put that on the place mat.

Step 4
- Put the speck of apple on your tongue and count to ten with your mouth closed.
- Take the piece of apple out and wipe your mouth with a serviette.
- You have earned the fourth reward star. We'll put that on the place mat.

Step 5
- Put the speck of apple in your mouth and count to five.
- Chew three times and wash it down with a drink of water.
- Fantastic! You have earned the fifth and last star for your place mat.
- You've already done one of the three lessons now, and so you deserve one of the three stickers for your taste-something-new plan!

That was the first tasting lesson

Altogether this will take about 10 minutes. Choose a set time of the day, when your child is well rested and open to trying, so not when she has just come home from the crèche and is very tired. If your child already dares to hold a speck of the food in her mouth, then you can go straight to the second tasting lesson. In that case do lesson three twice, so that the child has still tasted the food 15 times and has still earned three stickers.

THE SECOND TASTING LESSON
Step 1
- Put the piece of apple in your mouth.
- Chew it three times.
- Swallow, gone with a drink of water.
- Well done. You have earned the first reward star.
- We'll put that on the place mat.

Step 2
- Put the piece of apple in your mouth.
- Chew it three times.
- Swallow, gone.
- Then have a drink of water.
- Well done. You have earned the second reward star.
- We'll put that on the place mat.

Step 3
- Put the piece of apple in your mouth.
- Are you ready to begin? Go!

- Chew it so fast that it goes down all at once.
- Then have a drink of water.
- Well done. You have earned the third reward star.
- We'll put that on the place mat.

Step 4

- Now we are going to continue the game with the three pieces of apple on your plate.
- Put one of the three pieces of apple in your mouth.
- Are you ready to begin? Go!
- I'll give you 5 minutes to eat all three.
- Watch the timer.
- You can have a drink of water after each piece.
- Well done. You have earned the fourth reward star.
- We'll put that on the place mat.

Step 5

- Now you are going to eat a slightly bigger piece of apple three times.
- Are you ready to begin? Go!
- I'll give you 5 minutes to eat all three.
- Watch the timer.
- Chew it so fast that it goes down all at once.
- Then have a drink of water.
- Well done. You have earned the fifth reward star.
- We'll put that on the place mat.
- You'll find another sticker in the magic toadstool for managing to do this tasting lesson.
- Congratulations, you have finished the second tasting lesson! Stick your sticker on your taste-something-new plan and then be quick and look at your surprise message.

Watch your child

Observe your child carefully at every step to see if she can manage it. If she shows signs of fear just go back a step or distract her with a bright toy. That is the way to reduce the risk of aversion and it's the best way to motivate and encourage her. Sometimes it is necessary to use water longer to help with swallowing the food. Do not make a problem out of this. Patience is very important at this stage.

Stickers

You are actually well on the way. For children who go through the tasting lessons quickly and easily, you can move on to the next lesson. For those who are slower, keep practising lessons 1 and 2. Your child should decide for himself which tasting lesson he is going to start with. At the end of each tasting lesson, you put the reward stars your child earned back on the magic toadstool. There is one sticker to be earned for each lesson, which your child can stick on his taste-something-new plan. In total the book contains three stickers per category per tasting lesson. You decide when your child has earned a sticker and what he has to do for it.

Now it is time for the third and final tasting lesson. This involves different steps which all have an in-built play element. So you can make it into a competition by tasting yourself with your child. You can also set time limits, such as five pieces in 5 minutes.

THE THIRD TASTING LESSON

Step 1
- We are going to play a game to see who can taste, chew and swallow the piece of apple first (the size of the piece is the same as in lesson two).
- Get ready, go!
- Very well done! You have earned the first reward star.
- We'll put that on the place mat.

Step 2
- Now we'll take the timer.
- We'll each put five pieces on our plate.
- We're going to eat them up in 5 minutes.
- The time starts now!
- Very well done! You have earned the second reward star.
- We'll put that on the place mat.

Step 3
- Now we'll set the timer again.
- We'll each put eight pieces on our plate.
- We're going to eat them up in 8 minutes.
- The time starts now!
- Very well done! You have earned the third reward star.
- We'll put that on the place mat.

Step 4
- Now we are going to cut the apple into proper segments and bite pieces off the segments.
- Look I'll show you how with these two segments.
- The time starts now!
- Very well done! You have earned the fourth reward star.
- We'll put that on the place mat.

Step 5

- The last part of the lesson is to take a bite out of a whole apple.
- Look I'll show you.
- Now you do it.
- Fantastic! You have earned the fifth and last star for your place mat.
- Now look in the magic toadstool and see what your surprise message says.

What to do after the last tasting lesson

Your child has now learned to eat apple. From now on, give her apple three times a week and gradually increase the amount. Take it at your child's own pace.

It is sometimes a good idea to take it slowly for a while with the amount. When your child is ready for something new, choose what food to try next from the taste-something-new plan. Once your child has worked through the whole plan, he or she is officially crowned as a Food Prince or Food Princess.!

How to start with a slow eater

If your child eats sandwiches very slowly, cut them up into smaller portions. Use a timer and set it for 1 minute per bite-sized portion. Encourage your child to chew it up and swallow it before the bell rings. 'Well done, you finished that before the bell, Next bit', etc. One star for the place mat can be earned for every five bites. You keep control over the whole sandwich. You give him one little piece at a time on the plate. In this way, the amount of food seems more manageable to your child.

Hold the timer in your hand for the first few bites, so that your child can be guaranteed to finish before the bell goes. This is a good incentive and it gives him self-confidence. Check that his mouth is completely empty before you give him another piece. Then increase the number of pieces of bread (from two to four to six, etc.) that you put on your child's plate and that he has to eat up in a set time.

How to reward a slow eater

Your child gets a star if he eats up the agreed amount within the set time. Once your child has learned to eat his sandwich within a reasonable time (half an hour maximum), he gets his magic toadstool with the surprise message. This approach can also be used, of course, for other meals not just sandwiches.

How to start with a picky eater

A picky eater will investigate his food in minute detail and only pick out what he likes best. Teach your child that he has to eat the meat, potato and vegetables (or other foods on the plate) in turn, so that he does not eat one kind of food up first and leave the rest on the plate. You can also guide a picky eater by saying how many mouthfuls he still should eat from a one-pan meal. Always remember not to offer adult portion sizes.

1 Take a bite, have a drink; take a bite, have a drink.
2 Bit of meat, bit of potato, bit of vegetable, then bit of meat again, etc.

DOS AND DON'TS
How to start the day without stress

For some picky children breakfast, as the first meal of the day, is what they have most problems with and they struggle to swallow bread or toast. In that case, you could give them muesli or cornflakes with milk or yoghurt, or porridge.

What if your child tries to use food to manipulate you?

In that case, use the 20-minute method. This means that you do not allow the meal to become an endless drama. Instead you create a positive, orderly ritual within defined limits. You sit down together at the table, start to eat, and after 20 minutes the meal is over. Naturally you announce this clearly beforehand. Then you clear the table without any fuss. You give a desert, but no more than one. If your child is sorry about refusing to eat or wants to eat his dinner after all, you tell him firmly that he will have to wait for the next meal. By being firm and clear on this, you counteract the arbitrary wilfulness that a child of this age can display with regard to food (especially hot meals).

What should you do and what is it best not to do at mealtimes? We have a list of practical tips for healthy eating and drinking habits for you.

Do

Let you child decide how much to eat.

Don't

Push your child to eat more

Why?

You decide what to put on the table, but your child shows you how much food he needs. Pushing an infant to drink the whole content of his bottle or to eat a whole jar of food is a misguided approach. You yourself do not always consume the same amount of food and drink. Accept that a child will eat varying amounts each day. Urging a child to eat more increases the risk that he will refuse food. A small child cannot tell you when he has had enough. Bottle-fed infants are often given a standard measured quantity of milk, but you would do better to observe your own baby. Is your baby thriving? Is he alert and lively? If so, do not worry if there is milk left over. When parents worry about the daily calorific intake of their children, they start unconsciously pushing them to eat more, with exactly the opposite result. The child develops a dislike for eating and drinking.

Do

When he is ready for solid food, let your child experiment with a rusk or a crust of bread on a regular basis.

Don't

Interfere with your child while he is experimenting with the new food.

Why?

Children have something to eat on average five times a day. Let your child discover for himself what he can do with a bread crust: chew on it, suck on it or nibble it. Accept that his first attempts with solid foods (bread sticks, crusts) often result in retching. That is normal and it is good for the oral motor development. Stay close by for safety reasons. Children between the ages of one and two have a strong instinct to imitate. So take a roll yourself and bite bits off. Do it casually in front of your child. Say out loud how lovely your roll is. When you are walking with your child in the pushchair, give him something to eat to hold in his fists. By taking something yourself, your child will copy you. The things that you do not put too much emphasis on become the things they want. You need to subtly prompt your child to imitate.

Do

Offer small, manageable portions at mealtimes.

Don't

Allow your child to play with food at the table.

Why?

If you see that your child is not eating his food, but is playing with it or throwing it around, then take it away. Do not give it just for the sake of letting him have it. In this way you are giving a signal that food is not for playing with. By giving food in small doses you can see exactly whether he is eating it or not. It is a fact that children love to play with food. As young as they are, they will point to what they want in the fridge, and then refuse to eat it.

When you sit down to the table with your child, put a tiny dot of food on his plate. That stimulates his appetite. When that's gone, give him another bit of the same food. In that way, he will gradually get used to the flavour. Do not think in terms of adult portions. It is not just about the need for food at this stage, it is about the learning experience. There is nothing wrong with an eight-month-old baby who spits out his vegetables. He just has to get used to the flavours. So keep practising.

Do

Take into consideration the preferences and dislikes of children over the age of 3 years.

Don't

Stick to so-called 'general rules'.

Why?

Some children continue to eat puréed food for a long time. Your child may have had an unpleasant experience with food that had not been puréed. She may have experienced a persistent retching response to smooth food with more solid bits in it, such as yoghurt with bits of fruit. Your child may have developed a negative association with this kind of food. After all, there are even some adults who strongly dislike foods of this texture and this may be genetically determined. Be understanding about this. An aversion to a particular type of food begins with the acknowledgement of it by the parents. Do not say 'my child will just have to learn to like it' because you think that it is one of the 'general rules'. Quite the reverse – you can easily move from smooth food to thicker smooth food to completely solid food. It is not necessary to eat that kind of lumpy food in order to learn to eat solid food, and so you should not try to force it. Some children are able to go straight from purée to solid pieces – from baby cereal to bread and from smooth mash to potatoes, meat and vegetables served separately. In that case, you can miss out the lumpy stage altogether. Treat the yoghurt with fruity bits for what it is, and give your child smooth yoghurt and pieces of apple separately.

Do

Keep on trying.

Don't

Let your child (of eight months old) have his own way if he does not respond positively to new flavours right away.

Why?

Repetition is very important when children are learning to get used to new flavours. On average, a child will have to taste something ten to fifteen times to learn to enjoy something new. Even if the child is not keen or perhaps puts up strong resistance, you should try again another time and keep on trying. You must not give your child his own way on this. One thing that can help when introducing new flavours is to distract your baby with bright toys with lights and sound effects. Thanks to these distraction techniques, the baby experiences the new flavours unconsciously. A child of three or older can take on the step-by-step taste-something-new game, and so the distraction techniques are no longer needed for these older children.

Do

Take a step-by-step approach with each child.

Don't

Treat all children the same.

Why?

Some children naturally enjoy their food more than others. Some children are more sensitive to new flavours. These are usually alert children. They experience new flavours as being more extreme. Once they have got used to a variety of flavours, their parents report that they mainly go for spicy food. They prefer strong flavours like olives, prawns, herring and Chinese and Indian food. These children are less interested in food with a bland flavour, such as cauliflower or carrots. Parents often think that children like bland flavours. But that is not true. Try stir-frying cauliflower with some spices and see how your child reacts to it.

Do

Agree on some basic family rules for mealtimes.

Don't

Renegotiate the rules every day.

THE MOST COMMON PITFALLS

No matter how hard you try as a parent, sooner or later you will walk into a pitfall with your eyes wide open. A pitfall is a problem where you choose exactly the wrong solution. That is why we have summarised the most common pitfalls.

A child who loves sandwiches but is less keen on hot dinners is still well within the realms of what is normal. It only becomes a problem if the child really will only eat bread. If it has got that bad and he 'really will only eat …' you need to address the problem. Use the tasting lessons in this book. Give your child other foods, encourage him, and compliment him if he wants to try something new.

The child only wants to eat from those little packs

Individualism reigns supreme in our society. And the food industry has been quick to take advantage of this with a large number of products in mini packs: mini deserts, fruit squeezie pouches, and individually packed cheese snacks, to name just a few examples. All those small snacks and different brands of ready-to-serve jars can get children into the habit of only eating snacks and treats. The more normal (i.e. not associated with a particular brand) the constituents of a meal, the easier it will be for your child to deal with everyday meals. This is especially true if she sometimes goes to eat at grandma and granddad's where they do not have all these newfangled food products, of course.

The child makes every meal into a drama

What do you do if your child has an aversion to commonplace foods? No parent can remain unmoved if their baby or toddler starts screaming his heart out as soon as he sees the bib or the spoon. You want your child to eat, and your child obviously does not want to. Don't get drawn into this battle. Start with offering food on your finger instead of a spoon, accompanied by distraction techniques (see the section on *Eating and drinking between ages one and two*). Sometimes an episode of flu can cause a sudden aversion. Your child may take a dislike to hot meals because he was violently sick when eating a hot dinner. A negative reaction is then associated with hot food. Try to gradually get him to start eating it again. If this does not work, seek professional help.

TEN TOP TIPS

The 10 top tips to get through all the eating phases with the minimum of fuss.
1 Every child goes through the eating phases in his own unique way.
2 Stick to the three basic concepts (intuition, responsiveness and individualisation).
3 Learn to recognise your child's preferences for certain foods and drinks and take them into account when preparing meals.
4 Use distraction techniques with very young children.
5 Be patient (perseverance in the short term pays dividends in the long term).
6 Keep trying; taste can be learned.
7 Offer juice or milky drinks at set times of the day (don't let your child go around with a bottle or cup of juice all day long). Drink is also food, and it makes a child feel full so that he has no appetite at mealtimes.
8 When introducing new flavours and methods of eating, build in breaks if necessary.
9 Take it in small steps. Start with a tiny speck of a new flavour. Do not aim for too much variety – that makes young children unsettled.
10 Avoid battles at the table and find creative ways around them.

BUSY FAMILIES

6:00 p.m.: dinner time

When both parents work they often find that, after picking up the children, they still have to think what to have for dinner and who is going to do the shopping. That is not convenient. Apart from the fact that a child of one or two years old should ideally eat his evening meal at around 5:00 p.m., eating late is often rushed and stressful. At about 5:00 p.m. a young child can still summon up sufficient attention for the meal, and so will eat better. Furthermore, he will not have to go to bed on a full stomach.

PLANNING AND ORGANISATION

Anticipation is the key word. Plan your meals a (working) week ahead and do the bulk of your food shopping once a week. You can pick up fresh vegetables in between at your local convenience store. But going to the supermarket with your children every day is not to be recommended.

WHAT DO YOU PUT ON THE TABLE?

Do you find it an effort to put something tasty and original on the table every day? Well that's not necessary at all. You could cook enough for 2 days on alternate days. An average child will eat four or five different dinners and as a parent you should be content with that. For example, one pasta meal, three meals based around vegetables with meat or fish and one treat meal. You can eat a variety of staples with the vegetables, such as rice, pasta or potato. Be creative and flexible – try to think up variations that are healthy and tasty. Does your child like carrots? Then think up a tasty dish with carrots that you can repeat every 4 or 5 days, possibly with minor adaptations. The child recognises carrot, likes it and eats with relish.

When we talk about treats we usually mean pizza, pancakes and chips. Do you feel guilty about this kind of convenience food? That is not necessary at all – as long as you do not confine yourself to ready-to-eat products. With pizza and pancakes that you make yourself, you can think up healthy combinations with fresh vegetables, meat, fish, vegetarian products or eggs.

WHAT DO YOU PUT ON THE TABLE?

Choose something from each column when preparing a hot dinner and vary these to your heart's content

Pasta	Chicken	Broccoli
Rice	Fish	Carrot
Potato	Meat	Beans
Bread	Vegetarian	Pulses
	Egg or cheese	Tomato

A GOOD EXAMPLE LEADS TO GOOD HABITS

Even though you are really too tired to cook sometimes or feel uninspired, the way you approach food now, in the early years, really is important, simply because children love to copy. That is why it is important that eating is associated with a pleasant atmosphere and socially rewarding behaviour. Do not let your children get into the habit of snacking. If you let them have food and drink all day long without having set meals, they will be unlikely to eat proper meals when they leave home and are looking after themselves. They won't cook very often and they will be more likely to eat fast food out on the street or have a ready meal on their lap at home. Let children help you with preparing food from a young age. Take time for proper meals. That teaches children to appreciate food. Eating is a social occasion to be enjoyed together in a relaxed atmosphere *and* at the table – not on the sofa in front of the TV.

Sharing knowledge: a dietician's perspective on assessment and intervention

Dorthe Wiuf Nielsen
Klinisk Diætist, Copenhagen, Denmark

ASSESSMENT OF NUTRITIONAL STATUS

Assessment of nutritional status is important when working with children and especially when the children are sick or chronically ill.

Normal nutritional assessment includes objective evaluation, evaluation of the dietary intake, biochemical data, anthropometry as height and weight measurements and evaluation on growth charts, especially height for age and weight for height. (Gibson, Nutritional assessment)

Nutritional screening for malnutrition

Nutritional screening for malnutrition is a method to identify children in risk for malnutrition or obesity and a way to manage assessment of nutritional status. Every child who arrives at a hospital and is admitted on to a ward as an inpatient should be nutritional screened within the first 24 hours for malnutrition and risk of malnutrition. Examples of nutritional screening tools include the following.

The nutritional screening tool has five questions:

1 Has there been weight loss of more than 10% in children from 10 kg or more than 5% in young infants up to 10 kg?
2 Does the child's growth chart show any deviation from the expected trajectory for height and weight?
3 Is the dietary intake below 75% of the normal intake for age?
4 Is the child in need of any surgery?
5 Has the child a chronic illness which requires high calorific energy levels?

If there is just affirmative answer, the child presents a nutritional risk and the clinical dietician should be involved. More acute investigations and surgery may mean that some of the anthropometric measurements must be repeated afterwards.

Important factors for the nutritional status of the child

A nutritional screening tool should be followed by an identification of other important factors for the child's nutritional status. These include:

- chewing and swallowing
- oral-motor difficulties
- drinking and eating possibilities
- allergies
- dental problems
- communication issues (i.e. how does the child communicate hunger?)
- medication (medication may influence the child's appetite and lead to nausea and/or vomiting, as well as other factors, such as excess saliva production, absorption/malabsorption, constipation and diarrhoea.

FOOD AND CLINICAL NUTRITION FOR SICK CHILDREN

Favourite dishes

When working with food and clinical nutrition for sick children it is important to give the children the possibility to eat what kind of food they like and at what time they prefer to have it. This can be easier to achieve when there are kitchens on the children's wards and a nutritionally educated person is available to ensure favourite dishes can be made (this is always the best place to begin) and good, calorie and energy dense foods is on offer.

Energy dense food, fortifications, energy drinks, nutritional supplements

Sick children normally need energy-dense nutrition. It is difficult for them to eat enough for their energy needs and recommended energy needs are often higher when they are sick. The use of energy-dense foods and drinks which include fats and sugars will help ensure a better energy percent composition and will help meet needs.

Tube feeding and parenteral nutrition

In many cases it can be necessary to give supplemented feed or whole enteral nutrition in a tube for enteral nutrition. If the child cannot take enough food orally or is at nutritional risk then enteral nutrition must start.

If the problem is expected to be of more than 3 months duration, a percutan endoscopic gastrostomi (PEG) is likely to be placed into the child's stomach instead of a nasogastric tube. In these cases it is easier to continue oral stimulation and to give food and drink by mouth. A nasogastric tube can adversely affect the child's willingness to take food orally. However, the PEG, like the tube, can make the re-introduction of oral feeding difficult, not least because of the child's feeling of satiety and being physically full.

Despite the drawbacks, enteral nutrition is essential in many severe cases to ensure survival and a normal growth and developmental trajectory that are as normal as possible for each individual child.

Parenteral nutrition, either as a supplement to enteral nutrition or oral eating or in total, can be useful in severe situations, especially if there is a gastro-intestinal problem with the bowels, digestion or absorption.

In these cases a thorough evaluation must be carried out to determine whether it is possible to provide nutrition gastrointestinally, orally or enterally by tube prior to making the decision to provide parenteral nutrition.

MULTI-PROFESSIONAL FEEDING CLINICS

The multi professional team

To ensure and to optimise the energy intake for the child it is important to have a multi-professional feeding team. This may include doctors, nurses, clinical dieticians, social workers, physiotherapists, occupational therapists, psychologists, play therapists, speech and language therapists and dentists. Good teamwork is critical to success.

Cooperation in the multi professional feeding team

- Regular meetings of all team members.
- Regular meetings between the team and the child's parents, with flexibility to include others as and when appropriate (e.g. nursery staff and teachers).
- The activities of individual members of the team are coordinated.
- Individualised treatment plan for each child.

OUTCOMES: THE EXPERIENCE IN DENMARK

- Clinical experience suggests that multi-professional feeding clinics are important in helping children learn to eat and drink normally again.
- Tertiary services can offer families a 'fresh start' where the focus is on the feeding and eating difficulties, the environment is different and there is a new staff group.
- The children need time, patience, a single room at a hospital and at least two nurses on the ward to each child.
- Experience suggests that with tube-fed children, it might be beneficial to wait before removing the tube until the child is able to take food orally.
- We have also observed that it is probably best to start intensive feeding therapy after the child has first experienced some time with better nutrition, for example, through tube feeding, so that the child's weight is not compromised at the beginning of the programme.

Index